Perspectives in Exercise Science and Sports Medicine
Volume 4: Ergogenics— Enhancement of Performance in Exercise and Sport

Edited by

David R. Lamb, Ph.D.
The Ohio State University

Melvin H. Williams, Ph.D.
Old Dominion University

WCB Brown & Benchmark

Copyright © 1991 by Wm. C. Brown Publishers

ALL RIGHTS RESERVED

No part of this publication may be reproduced, stored in a retrieval system, or transmitted, in any form or by any means, electronic, photocopying, recording, or otherwise, without the prior written permission of the publisher.

Library of Congress Cataloging in Publication Data:
LAMB, DAVID R., 1939–
PERSPECTIVES IN EXERCISE SCIENCE AND SPORTS MEDICINE
VOLUME 4: ERGOGENICS—ENHANCEMENT OF PERFORMANCE IN
EXERCISE AND SPORT

Cover Design: Gray Schmitt

Manufactured By: Edwards Brothers
                Ann Arbor, Michigan

ISBN: 0697-14977-3

Printed in the United States of America
10 9 8 7 6 5 4 3 2 1

Contributors

Gail Butterfield, Ph.D.
GRECC
Palo Alto V.A. Medical Center
Palo Alto, CA 94304

Priscilla Clarkson, Ph.D.
University of Massachusetts
Department of Exercise Science
Amherst, MA 01003

Andrew Coggan, Ph.D.
School of Health, Physical Education
and Recreation
The Ohio State University
Columbus, OH 43210

Robert Conlee, Ph.D.
Department of Physical Education
Brigham Young University
Provo, UT 84602

David Costill, Ph.D.
Ball State University
Human Performance Laboratory
Muncie, IN 47306

Edward Coyle, Ph.D.
Human Performance Lab
University of Texas
Austin, TX 78712

Lynis Dohm, Ph.D.
Department of Biochemistry
School of Medicine
East Carolina University
Greenville, NC 27834

Edward R. Eichner, M.D.
University of Oklahoma
Health Sciences Center
Oklahoma City, OK 73190

Carl V. Gisolfi, Ph.D.
Department of Exercise Science and
Physical Education
University of Iowa
Iowa City, IA 52242

Steven Gregg, Ph.D.
The Quaker Oats Company
Barrington, IL 60010

George Heigenhauser, Ph.D.
Department of Medicine [MUMC
3U27]
McMaster University
Hamilton, Ontario L8N3Z5,
Canada

Robert Hickson, Ph.D.
Department of Physical Education
University of Illinois
Chicago, IL 60680

Linda Houtkooper, Ph.D.
University of Arizona
Tucson, AZ 85721

Howard Knuttgen, Ph.D.
Center for Sports Medicine
Greenberg Sports Complex
Pennsylvania State University
University Park, PA 16082

Richard Kreider, Ph.D.
Human Performance Laboratory
Old Dominion University
Norfolk, VA 23508

Chester Kyle, Ph.D.
Sports Equipment Research
Associates
Weed, CA 96094

David Lamb, Ph.D.
School of Health, Physical Education
and Recreation
The Ohio State University
Columbus, OH 43210

Peter Lemon, Ph.D.
Applied Physiology Research Lab
Kent State University
Kent, OH 44242

John Lombardo, M.D.
Department of Internal Medicine
Division of Family Medicine
The Ohio State University
Columbus, OH 43210

Ronald Maughan, Ph.D.
University Medical School
Department of Environmental and
Occupational Medicine
Foresterhill
Aberdeen, AB9 2ZD
Scotland

Robert Murray, Ph.D.
The Quaker Oats Company
Barrington, IL 60010

Ethan R. Nadel, Ph.D.
John B. Pierce Foundation Laboratory
New Haven, CT 06519

Scott Powers, Ph.D.
Center for Exercise Science
University of Florida
Gainesville, FL 32611

Robert Robertson, Ph.D.
Human Energy Research Lab
University of Pittsburgh
Pittsburgh, PA 15261

Michael Sawka, Ph.D.
US Army Research Institute of
Environmental Medicine
Natick, MA 01760

Michael Sherman, Ph.D.
School of Health, Physical Education,
and Recreation
The Ohio State University
Columbus, OH 43210

Lawrence Spriet, Ph.D.
School of Human Biology
University of Guelph
Guelph, Ontario N1G2W1
Canada

John R. Sutton, M.D.
Department of Biological Sciences
Cumberland College of Health
Sciences
Lidcombe, NSW
Australia 2141

Ronald L. Terjung, Ph.D
S.U.N.Y. Health Sciences Center
at Syracuse
Department of Physiology
Syracuse, NY 13210

Melvin Williams, Ph.D.
Human Performance Laboratory
Old Dominion University
Norfolk, VA 23508

Jack Wilmore, Ph.D.
Human Performance Lab
University of Texas
Austin, TX 78712

iv

Acknowledgment

The Quaker Oats Company and The Gatorade Sports Science Institute are proud to have facilitated the publication of this fourth volume in the series *"Perspectives in Exercise Science and Sports Medicine."* The symposium on "Ergogenics—Enhancement of Performance in Exercise and Sport" and this publication represent contributions of eminent sports scientists and consequently the highest quality of scientific endeavor.

We at The Quaker Oats Company and Gatorade Sports Science Institute will continue our ongoing support of research and education in exercise science and sports medicine. By working with the scientific community, we hope to make a significant contribution to the science and medicine of exercise and sports.

Peter J. Vitulli
President
Grocery Specialties Division
The Quaker Oats Company

Foreword

The American College of Sports Medicine is proud to be associated with the Quaker Oats Company and Gatorade Thirst Quencher in publishing the series entitled *Perspectives in Exercise Science and Sports Medicine*. The proceeds of the *Perspectives* series have been generously donated to the American College of Sports Medicine Foundation, and I look forward to a continued and productive association between the college and The Quaker Oats Company in fostering interest in and generating knowledge about exercise, sport, and physical activity as vital concerns in optimizing long-term health.

The fourth volume, *Ergogenics—Enhancement of Performance in Exercise and Sport*, addresses an aspect of exercise science and sports medicine that is fraught with myths, half truths, misunderstandings, and outright fraud. This area is of particular concern to the college and its members as well as to the many others around the world involved in exercise and sports such as competitors, enthusiasts of all ages including young people and their parents, coaches, scientists and administrators. While the issues of steroids, blood doping and growth hormone as ergogenic aids have captured much of the public's interest, much still needs to be learned not only about these but also the many other, although perhaps less publicly controversial, ergogenic aids. The objective, authoritative, and no-nonsense approach to the topic by the authors of the chapters in this book will do much to help clarify the many complex issues by accurately and meaningfully interpreting the literature on ergogenics.

Neil Oldridge, Ph.D.
President
American College of Sports Medicine

Preface

Successful performance in sports is dependent primarily upon two major factors—genetic potential and state-of-the-art training. Elite international class athletes have been endowed with those physical, physiological, and psychological characteristics determinant of superior sports performance, but they have also maximized this inherited potential through appropriate biomechanical, physiological, psychological, and nutritional training. However, given the social prestige and economic benefits associated with successful sports performance, athletes today are constantly searching for a means to obtain a competitive edge over their opponents beyond training, often by the use of ergogenics.

Ergogenics are thought to enhance sports performance by a variety of means, but ultimately by exerting a favorable effect upon human energy utilization. In this regard, ergogenics may be used in attempts to improve the athlete's ability to produce energy at a faster rate, to sustain optimal energy production for a longer period of time, to modify negative psychological processes that may interfere with the proper application of energy, or to enhance biomechanical applications by increasing propulsive forces or reducing resistive forces.

Ergogenics have been used by athletes for centuries, but their use at all levels of athletic competition appears to have increased tremendously over the past 40 years. Some effective ergogenics are safe and legal, whereas others are potentially harmful and illegal. For example, carbohydrate loading, an innocuous dietary modification, has been used safely and legally by thousands of athletes in preparation for ultraendurance events. On the other hand, anabolic steroids, potent pharmacological agents, may convey serious medical risks and are banned by various athletic governing bodies, such as the International Olympic Committee. Sports scientists throughout the world are constantly investigating the safety and efficacy of various ergogenics.

In June, 1990, 27 scientists who have been active in ergogenic research met in Maui, Hawaii, in an interactive conference to discuss the major ergogenics used by athletes. Prior to the conference, scientists developed 10 review papers, each of which was formally reviewed by one or more of the other conferees and subsequently revised. Following presentation of the revised papers at the conference, all attending scientists made additional comments, which were also incorporated into the final version.

Thus, this fourth volume of PERSPECTIVES IN EXERCISE SCIENCE AND SPORTS MEDICINE represents a contemporary, detailed analysis of the available scientific literature dealing with the efficacy and safety of the major ergogenics used by athletes. It should be useful to the sport scientist involved in ergogenic research, as well as to the practitioner who has a basic understanding of the sport sciences. Each chapter incorporates not only the theoretical background and research relative to the efficacy of the ergogenic but also the medical and legal implications and recommendations for use.

The first four chapters deal with purported nutritional ergogenics. Of the energy nutrients, carbohydrate has been shown repeatedly to enhance performance in prolonged endurance events. In Chapter 1, Dr. Sherman discusses the strategies underlying carbohydrate feedings both before and after exercise, while in Chapter 2, Dr. Maughan reviews the benefits of carbohydrate replenishment during exercise. In addition, Dr. Maughan comments on the role of electrolyte supplementation during prolonged exercise.

Protein has historically been considered to be a nutritional ergogenic for strength in athletes, but in recent years protein and amino acid supplements have also been marketed for endurance athletes. In Chapter 3, Dr. Butterfield addresses the research findings relative to protein and amino acid supplementation and exercise performance. Although vitamins and minerals are not sources of human energy, they are intimately involved in physiological processes important to energy production during exercise. An extensive overview of the ergogenic effect of vitamins, iron, and various trace minerals is provided by Dr. Clarkson in Chapter 4.

Chapters 5 and 6 discuss ergogenics designed to complement physiological processes important to success in anaerobic or aerobic exercise endeavors. Sodium bicarbonate is a physiologically important buffer that is thought to benefit performance in sports involving anaerobic glycolysis and, in Chapter 5, Dr. Heigenhauser effectively reviews and criticizes the available literature, also providing some interesting viewpoints on possible mechanisms of action. In Chapter 6, Dr. Spriet addresses the subject of blood doping, which seems to be one of the most effective, but illegal, ergogenic aids for aerobic endurance athletes. Dr. Spriet presents a refreshingly new approach in his detailed and updated review of the role blood doping plays relative to oxygen transport and enhanced aerobic endurance performance.

The next three chapters focus upon eight pharmacological agents that have been theorized or found to be ergogenic for various athletic endeavors. Strength and power athletes attempt to increase muscle mass by a variety of means, and anabolic steroids appear to be one of the most used and abused ergogenics by these athletes. Also, with the increased availability of human growth hormone via genetic engineering, there is increasing concern by medical practitioners of its use by athletes for similar purposes. In Chapter 7, Dr. Lombardo discusses the efficacy and safety of these two agents.

Most pharmacological stimulants, such as amphetamines, are banned from use by athletes during competition. However, some stimulants, such as caffeine, are consumed as natural ingredients in beverages like coffee, while other stimulants, such as cocaine, are taken for their ability to elicit altered states of consciousness. All three of these drugs have potential ergogenic qualities, and their effectiveness and medical risks are reviewed by Dr. Conlee in Chapter 8.

Although alcohol and marijuana are considered primarily as social drugs, and beta blockers are utilized almost exclusively for medical purposes, they have been considered to be ergogenic for athletes under certain circumstances, particularly to reduce excess anxiety in sports necessitating a relaxed state of mind. In Chapter 9, Dr. Williams reviews the available literature regarding the ergogenic effect of these drugs, including the possible effects associated with the social use of alcohol and marijuana and the medical use of beta blockers.

As we are all aware, the individual with the best talent and training does not always win in sports. In some sports, the equipment used may be the key to success. Who can forget the tremendous advantage the United States possessed with its catamaran in the recent Americas Cup competition? The final chapter, by Dr. Kyle, provides an excellent example of the application of mechanical and biomechanical ergogenics to sports. Although the first nine chapters concentrate on ergogenics designed to enhance the production and control of human energy, Chapter 10 demonstrates the difference that equipment may make in determining the outcome of an athletic contest. Dr. Kyle details the research involved in developing the ideal bicycle, which, coupled with proper techniques and strategy, may provide a competitive advantage, as evidenced by Greg Lemond in the final day of the 1989 Tour de France.

This series, PERSPECTIVES IN EXERCISE SCIENCE AND SPORTS MEDICINE, represents only one of the many contributions that The Quaker Oats Company and Gatorade Thirst Quencher have made to foster exercise science and sports medicine. There are numerous people in the Quaker Oats Company that participated in this endeavor, but Robert Murray and William Schmidt deserve special recognition. Without their support, ideas, and encouragement this scientific contribution would not have been possible.

We acknowledge the crucial contribution of Leslie Finnin and her colleagues at McCord Travel. The conference in Maui was such a pleasant experience because Leslie worked behind the scenes to prevent and resolve problems before they became major issues. We also appreciate the efforts of Butch Cooper and Kendal Gladish of Benchmark Press for producing such a high-quality finished product.

David R. Lamb
Melvin H. Williams

Contents

Introductory Notes on Validation and Applications of Ergogenics

Robert J. Robertson, Ph.D.

The literal definition of ergogenic is "work producing," but a more specific definition is needed when the term is applied to exercise and sport. To the sport practitioner (i.e., the athlete, coach, trainer, and team physician), an ergogenic is often defined as a procedure or agent that enhances energy production, energy control, or energy efficiency during sport performance, and thus provides the athlete with a competitive edge beyond that which may be obtained through normal training methods (Williams, 1989). To the exercise scientist, an ergogenic is defined as an experimental procedure or agent that increases exercise performance in comparison to a placebo condition.[1]

This book discusses a broad range of ergogenics that have been used in competitive sports. Each ergogenic is examined within the context of: 1) performance enhancement, 2) mechanisms of action, and 3) mode of application.

It is recognized that some procedures initially thought to enhance sport performance are found upon closer inspection to actually produce the opposite effect, resulting in a performance decrement. These procedures are termed *ergolytic* (Eichner, 1989). Where possible, a clear distinction is made between ergogenic and ergolytic procedures throughout the chapters of this book. However, this distinction is not always easily made because some procedures that have marked ergogenic effects when applied properly become ergolytic when improperly administered. The consumption of alcohol is a good example of a procedure that can have ergogenic or ergolytic effects, depending on the type of sport performance involved or the dose used.

---

[1]Improvement in exercise performance is evidenced by: (1) a longer time to reach exhaustion, (2) production of more work at a given exercise intensity, and/or (3) attainment of a greater average power output for a given duration.

CLASSIFICATION OF ERGOGENICS

Ergogenics are generally classified as physical, mechanical, bio-mechanical, nutritional, physiological, psychological, or pharmacological substances or treatments (Morgan, 1972; Williams, 1989). The ergogenics discussed in this book are representative of many of these classifications. For example, carbohydrate, electrolyte, vitamin, and protein supplementations are classified as nutritional ergogenics. Caffeine, alcohol, amphetamines, beta-blockers, and anabolic steroids are pharmacological ergogenics. Blood doping and bicarbonate loading may be regarded as physiological procedures, whereas bicycle design involves mechanical ergogenics. It is important to note that some ergogenics fall under more than one classification; e.g., sodium bicarbonate supplementation can be considered as a physiological, nutritional, or pharmacological procedure. Further, many ergogenic procedures may exert psychological effects in addition to their primary modes of action. Thus, multiple classifications may be necessary to characterize a particular ergogenic.

Ergogenics can also be classified according to the times of their use relative to the onset of training and competition; i.e., an ergogenic can be employed during training, during competition, or during both training and competition. Anabolic steroids are usually taken during the pre-competitive training period to enhance the normal adaptive responses to a resistance exercise stimulus, while bicarbonate loading exerts its greatest ergogenic effect when administered very close to the start of a competitive event. Carbohydrate supplementation can be employed during both training and competition.

ERGOGENICS RESEARCH

Scientific study of proposed ergogenic procedures is undertaken for two interrelated purposes. First, it is necessary to incontrovertibly identify the ergogenic or ergolytic properties of a procedure prior to its sport application. Information regarding the magnitude and duration of the ergogenic effect must be derived through controlled laboratory and field experimentation to accurately evaluate the merits and/or limitations of a particular ergogenic. For example, systematic research has shown that the optimal ergogenic effect of bicarbonate loading occurs when sodium bicarbonate is ingested at a dose of 0.3 g/kg body weight 2–3 h prior to competition. Lower doses of sodium bicarbonate or those taken too far in advance of competition are ineffective.

Second, ergogenic procedures are used in laboratory protocols to study the rate-limiting mechanisms for exercise performance. In this context, the ergogenic procedure is used to perturb a particular physiological, psychological, and/or biomechanical process that is critical to a successful exercise performance. It is then possible to answer questions regarding the importance of specific physiological, psychological, and/or biomechanical events in determining the upper limit of exercise capacity. The effects of training, gender, and environment on these same rate-limiting physiological, psychological, and/or biomechanical events can also be identified using this experimental paradigm. As an example, the ingestion of sodium bicarbonate by subjects under controlled conditions enables exercise scientists to examine the role of acid-base regulation in determining the upper limits of high-intensity exercise performance. The scientific study of ergogenics as described in this book contributes directly to the knowledge base underlying rate-limiting factors in exercise performance.

CRITERIA FOR VALIDATION AND APPLICATION OF PURPORTED ERGOGENICS

When evaluating experiments on ergogenics, the criteria listed in Table 1 are among those that should ordinarily be satisfied. When such criteria are met, one can have a reasonable degree of confidence that a given ergogenic was appropriately validated.

Optimal performance benefits are derived when an ergogenic is applied according to criteria that reflect: 1) the appropriate schedule of administration (i.e., timing and frequency) and 2) the optimal dose-response relation.

Two factors must be considered when determining the optimal schedule of administration of an ergogenic. First, it is necessary to determine the appropriate timing of the ergogenic application relative to the onset of competition. For example, sodium bicarbonate

TABLE 1. *Some experimental criteria that should ordinarily be employed to validate an ergogenic procedure*

Double-blind presentation of both treatment and placebo conditions
Random assignment of subjects to treatments
Repeated measures design, if appropriate
Counterbalanced order of treatments
Familiarization trials for the criterion test(s)
Euhydration throughout all treatments and tests (unless dehydration or hypohydration is an experimental variable)
Thermoneutral test environment (unless the thermal condition is an experimental variable)
Control for level of fitness, training, and athletic experience of subjects
Appropriate statistical analyses

appears to be most effective when used 2–3 h prior to the start of a competitive event. In contrast, blood doping may take place as much as 1–2 weeks prior to competition without loss of its ergogenic properties. Second, caffeine and certain other ergogenics are administered only once for a given competition, whereas others, such as carbohydrate drinks, must be administered prior to and intermittently throughout a competitive event to achieve optimal efficacy.

The optimal dose-response relation must be identified for a given set of performance conditions. Such conditions include but are not limited to: 1) type of sport; 2) time during competitive season; 3) caliber of athlete; 4) caliber of the competition; 5) maturational level of the athlete; 6) age, height, weight, and gender of the athlete; and 7) prior experience with the ergogenic.

THE DECISION TO USE AN ERGOGENIC

When considering the use of an ergogenic, it is important that the sport practitioner ascertain unequivocally that the procedure is *safe*, *legal*, and *effective* (Robertson, Metz, Goss & Stanko, 1990). The algorithm presented in Figure 1 describes this decision-making process. The first step is to determine whether the use of the ergogenic produces short- and/or long-term side effects that pose a medical risk to the athlete. The safety of the procedure must always be balanced against the ergogenic benefits derived. In this way, a risk:benefit ratio is established for each ergogenic, providing a scientific and clinical basis for decisions regarding its use. Second, the legality of the procedure must be considered. While some ergogenics are both effective and safe, their use may be judged by athletic governing organizations to provide an unfair performance advantage. Consequently, they are banned from use during training and competition. The sport practitioner is encouraged to consult the "rules of competition" of the individual sport organization prior to using a particular ergogenic procedure. The third step is to determine through published findings of rigorously controlled laboratory and field experiments whether or not the procedure is effective in improving performance in a specific sport or exercise setting. Both ergogenic and ergolytic properties of the procedure must be considered at this point.

In summary, the decision to use an ergogenic in competitive sport must consider the following questions: Is it safe? Is it legal? and Is it effective? It is only when the answer to each question is *yes* that the ergogenic procedure can be considered as an appropriate aid to sport performance.

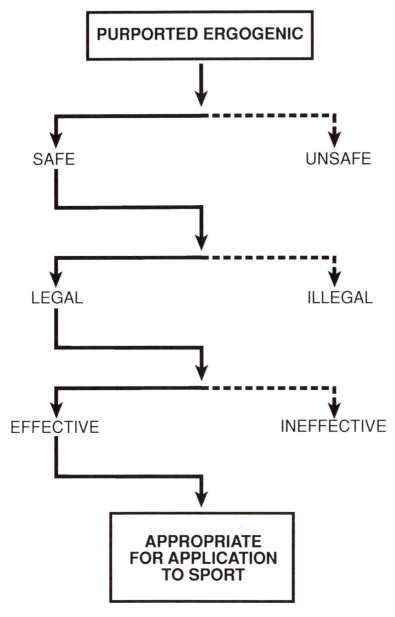

FIGURE 1: *Algorithm for deciding whether or not a purported ergogenic is appropriate for application to sport.*

REFERENCES

Eichner, E. R. (1989) Ergolytic Drugs. *Sports Science Exchange* Vol. 2, No. 15. Chicago: Gatorade Sports Science Institute.

Morgan, W. P. (1972). *Ergogenic Aids and Muscular Performance.* New York: Academic Press.

Robertson, R. J., Metz, K. F., Goss, F. L., and Stanko, R. T. (1990). Ergogenic aids: blood doping, bicarbonate ingestion, and carbohydrate supplementation. *Synopsis of Sports Medicine and Sports Science* Vol. 2. Hong Kong: The Chinese University of Hong Kong.

Williams, M. H. (1989). *Beyond Training. How Athletes Enhance Performance Legally and Illegally.* Champaign, IL: Human Kinetics.

1

Carbohydrate Feedings Before and After Exercise

W. MICHAEL SHERMAN, PH.D.

INTRODUCTION

The body's carbohydrate stores often limit the ability of athletes to train and compete in events requiring energy expenditure at 65–80% $\dot{V}O_2$max for longer than 60 to 90 min (Sherman & Lamb, 1988).

1

When the muscle glycogen content or blood glucose concentration is low during prolonged exercise, the intensity must be reduced or exercise stopped. It is well known that dietary carbohydrates significantly influence the body's carbohydrate reserves. This knowledge has stimulated experimentation with nutritional manipulations that have the potential to optimize bodily carbohydrate levels and improve training capacity and sport performance. This paper will discuss the ergogenic effects of nutritional manipulations that may favorably alter carbohydrate reserves during the hours preceding and following exercise.

DIETARY HABITS OF ATHLETES

Athletes who train and compete in activities limited by carbohydrate reserves often consume diets that may compromise "optimal" training and performance. Evaluation of athletes' diets reveals consumption of roughly 210 kJ $\cdot$ kg^{-1} $\cdot$ day^{-1} (50 kcal $\cdot$ kg^{-1} $\cdot$ d^{-1}) containing 15% of the energy as protein, 49% of the energy as carbohydrate, and 36% of the energy as fat (Brotherhood, 1984).

Because increased dietary carbohydrate energy can increase bodily carbohydrate stores, athletes have been advised to consume greater than 70% of energy as carbohydrate (Costill & Miller, 1980; Sherman & Lamb, 1988). Despite this advice and despite attempts to consume a high-carbohydrate diet, many athletes continue to consume less carbohydrate than recommended. For example, members of the Irish Olympic road race squad consumed only 51% carbohydrate (Johnson et al., 1985); USA Olympic marathon trials athletes consumed only 49–54% carbohydrate (Deuster et al., 1986); female cyclists in a 12 d cycling stage race consumed only 51% carbohydrate (Grandjean, Footnote 1); 15 males in a 20 d, 500 km footrace consumed only 51% carbohydrate (Peters et al., 1986); and intensely training triathletes consumed 60% carbohydrate (Burke & Read, 1987).

Obviously, athletes typically consume less than recommended quantities of carbohydrate. Such athletes may be nutritionally jeopardizing their training capacity and, because they may not be able to continue a progressive training program, they may be competing suboptimally. These observations suggest that athletes must be educated to make "wise" food choices to optimize dietary carbohydrate energy and thereby improve athletic potential.

CARBOHYDRATE FEEDINGS BEFORE EXERCISE

Rationale for Carbohydrate Feedings Before Exercise

The less than "optimal" content of carbohydrate in athletes' diets may lead to early fatigue. Fatigue during endurance exercise is often attributed to muscle glycogen depletion, to hypoglycemia (blood glucose <3.3 mM), or to a more modest decline in blood glucose. These substrates are used significantly for muscle metabolism when the exercise intensity is 65–80% $\dot{V}O_2$max for longer than 60–90 min (Bergstrom et al., 1967). When muscle glycogen reaches low levels (<50 mmol/kg wet weight), exercise has to be stopped or the intensity must be significantly reduced (Saltin & Karlsson, 1971).

There is a direct relationship between carbohydrate consumption and muscle glycogen content (Costill et al., 1981) as well as between the preexercise muscle glycogen content and exercise time to exhaustion (Ahlborg et al., 1967). Therefore, consuming a high-carbohydrate diet should increase muscle glycogen and improve endurance capacity. When the diet is chronically low in dietary carbohydrate, the preexercise muscle glycogen concentration will be lower than the optimal level, and high-quality training may not be maintained (Simonsen et al., 1990).

Some athletes experience fatigue when the blood glucose concentration is moderately reduced by endurance exercise. These athletes are "sensitive" to a lowering of blood glucose (Coyle et al., 1983). Alternately, other athletes do not fatigue until exhibiting a "hypoglycemic" concentration of blood glucose (<3.3 mM)(Coyle & Coggan, 1984). Also, the lowering of blood glucose during exercise may be accelerated in athletes exercising after an overnight fast that depletes liver glycogen (Hultman, 1978), and this may result in early fatigue. Furthermore, fasting is detrimental to performance (Loy et al., 1986; Gleeson et al., 1988).

Athletes nutritionally compromise their exercise potential if they consume insufficient dietary carbohydrate to maintain muscle glycogen, or if they fast before exercise and thereby reduce liver glycogen stores. A carbohydrate preexercise meal has the potential to increase the liver (Nilson & Hultman, 1974) and muscle glycogen concentrations (Coyle et al., 1985), delay the time at which those carbohydrate reserves become low, and thereby improve performance. Similarly, because athletes generally consume suboptimal amounts of dietary carbohydrate, consuming carbohydrates *immediately* after exercise may speed the replenishment of liver and muscle glycogen metabolized by exercise, allowing those carbohydrate reserves to recuperate faster and thereby allowing the athlete to recover more quickly (Brewer et al., 1988).

The following sections will consider: a) our understanding of the efficacy of carbohydrate feedings during the hours before exercise on metabolism and performance, and b) our understanding of the efficacy of postexercise carbohydrate feedings on optimizing liver and muscle glycogen synthesis after exercise. Only publications in which human beings were used as subjects are reviewed in this analysis.

Metabolism of Carbohydrates Ingested Before Exercise

Carbohydrate ingested during the hours before exercise can be oxidized by active muscle. For example, Ravussin et al. (1979) reported that 40% of a 100 g glucose feeding consumed 1 h before exercise was oxidized during exercise at 35% $\dot{V}O_2$max for 2 h, and Jandrain et al. (1984) noted that 70% of a similar dosage was used during exercise at 45% $\dot{V}O_2$max for 4 h. The amount of glucose oxidized during low-intensity exercise preceded by a carbohydrate feeding is not affected by the preexercise muscle glycogen level (Ravussin et al., 1979). Therefore, carbohydrate in preexercise feedings is available for muscle oxidation during exercise and may provide an important substrate during exercise.

Metabolic Responses During Exercise

Blood Substrates and Hormones. Ingestion of foods before exercise may alter the blood concentrations of substrates and hormones, and these perturbations may subsequently alter the "normal" metabolic responses during exercise. When athletes consumed 75 g glucose 45 min before running for 30 min at 70% $\dot{V}O_2$max, blood glucose was significantly elevated at the start of exercise and declined by 50% after 15 min to 3.5 mM, a value significantly lower than for the placebo trial (Costill et al., 1977). Preexercise carbohydrate feedings have also evoked a decline in blood glucose below placebo levels early in exercise in other studies (Figure 1-1, lines B and C) (Koivisto et al., 1981; Hargreaves et al., 1987; Koivisto et al., 1985; Levine et al., 1983; Coyle et al., 1985; Sherman et al., 1989; Peden et al., 1989). For some studies, however, blood glucose soon returned to values similar to those for placebo (Figure 1-1, line B) (Koivisto et al., 1985; Levine et al., 1983; Coyle et al., 1985; Hargreaves et al., 1987; Sherman et al., 1989) or to values greater than those under placebo conditions (Figure 1-1, line C) (Peden et al., 1989).

In other studies using preexercise carbohydrate feedings, blood glucose was not affected relative to placebo during exercise, despite initially high insulin levels (Fielding et al., 1987; Gleeson et al., 1986; Devlin et al., 1986). Conversely, blood glucose may rise significantly during exercise preceded by a preexercise carbohydrate feeding (Figure 1-1, line D), even when the blood insulin concentration is elevated (Bonen et al., 1981; Wright & Sherman, 1989; Peden et al., 1989). Figure 1-1 provides a schematic representation of the possible

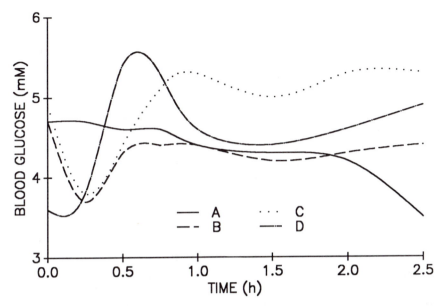

FIGURE 1-1. *Blood glucose responses that occur during exercise following a preexercise meal. When glucose declines during exercise, liver glucose production is less than muscle glucose uptake and when glucose rises, liver glucose output exceeds muscle glucose uptake. Possible blood glucose responses follow: A) when fasted, blood glucose gradually declines (Sherman et al., 1989); B) when moderately trained subjects consume carbohydrate 4 h before exercise (4.5 g/kg), blood glucose will decline and recover to normal levels (Sherman et al., 1989); C) when trained subjects consume carbohydrate 1 h before exercise (1 or 2 g/kg) blood glucose will initially decline but increase to above-normal levels (Peden et al., 1989); and D) when well trained subjects consume carbohydrate 3 h before exercise (5 g/kg), blood glucose will rise and then slowly decline (Wright and Sherman, 1989).*

fluctuations in blood glucose during exercise after preexercise carbohydrate feedings.

The fall in blood glucose during exercise preceded by carbohydrate feedings is primarily attributed to the elevated insulin concentration at the onset of exercise or to a persistent effect of the elevated insulin levels during the period before exercise (Costill et al., 1977; Bonen et al., 1981; Coyle et al., 1985). This also is supported by the strong correlations between the preexercise glucose and insulin concentrations and the fall in blood glucose and insulin during exercise (Ahlborg & Felig, 1982; Koivisto, et al., 1981). On the other hand, when the blood glucose concentration is not affected, returns to normal, or surpasses normal levels during exercise preceded by carbohydrate feedings, either liver glycogenolysis or intestinal absorption of glucose must have produced a glucose appearance rate that exceeded tissue glucose uptake. Therefore, preexercise carbohydrate feedings may improve exercise performance by delaying the normal decline in blood glucose. Stimulation of liver glycogenolysis or persistent gastric emptying and intestinal absorption of the carbohydrate could account for such a delay.

Preexercise carbohydrate feedings usually increase blood insulin levels (Sherman et al., 1989; Peden et al., 1989; Wright et al., 1989) and suppress the normal rise in blood glucagon (Ahlborg & Felig, 1977). Preexercise carbohydrate feedings do not alter the typical elevations in blood growth hormone and cortisol during exercise (Koivisto et al., 1981). The hormonal milieu associated with preexercise carbohydrate feedings suppresses the normal increase in blood free fatty acid concentration and oxidation (Sherman et al., 1989) and suppresses liver gluconeogenesis (Ahlborg & Felig, 1977).

Because the insulin response to a given dose of fructose is significantly less than for an equivalent amount of glucose, fructose is often advocated as a preexercise carbohydrate source. The lower insulin response to fructose should minimize changes in blood glucose during exercise. The preexercise consumption of fructose produces a blood insulin concentration that is less at the start of exercise than that resulting from ingestion of an equivalent amount of glucose. The changes in blood glucose during exercise preceded by fructose ingestion is usually similar to that observed in a placebo trial (Levine et al., 1983; Fielding et al., 1987; Koivisto et al., 1985; Koivisto et al., 1981; Hargreaves et al., 1987). However, the question remains open as to whether the smaller changes in blood glucose and insulin after preexercise fructose ingestion provide a greater ergogenic effect than an equivalent preexercise glucose feeding (see below).

Muscle Glycogen and Blood Glucose. Studies of preexercise carbohydrate feeding have shown that such feedings increase total carbohydrate oxidation (Costill et al., 1977; Coyle et al., 1985), and it was initially reported that muscle glycogen degradation was significantly increased as well (Costill et al., 1977). If the body's carbohydrate reserves limit training and performance capacity at 65–80% VO_2max, it would obviously be unwise to institute nutritional strategies that accelerate carbohydrate degradation unless the dietary manipulation provides carbohydrate at a rate equal to or greater than the increase in the rate of carbohydrate degradation. However, the studies that initially documented elevated carbohydrate oxidation did not test exercise performance, but only examined the metabolic responses during exercise. Most subsequent studies showed that preexercise carbohydrate feedings do not affect the rate of muscle glycogen utilization during exercise (Table 1-1) (Ahlborg & Bjorkman, 1987; Coyle et al., 1985; Fielding et al., 1987; Koivisto et al.,

TABLE 1-1.* Effects of Preexercise Feedings on Muscle Glycogen Degradation During Exercise

Reference	Number of Subjects (n)	V̇O₂max (L/min)	Time of feeding Before Exercise (h)	Amount fed (g/kg bw)	Intensity of Exercise/ Duration (% V̇O₂max/min)	Rate of Glycogen Use (mmol/kg/min)	Sparing of Glycogen
Ahlborg & Bjorkman, 1987	6	3.8	0.83	2.9	30%/ 40	G = 1.2 Pl = 0.8	NO
Coyle et al., 1985	7	4.7	4.0	2.0	70%/105	G = 0.9 Fr = 0.6	NO
Devlin et al., 1986	8	3.7	0.5	0.6	68%/Exh	SF = 1.1 Pl = 1.0	NO
Fielding et al., 1987	6	4.8	0.5	1.1	55%/120	G = 0.8 Fr = 1.2 Pl = 0.9	NO
Hargreaves et al., 1987	6	4.6	0.75	1.0	75%/Exh	G = 1.0 Fr = 1.3 Pl = 1.1	NO
Koivisto et al., 1985	8	4.3	0.75	1.0	55%/120	G = 1.6 Fr = 1.7 Pl = 1.4	NO

* from Sherman & Wright, 1989, with permission; values are means; L/min = liters oxygen consumed per minute; min = minute; g/kg bw = grams/kilogram body weight; %V̇O₂max/min = percent of maximal oxygen consumption/minutes of exercise; mmol/kg/min = millimoles glucose units/kilogram/minute; G = glucose, Fr = fructose, Pl = placebo, SF = snack food.

1985; Devlin et al., 1986; Hargreaves et al., 1987). An exception was a report by Levine et al. (1983) that a preexercise fructose feeding decreased glycogen utilization by 55% during 30 min of running at 70% $\dot{V}O_2$max. However, the study of Hargreaves et al. (1987), which required subjects to exercise at 75% $\dot{V}O_2$max until exhausted, found that glycogen degradation and time to exhaustion were similar for preexercise glucose and fructose feedings.

Because blood glucose concentration is a function of the splanchnic release of glucose and the muscle uptake of glucose, and because preexercise carbohydrate feedings alter the substrate and hormonal milieu, it is reasonable to assume that carbohydrate feedings alter the factors that influence the blood glucose concentration. Indeed, both Ahlborg & Felig (1977) and Ahlborg & Bjorkman (1987) observed significantly elevated muscle glucose uptake, and Ahlborg & Felig (1977) observed significantly elevated splanchnic glucose release from glycogenolysis and decreased liver gluconeogenesis after preexercise carbohydrate feedings. Thus, because muscle glycogen sparing typically does not occur with preexercise carbohydrate feedings (Table 1-1), it is probable that enhanced glucose availability and oxidation can at least partly account for any observed enhancement of exercise performance.

Preexercise Carbohydrate Feedings: Effects on Performance

Because several early studies using preexercise carbohydrate feedings have observed precipitous declines in blood glucose, increased glycogen utilization, and greater total carbohydrate oxidation, professionals who advise athletes about nutritional practices have traditionally recommended that their athlete clients refrain from carbohydrate ingestion during the hours before endurance exercise (Grandjean, Footnote 2). However, scrutiny of more recent studies should significantly alter this traditional recommendation. A summary of the results of these studies appears in Table 1-2.

High-Intensity Aerobic Exercise. Five studies examined the effects of preexercise carbohydrate feedings on exercise performance at intensities > 80% $\dot{V}O_2$max. Foster et al. (1979) reported a 19% reduction in exercise time to exhaustion at 80% $\dot{V}O_2$max but no effect at 100% $\dot{V}O_2$max when subjects consumed 1.1 g glucose/kg (Footnote 3) 30 min before exercise. Foster et al. (1979, p. 2) ascribed the early fatigue to glycogen depletion, although glycogen was not measured; furthermore, the criterion for fatigue is clouded by the statement, ". . . exhaustion was . . . subjectively determined and usually was manifested as an unwillingness on the part of the subject to continue the ride, rather than a physical inability to turn the pedals." Both McMurray et al. (1983) and Keller and Schwarzkopf

(1984) found that preexercise carbohydrate ingestion had no effect on time to exhaustion at 85% $\dot{V}O_2$max, or on the cumulative exercise time for well-trained runners performing intermittent exercise at 85% $\dot{V}O_2$max, respectively. These findings should be viewed with caution because the aspartame-containing placebo treatment decreased performance by 20% vs. water (McMurray et al., 1983), and because the Keller and Schwarzkopf (1984) study used a single blind design.

Lamb et al. (1986) required wrestlers to perform two sets of simultaneous, maximal arm and leg cranking exercise until fatigue. This was preceded by ingestion of 750 mL of either a placebo, a solution containing 37.5 g glucose, or a solution containing 150 g of maltodextrins 30 min before exercise. The performance times for the first set averaged roughly 138 s, whereas the performance times for the second set averaged roughly 27 s. Neither the performance times for the individual sets nor their combination were significantly different among trials.

Based on these studies, there is little reason to believe that preexercise carbohydrate feedings impair exercise capacity at intensities above 80% $\dot{V}O_2$max. However, the effect of preexercise carbohydrate feedings on endurance in an exercise session that includes many repetitions of high-intensity exercise is unknown. Such exercise depletes muscle glycogen, and preexercise feedings may slightly increase muscle glycogen before exercise (Coyle et al., 1985) or may elevate blood glucose to match an elevated rate of muscle glucose uptake when glycogen stores are depleted (Coyle et al., 1986; Gollnick et al., 1981).

Moderate Intensity Aerobic Exercise. Nine studies have examined the effects of preexercise carbohydrate feedings on endurance for prolonged exercise. Of these, three have observed no effects, whereas six have observed improved endurance after preexercise carbohydrate feedings. No studies have reported negative effects of preexercise carbohydrate feedings on performance.

Negative Effects. Only anecdotal reports exist about the potentially negative effects of preexercise carbohydrate feedings on performance of prolonged exercise. Apparently, some people are sensitive to the lowering of blood glucose that occurs during the initial 15 min of exercise preceded by carbohydrate ingestion (Figure 1-1, lines B and C). This "sensitivity" may result in lethargy, nausea, light-headedness, and the inability to continue exercise. However, it should be emphasized that more than 125 subjects have been used in studies of preexercise carbohydrate feedings and no one has reported negative effects of such feedings. It is possible that neither the investigators nor the subjects were responsive to these symptoms and failed to note their occurrences. Nonetheless, of >30 sub-

TABLE 1-2. Ergogenic effects of preexercise carbohydrate feedings.

Reference	Number of subjects (n)	V̇O₂max (mL/kg/min)	type of subject	time ingested before exercise (min)	treatments content	amount (g/kg)	exercise protocol intensity & duration (% V̇O₂max & min)	mode	Results (% change vs. placebo)
HIGH INTENSITY EXERCISE									
Foster et al. (1979)	16	50	cyclists	30	water glucose meal	0 1.1 0.2	100% until exhaustion (SR) and 80% until exhaustion (LR)	cycling	−4% SR −19% LR* −0% SR −0 % LR
McMurray et al. (1983)	6	?	runners	45	water placebo glucose fructose	0 0 1.5 1.5	85% until exhaustion	running	−20%* −3% −6%
Keller & Schwartzkof (1984)	5	71	runners	60	placebo glucose	0 1.5	85% until exhaustion 2:1 min, work:rest	cycling	−25%
Lamb et al. (1986)	9	?	wrestlers	30	placebo glucose maltodextrins	0 0.5 2.0	2 maximal output sessions 15 min break simultaneous arm & leg cranking		+13% +0%
MODERATE INTENSITY EXERCISE									
Koivisto et al. (1981)	9	60	volleyball	45	placebo glucose fructose	0 1.0 1.0	75% until exhaustion	cycling	−3.6% −1%
Gleeson et al. (1986)	6	47	nonathletes	45	placebo glucose glycerol	0 1.0 1.0	73% until exhaustion	cycling	+14%* −10%

Study	n	Subjects	min	Treatment	CHO	Exercise protocol	Exercise	Change
Devlin et al. (1986)	8	nonathletes	30	placebo snack food#	0 0.6	70% until exhaustion 15:5 min, work:rest	cycling	+8%
Neuffer et al. (1987)	10	cyclists	5 SF@4h	placebo glucose snack food (SF)@ SF + glucose	0.6 0.6 3.4	77% for 45 min then isokinetic work test	cycling	+10%* +11%* +22%*
Hargreaves et al. (1987)	6	cyclists	45	placebo glucose fructose	0 1.0 1.0	75% until exhaustion	cycling	0% +2%
Okano et al. (9188)	12	athletes	60	placebo fructose fructose	0 0.9 1.3	62% for 90 min, 72% for 30 min, 81% for 30 min, continue to exhaustion	cycling	+7%* +17%*
Sherman et al. (1989)	10	conditioned	240	placebo maltodextrins maltodextrins Exceed	0 0.6 2.0 4.5&	4 X 15:5 min, 70%:60% Time trial performance	cycling	0% 0% +13%*
Wright & Sherman (1989)	9	cyclists	180	placebo Exceed	0 5&	70% until exhaustion Work capacity test every 40 min	cycling	+18%* +18%*
Peden et al. (1989)	9	cyclists	60	placebo Exceed Exceed	0 1& 2&	70% for 90 min Time trial performance	cycling	+14%* +14%*

and @ = snack food contained 260 kcal with 43 g carbohydrate, 9 g fat, and 3 g protein; & = Exceed contains 70% maltodextrins, 15% glucose, and 15% sucrose; * = significantly different from placebo treatment.

jects used in preexercise feeding trials at The Ohio State University, neither the investigators nor the subjects could document such symptoms during trials when blood glucose initially declined during exercise following a preexercise carbohydrate feeding.

Indeterminate Effects. Koivisto et al. (1981) fed either glucose or fructose (1 g/kg) or a placebo to trained volleyball players 45 min before cycling to exhaustion at 75% $\dot{V}O_2$max. Times to exhaustion were similar among the trials (29.9 min). These unusually short endurance times may be related to the fact that the exercise test was not specific to the type of training engaged in by the athletes. In untrained subjects, Devlin et al. (1986) determined the effects of consuming a snack bar (0.6 g carbohydrate/kg) or *liquid* placebo 30 min before interval cycling at 70% $\dot{V}O_2$max until exhaustion. There was no difference in time to exhaustion between the trials (52 min vs. 48 min, respectively). It may be argued that the placebo should have been a snack bar containing no carbohydrate and that the amount of carbohydrate was too small to produce an effect. Furthermore, during exercise the 8 mM blood lactate concentration might have contributed to fatigue in the untrained subjects. Hargreaves et al. (1987) fed subjects a placebo or solutions containing 1 g/kg fructose or glucose 45 min before exercising to exhaustion at 75% $\dot{V}O_2$max. Exercise time was similar among trials (92 min). Flynn et al. (1989) did not test the effects of preexercise carbohydrate feedings on performance because there was not a placebo trial; however, they did compare the effects of ingesting a mixed solid/liquid preexercise meal (3.5 g carbohydrate/kg) consumed either 4 or 8 h before 120 min of cycling at 65% $\dot{V}O_2$max. This was followed by cycling on an isokinetic ergometer during which the subjects were instructed to produce as much work as possible for 15 min. All subjects completed the 2 h rides, and isokinetic work production was similar between trials (217 vs. 218 kJ, respectively).

Positive Effects. Gleeson et al. (1986) published the first evidence that preexercise carbohydrate feedings improve performance. Subjects consumed a liquid carbohydrate beverage (1 g/kg) or placebo 45 min before cycling to exhaustion at 73% $\dot{V}O_2$max. The preexercise carbohydrate feeding significantly extended time until exhaustion by 9 min.

Since this report, several studies have examined the effects of the timing, amount, and constitution of the preexercise feeding on performance. Neufer et al. (1987) examined the effects on performance of consuming liquid or solid carbohydrate 5 min before exercise, or consuming solid carbohydrate both 4 h and 5 min before exercise. The subjects' baseline muscle glycogen stores were reduced to 104 mmol/kg by a 12 h fast and a low carbohydrate diet.

The 5 min preexercise feedings provided 0.6 g carbohydrate/kg, whereas the 4 h preexercise feeding provided 2.8 g carbohydrate/kg. Total preexercise carbohydrate feeding was 3.4 g/kg. The 10 subjects cycled 45 min at 77% $\dot{V}O_2$max and then cycled on an isokinetic cycle ergometer to assess the amount of work that could be accomplished in 15 min. The solid and liquid 5 min preexercise feedings resulted in significantly more average work (175 kJ) than placebo (159 kJ), whereas the combination of the solid 4 h plus 5 min preexercise feeding resulted in significantly more average work production than all other trials (194 kJ). Thus, the preexercise carbohydrate feedings resulted in an average 14% greater work output compared to placebo when the subjects' initial muscle glycogen levels were lower than normal.

Okano et al. (1988) tested the effectiveness of 0.9 g/kg or 1.3 g/kg preexercise liquid fructose on endurance performance at 63% $\dot{V}O_2$max. The preexercise fructose feedings increased time to exhaustion by 13 min compared to a placebo trial. Additionally, the larger dose of fructose resulted in a significant 13 min extension of exercise time versus the lower dose of fructose. These results differ from those of a somewhat similarly designed study by Hargreaves et al. (1987). One possible explanation for the different results is that the two studies used different exercise intensities—63% vs. 75% $\dot{V}O_2$max for Okano et al. (1988) and Hargreaves et al. (1987), respectively.

A series of recent studies by Sherman and colleagues (Sherman et al., 1989; Peden et al., 1989; Wright & Sherman, 1989) have examined the effects on performance of the timing and amounts of preexercise carbohydrate feedings in subjects with different training levels. In the first study (Sherman et al., 1989), moderately trained cyclists consumed either a placebo, 0.6, 2.0, or 4.5 g carbohydrate/kg 4 h before 95 min of interval exercise. This was followed by a cycling time trial for which the subjects were blinded to time and asked to complete as fast as possible, the distance equivalent to an additional 45 min of cycling at 70% $\dot{V}O_2$max. A *shorter time* to complete this distance, therefore, indicates that the subjects maintained higher exercise intensities for the time trial and improved their performances. The subjects completed the time trials for the 0, 0.6, 2.0, and 4.5 g carbohydrate/kg doses in 52, 53, 53, and 42 min, respectively. These results demonstrate an ergogenic effect for consuming 320 g (equivalent to 4.5 g carbohydrate/kg) liquid carbohydrate in a 4 h preexercise feeding.

In another study, trained subjects who were able to maintain 70% $\dot{V}O_2$max during the 90 min before a time trial similar to that used by Sherman et al. (1989), completed the time trial 7 min faster than the placebo trial (47 min) when fed solutions containing either 1 g glucose or 2 g maltodextrins/kg body weight 1 h before exercise (Peden et al., 1989). Also, using well trained cyclists, Wright and Sherman (1989) determined the separate and combined effects of liquid carbohydrate feedings 3 h before exercise (5 g maltodextrins/ kg) and/or during exercise (0.2 g maltodextrins/kg every 20 min). The cyclists exercised at 70% $\dot{V}O_2$max until the pedalling cadence dropped to that which elicited 50% $\dot{V}O_2$max. Additionally, every 45 min they completed a test that required them to pedal as fast as possible the distance they would travel in 3 min at 90% $\dot{V}O_2$max. The preexercise feeding permitted the cyclists to generate 18% more work for the work tests and to exercise for 36 min longer than for the placebo trial (201 min). Furthermore, when the preexercise carbohydrate feedings were combined with feedings during exercise, the cyclists generated 46% more work during the work tests and exercised 89 additional minutes compared to placebo.

Conclusions, Recommendations, and Precautions

Because the body's carbohydrate stores may be reduced by poor eating habits and training practices, training and performance can be compromised. Preexercise carbohydrate feedings may increase carbohydrate reserves by promoting liver and muscle glycogen synthesis or providing an absorbable source of blood glucose during exercise that should improve training and performance capabilities. Based on this rationale and the review of literature, the following observations, recommendations and precautions are warranted:

a. preexercise feedings may elevate the liver or muscle glycogen concentrations and/or may provide an absorbable source of glucose;

b. the preexercise feeding should contain 1–5 g carbohydrate/ kg body weight and should be consumed 1–4 h before exercise;

c. the sources of carbohydrates fed 4 h before exercise may be easily digestible, solid high carbohydrate foods, but when fed 1 h before exercise, they should be in liquid form;

d. endurance athletes who train in the morning after an overnight fast, whose schedules preclude normal eating patterns, or who cannot sustain a diet containing 60–70% of their food energy as carbohydrate should use preexercise carbohydrate feedings to optimize exercise capacity;

e. athletes should incorporate preexercise feeding strategies into their training and use them in competition only when they are comfortable with them;

f. metabolic responses to preexercise feedings may differ, depending upon the training state of the athlete and the type and quantity of carbohydrate consumed;

g. following a preexercise carbohydrate feeding, some athletes may experience a lowering of blood glucose to which they are sensitive (i.e., it causes fatigue), and these athletes may not benefit from preexercise feedings; however, for the 125 subjects tested in the indeterminate and positive studies (Table 1-2), there were no reports that individuals were sensitive to the lowering of blood glucose.

CARBOHYDRATE FEEDINGS AND GLYCOGEN SYNTHESIS AFTER EXERCISE

When athletes undertake strenuous training or competition that significantly reduces liver and muscle glycogen, it is necessary to replenish those carbohydrate reserves so that subsequent exercise performance is not impaired. This section will examine various nutritional strategies designed to replace body carbohydrate reserves after exercise. Because very few studies have examined the recovery of exercise capacity as glycogen stores are resynthesized after exercise, it is assumed that nutritional strategies causing the highest rate of glycogen synthesis will result in a greater exercise capacity than nutritional strategies causing a slower rate of glycogen synthesis.

Replenishment of Liver Glycogen

Fructose *may be* a better carbohydrate source to replenish liver glycogen than glucose. Nilson & Hultman (1974) infused or fed glucose or infused fructose in the postabsorptive state. The rate of liver glycogen synthesis was similar for infused and ingested glucose; however, fructose infusion increased liver glycogen synthesis 3.7-fold above that for glucose. The greater rate of glycogen synthesis from fructose than from glucose may be due to a higher liver fructose kinase activity than glucose kinase activity (Heinz, 1972). Thus, consuming fruits or fructose-containing beverages after exercise *may* promote greater liver glycogen synthesis than will foods or beverages containing only glucose. There are no fructose versus glucose oral feeding studies that have confirmed this effect shown with infusion.

Liver Versus Muscle Glycogen Synthesis

Both liver and muscle must replenish glycogen after exercise, but which tissue predominates? Maehlum et al. (1978) suggested that most of a glucose load ingested after exercise escapes the splanchnic bed and contributes to muscle glycogen synthesis. Also, Krzentowski et al. (1982) suggested that the enhanced splanchnic glucose release during recovery is contributed to by elevated glucagon and lower insulin concentrations following exercise. Furthermore, 90% of an oral glucose load in postprandial resting subjects is disposed of as muscle glycogen (Ferrannini et al., 1985). Therefore, muscle glycogen synthesis apparently predominates over liver glycogen synthesis during recovery from exercise.

Time-Course of Muscle Glycogen Replenishment

Although two studies suggest that 48 h is required to "normalize" muscle glycogen after exercise (Piehl, 1974; Piehl et al., 1974), at least five separate studies observed repletion of muscle glycogen by 24 h after exercise (Ahlborg et al., 1967; Bergstrom et al., 1972; Kochan et al., 1979; MacDougall et al., 1977; Keizer et al., 1987). The subjects in these studies undertook prolonged exercise that exhausted stores of muscle and presumably liver glycogen. Subjects consumed between 9 and 16 g carbohydrate/kg in 24 h. Similarly, when subjects depleted muscle glycogen with intense interval exercise but consumed 4.8 g carbohydrate/kg beginning 2 h after exercise, muscle glycogen was normal 24 h after exercise (MacDougall et al., 1977).

When no carbohydrate is consumed after exercise, very little glycogen synthesis occurs (MacDougall et al., 1977; Ivy et al., 1988a). Similarly, there is a strong relationship between the amount of dietary energy as carbohydrate and the amount of glycogen synthesized in a 24 h period (r=0.84; Costill et al., 1981). A diet consisting of simple carbohydrates induces greater synthesis of glycogen than a complex carbohydrate diet during the first 6 h after exhaustive exercise (Kiens et al., 1990). On the other hand, there is no difference in glycogen synthesis between a simple or complex carbohydrate diet 20, 32, or 44 h after exhaustive exercise (Kiens et al., 1990). Therefore, when at least 9 g carbohydrate/kg are consumed after exercise, muscle glycogen should be replenished in 24 h.

Amount and Timing of Carbohydrate Ingestion

While the previously cited studies investigated muscle glycogen synthesis over a 24 h period or longer, many recent studies have determined the appropriate timing and amount of ingested carbohydrate to optimize glycogen synthesis within the first 10 h after exercise (Table 1-3). Blom et al. (1987a) depleted muscle glycogen and fed subjects 0.35, 0.7, or 1.4 g glucose/kg every 2 h for a total of 6 h beginning immediately after exercise. The rate of glycogen synthesis was the same, regardless of the amount of glucose in-

TABLE 1-3. Postexercise carbohydrate intake and muscle glycogen synthesis.

Reference	Number of subjects (n)	mode	Exercise time (min)	intensity (%V̇O₂max)	post-exercise glycogen (mmol/kg)	Beverages type & composition	duration of feedings (h)	number of feedings	amount of CHO fed (g/kg/feeding)	Glycogen synthesis (mmol/kg/h)
Keizer et al. (1987)	8	cycling		MPWC test	18	solid *	5	4	3.3	6.8
			2:2	90% to exhaustion	18	liquid Powerback	5	4	3.3	6.3
			2:2	80% to exhaustion						
			2:2	70% to exhaustion						
Blom et al. (1987a)	5	cycling	20:10	75% to exhaustion	32	liquid glucose	6	3	0.35	2.7
	5				15	liquid glucose	6	3	0.70	6.8
	5				23	liquid glucose	6	3	1.40	5.7
	5				8	liquid sucrose	6	3	0.70	6.3
	7				23	liquid fructose	6	3	0.70	3.3
Ivy et al. (1988a)	12	cycling	8:2	68%;88% to exhaustion	36	liquid Excell#+	4	2	1.0	6.0
					31	liquid Excell$+	4	1	1.0	4.1
					31	placebo	4	0	0	3.2
Ivy et al. (1988b)	8	cycling	4 x 15:15	62%;75%	36	placebo	4	2	0	0.5
					36	liquid Exceed +	4	2	1.5	4.6
					32	liquid Exceed +	4	2	3.0	5.2
					27	solid &	4	2	1.5	5.5
Reed et al. (1989)	8	cycling	4 x 15:15	62%;72%	24	liquid Exceed +	4	2	1.5	5.1
					31	glucose infused			3.2	5.6
Vollestad et al. (1989)	6	cycling	20:10	75%;rest to exhaustion	23	liquid glucose	3	3	~	10.0
Blom (1989)	5	cycling	3 x 20:10	75%;rest to exhaustion	22	liquid glucose	3	3	~	9.3
					14	glucose infused			3.5	8.3

* = solid food was whole wheat bread with jam, honey, bananas; @ = Powerback contains 1.3% glucose, 0.7% fructose, 0.5% maltose, 53% sucrose, and 45% maltodextrins; # = feedings were 5 min before exercise stopped or immediately after exercise; $ = carbohydrate feeding 2 h after exercise; & = solid foods were rice cakes, banana cakes and supplemental glucose; + = Excell and Exceed contains 70% maltodextrins, 15% glucose, and 15% sucrose; ~ = first feeding immediately after exercise 1.4 g/kg and then two additional feedings containing 0.7 g/kg.

gested, and averaged 5.2 mmol·kg^{-1}·h^{-1}. A second group of subjects in a similar design consumed 0.7 g/kg of either sucrose or fructose. Glycogen synthesis was 6.3 mmol·kg^{-1}·h^{-1} for sucrose but was only 3.3 mmol·kg^{-1}·h^{-1} for fructose. Blom (1989) also fed subjects a total of 2.8 g carbohydrate/kg or infused a similar amount of glucose during a 3 h postexercise period. The rate of glycogen synthesis was similar for the two routes of carbohydrate administration and averaged 8.8 mmol·kg^{-1}·h^{-1}.

In a similarly designed study, Vollestad et al. (1989) examined fiber-type-specific glycogen synthesis when subjects consumed a total of 2.8 g carbohydrate/kg during the 3 h after exercise. Although the rate of glycogen synthesis was 65% slower in the slow twitch fibers during the 0–90 min postexercise period, thereafter the rate of glycogen synthesis was similar among fiber types (10.0 mmol·kg^{-1}·h^{-1}).

In a similar series of studies, Ivy et al. determined the effects of timing (1988a), amount (1988b), or type (Reed et al., 1989) of postexercise carbohydrate ingestion on the rate of muscle glycogen synthesis. Subjects depleted glycogen with intermittent high- and low-intensity exercise for all three studies. To determine the effects of timing of postexercise carbohydrate ingestion on glycogen synthesis, the subjects consumed either a placebo, 1 g glucose/kg immediately after and 2 h after exercise, or 1 g glucose/kg only 2 h after exercise (Ivy et al., 1988a). Muscle biopsies taken immediately after and 4 h later revealed that the glycogen synthesis rate was 6.0 mmol·kg^{-1}·h^{-1} when subjects were fed immediately after exercise. When no carbohydrate was consumed for 2 h after exercise, the rate of glycogen synthesis was only 3.2 mmol·kg^{-1}·h^{-1}. When carbohydrate was ingested 2 h after the exercise, the glycogen synthesis rate was higher (4.1 mmol·kg^{-1}·h^{-1}), but was still significantly less than when carbohydrate was ingested immediately after exercise (Figure 1-2). The results of Bonen et al. (1985) are comparable to those of Ivy et al. (1988a).

To determine if the amount of carbohydrate ingested after exercise influences the rate of glycogen synthesis during the first 4 h of recovery, Ivy et al. (1988b) fed subjects a placebo or either 1.5 or 3.0 g glucose/kg immediately after and also 2 h after exercise. The rates of glycogen synthesis for the 4 h period were 0.5, 4.6, or 5.2 mmol·kg^{-1}·h^{-1} for the placebo and two carbohydrate feeding trials, respectively. Ivy et al. (1988b) concluded that consuming 1.5 g carbohydrate/kg at 2 h intervals was sufficient carbohydrate to fully stimulate postexercise glycogen synthesis. This interpretation is consistent with the findings of Keizer et al. (1987), who fed subjects 3.3 g liquid or solid carbohydrate in 4 feedings for the 5 h after

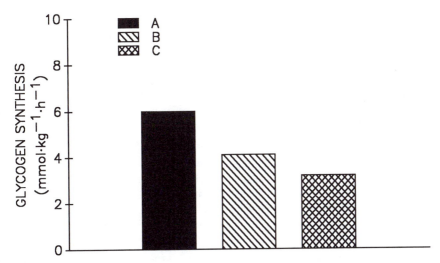

FIGURE 1-2. *Effects of the timing of carbohyhdrate ingestion on muscle glycogen synthesis following exercise (Ivy et al., 1988a). A) when carbohydrate is consumed immediately after exercise stops, glycogen synthesis is rapid; B) when carbohydrate consumption is delayed for 2 h after exercise stops and then consumed, glycogen synthesis is restored but not to rapid levels; and C) when no carbohydrate is consumed, glycogen synthesis is very slow.*

exercise and observed an average glycogen synthesis rate of 6.5 mmol·kg^{-1}·h^{-1}. Finally, Reed et al. (1989) also determined the effects of liquid or solid carbohydrate feedings or infusion of a comparable amount of glucose (225 g) on the postexercise rate of glycogen synthesis. Regardless of the physical form of carbohydrate, glycogen synthesis averaged 5.4 mmol·kg^{-1}·h^{-1}.

The studies by Blom and colleagues (1987a; 1987b; 1989), Vollestad et al. (1989), Ivy et al. (1988a; 1988b), Reed et al. (1989), and Keizer et al. (1987) suggest that when carbohydrate beverages are consumed during the 3 to 6 hours after exercise, glycogen synthesis will be between 5 and 10 mmol·kg^{-1}·h^{-1}. Although this may not represent the maximal capacity of muscle glycogen synthesis, glucose infusions (Bergstrom & Hultman, 1967) and hyperinsulinemic clamp procedures (Bourey et al., 1990) that produce glycogen synthesis rates between 12 and 25 mmol·kg^{-1}·h^{-1} are not ethical and probably not practical methods to stimulate postexercise glycogen synthesis.

Carbohydrate feedings consumed before the end or immediately after exercise will result in a glycogen synthesis rate between 5 and 10 mmol·$^{-1}$·h^{-1}. If carbohydrate feedings are delayed for several hours, the rate of glycogen synthesis will be very low (<3 mmol·$^{-1}$·h^{-1}); however, glycogen synthesis can be stimulated with delayed carbohydrate ingestion (4 mmol $\cdot$ $^{-1}\cdot h^{-1}$), but not to its maximal rate (6–10 mmol $\cdot$ $^{-1}\cdot h^{-1}$). Thus, athletes should consume between 0.7 and 2 g carbohydrate/kg every 2 h after exercise to promote glycogen synthesis. In practice, this means that athletes should consume high carbohydrate energy snacks at intervals throughout the day between training sessions.

Muscle Damage and Glycogen Synthesis

Low muscle glycogen concentrations have been observed during the 7 d after a marathon when subjects rested or undertook short, low intensity exercise (40% to 55% $\dot{V}O_2max$) while consuming a 6.8 g carbohydrate $\cdot kg^{-1}\cdot d^{-1}$ (Sherman et al., 1983). The evidence of muscle damage during those recovery days (Hikida et al., 1983) and "... the possible effect of muscular trauma on muscle glycogen synthesis ..." (Sherman et al., 1983, p. 1223) have led exercise physiologists to speculate that muscle damage impairs glycogen synthesis. However, there is a possibility that rest and daily low intensity exercise during the week after the marathon may have constituted an insufficient stimulus for glycogen synthesis. This is supported by the low activation state of glycogen synthase on the days after the marathon (Sherman et al., 1983).

While examining the effects of a prostaglandin inhibitor (flurbiprofen) on muscle soreness, Kuipers et al. (1985) determined muscle glycogen content before, immediately after, and 24 h after concentric and eccentric exercise. Unfortunately, these authors did not describe the amount of carbohydrate consumed after exercise. Nevertheless, muscle glycogen had returned to the preexercise concentration 24 h after concentric exercise, but was 18% lower than baseline after eccentric exercise. Kuipers et al. (1985, p. 338) speculated that, "... changes in muscle after eccentric exercise interfere with glycogen synthesis," despite the observations that, "In none of the subjects was a significant release of muscle enzymes found ... ," and, "Histological examination ... revealed minor changes ..."

Subsequently, Blom et al. (1987b) suggested that running is an "inappropriate" stimulus for glycogen synthesis because glycogen did not return to the preexercise supercompensated level after 3 d of rest while subjects consumed a high carbohydrate diet (8 g carbohydrate $\cdot kg^{-1}\cdot d^{-1}$). They also suggested that the eccentric phase of running results in damage that impairs glycogen synthesis although muscle damage was not assessed (Blom et al., 1987b). It is hard to reconcile this notion that running is a poor stimulus for glycogen synthesis with the fact that Sherman et al. (1981) and Roedde et al. (1986) observed glycogen supercompensation in runners.

Although the effects of running on glycogen synthesis are inconsistent, eccentric contractions *per se* appear to reduce the muscle's capacity to synthesize glycogen; however, the mechanism is unknown. The subjects in the study of Costill et al. (1990) performed either eccentric or concentric leg extensions followed by cycling exercise employed to lower muscle glycogen. They consumed a relatively low amount of carbohydrate, $4.3 \text{ g} \cdot \text{kg}^{-1} \cdot \text{d}^{-1}$, for the next 2 d. Twenty-four hours after exercise, muscle glycogen was the same in each of the legs (78 mmol/kg), but at 72 h the glycogen concentration in the eccentric leg was 32% lower than that in the concentric leg. Costill et al. (1990) theorized that the inflammation resulting from muscle damage induced by the eccentric contractions causes glycogen degradation and impairs glycogen synthesis.

Other studies have also reported low muscle glycogen levels during the days following eccentric exercise. O'Reilly et al. (1987, p. 253) found significantly lowered glycogen concentrations 10 d after eccentric exercise in subjects consuming a high carbohydrate diet. A potentially confounding variable for interpreting this study is the fact that the 10 d posteccentric- exercise biopsy was, ". . . taken near the scar left by the previous biopsy." Because the muscle biopsy is traumatic, it is possible that the biopsy itself may induce inflammation similar to that resulting from eccentric exercise and, if the muscle biopsies during eccentric studies are not obtained from alternating legs or from a site some distance away from the previous biopsy, there may be an effect of the biopsy itself on muscle glycogen. Indeed, Costill et al. (1988, p. 2245) suggested that, ". . . alterations in muscle glycogen storage persists for 10 days after the first biopsy, suggesting that care must be taken in selecting the site for repeated biopsies from the same muscle." Although it is not clear how discrimination of biopsy sites 1 or 3 cm apart (Costill et al., 1988) can be accurately determined, it would be advisable to obtain muscle samples 3 to 5 cm distal or proximal to the initial site when repeated muscle biopsies from the same muscle are required within a 10 d period.

Collectively, the literature indicates that eccentric exercise reduces muscle glycogen content, even when moderate or high carbohydrate diets are consumed. No study has elucidated the mechanism(s) by which damage from eccentric contractions affects muscle glycogen synthesis. However, Doyle and Sherman (Footnote 4) obtained evidence consistent with the hypothesis that muscle damage may adversely affect muscle glycogen resynthesis. They noted that the rate of muscle glycogen synthesis was similar in muscles of concentrically and eccentrically exercised legs immediately after exercise; however, glycogen synthesis was significantly lower 2 d later in the eccentrically exercised leg compared to the concentrically exercised leg. Presumably, muscle damage was limited immediately after exercise but was markedly greater in the eccentric leg 2 d after exercise.

Postexercise Carbohydrate Feedings and Performance

Many studies have examined the effects of carbohydrate ingestion on muscle glycogen synthesis, but few have examined the effects of the resulting glycogen levels on exercise capacity. It is generally assumed that nutritional strategies stimulating high rates of glycogen synthesis will result in a greater restoration of exercise capacity than strategies resulting in slower rates of glycogen synthesis.

Brooke and Green (1974) examined the effects of consuming various amounts of carbohydrate during a 40 min postexhaustion rest period on subsequent exercise capacity. Subjects were fasted and exercised at 70% $\dot{V}O_2$max to exhaustion (153 min) and then consumed either a low-energy drink (less than 20 kJ) or 1.49 mJ of either a semi-solid meal (rice pudding and sucrose) or a glucose syrup beverage (115 g glucose, 25% wt/vol). This double-blind (for the liquid drinks) study resulted in an exercise duration of 29 min following the low-energy drink. Relative to the low-energy drink, the semi-solid meal resulted in a 2-fold increase and the glucose syrup resulted in a 2.7-fold increase in exercise time to exhaustion. The criterion for exhaustion was a respiratory exchange ratio of 0.70, which is not a universally accepted criterion.

In a study of recovery from the marathon, Sherman and colleagues (1983, 1984) measured muscle glycogen, isokinetic muscular strength, and isokinetic work capacity before, immediately after, and 1, 3, 5, and 7 d after a marathon. Work capacity was assessed by measuring the work produced during a 50 contraction leg flexion/extension test at 180 °/s. The subjects were fed 800 g carbohydrate following the marathon and, for each subsequent day, consumed 425 g carbohydrate/d (60% energy from carbohydrate). Half the subjects rested and half exercised (20–45 min/d at 50–60% $\dot{V}O_2$max) during the postmarathon week. Immediately before the marathon, muscle glycogen was supercompensated (196 mmol/kg). It was significantly reduced immediately after the marathon to 25 mmol/kg and was only 80 and 125 mmol/kg 1 d and 7 d, respectively, after the marathon. Muscle glycogen was not appreciably different during the recovery week between the rested and exercised groups. After the marathon, isokinetic muscular strength and work capacity were reduced by more than 47%. Seven days after the marathon, although exercise capacity was recovered in the rested group, isokinetic strength was still significantly lower for both groups than before the marathon. Furthermore, the isokinetic strength of the exercised group was significantly lower than the rested group 7 d after the marathon, suggesting that exercise during the week after the marathon may have detrimentally affected recovery.

Keizer et al. (1987) determined the so-called maximal physical working capacity (MPWC) using an exercise:rest ratio of 2 min:2min for three sets of cycling at 90%, 80%, and 70% $\dot{V}O_2$max, respectively. The MPWC test reduced glycogen to an average of 18 mmol/kg (estimated from dry muscle weight), and during the next 22 h the subjects consumed 28,234 kJ energy containing 1.2 kg of carbohydrate. Muscle glycogen after 22 h equaled the baseline value of 77 mmol/kg. Nevertheless, MPWC remained significantly reduced by 7% even when the muscle glycogen had returned to normal. While this difference may be close to the test-retest variability for the MPWC test, the reduced exercise capacity at normal glycogen levels supports the idea that factors other than muscle glycogen influence muscle function (Young & Davies, 1984).

CONCLUSIONS, RECOMMENDATIONS, AND PRACTICAL APPLICATIONS

Because athletes train at intensities and for durations that utilize significant amounts of the body's carbohydrate reserves, it is important to replace carbohydrate stores quickly following exercise. Manipulations that increase the rate of restoration of the depleted carbohydrate reserves should theoretically result in better performance than those manipulations that result in a slower rate of carbohydrate synthesis. Therefore, based on this rationale and the review of literature, the following observations, recommendations and precautions are warranted:

a. fructose may induce more liver glycogen synthesis than glucose, whereas glucose induces more muscle glycogen synthesis than fructose;

b. after exercise, the majority of ingested glucose escapes the liver and is taken up by muscle for synthesis of muscle glycogen;

c. after exercise, glycogen will be restored in 24 h if between 9 and 16 g carbohydrate $\cdot kg^{-1} \cdot {}^{-1}$ are consumed;

d. to optimize muscle glycogen synthesis during the immediate hours following exercise:
   1) begin consumption of carbohydrate immediately after exercise;

2) consume at least 0.75 g carbohydrate $\cdot$ kg^{-1} $\cdot$ h^{-1};
3) consume either liquid carbohydrate *or* rapidly digested high carbohydrate foods;

e. eccentric exercise that causes muscle damage may reduce the muscle's ability to synthesize glycogen, especially 2–10 d after the eccentric exercise.

FOOTNOTES

1. Ann C. Grandjean, Chief Nutrition Consultant, USOC, Swanson Center for Nutrition, 502 S. 44th Street, Room 3007, Omaha, Nebraska, 68105, personal communication.
2. Ann C. Grandjean, Chief Nutrition Consultant, USOC Swanson Center for Nutrition, 502 S. 44th Street, Room 3007, Omaha, Nebraska, 68105, "Nutrition Knowledge and Practices of Professionals Working in Sports Nutrition," University of Kansas, 1987, thesis.
3. The terminology g/kg is indicative of ingestion of carbohydrate relative to body mass, e.g., g/kg body weight.
4. Doyle, J.A., and W.M. Sherman. (1991). Eccentric exercise & glycogen synthesis. *Med. Sci. Sports Exerc.* 23:Sxx, abstract.

BIBLIOGRAPHY

Ahlborg, G., and O. Bjorkman (1987). Carbohydrate utilization by exercising muscle following preexercise glucose ingestion. *Clin. Physiol.* 7: 181–195.

Ahlborg, G., and P. Felig (1982). Lactate and glucose exchange across the forearm, legs, and splanchnic bed during and after prolonged leg exercise. *J. Clin. Invest.* 69: 45–54.

Ahlborg, G., and P. Felig (1977). Substrate utilization during prolonged exercise preceded by ingestion of glucose. *Am. J. Physiol.* 233: E188–E194.

Ahlborg, B., J. Bergstrom, J. Brohult, L.-G. Ekelund, E. Hultman, and G. Maschio (1967). Human muscle glycogen content and capacity for prolonged exercise after different diets. *Foersvarsmedicin* 3: 85–99.

Bergstrom, J., E. Hultman, and A.E. Roch-Norlund (1972). Muscle glycogen synthase in normal subjects: basal values, effect of glycogen depletion by exercise and of a carbohydrate-rich diet following exercise. *Scand. J. Clin. Lab. Invest.* 29: 231–236.

Bergstrom, J., and E. Hultman (1967). Synthesis of muscle glycogen in man after glucose and fructose infusion. *Acta Med. Scand.* 182: 93–107.

Bergstrom, J., L. Hermansen, E. Hultman, and B. Saltin (1967). Diet, muscle glycogen and physical performance. *Acta Physiol. Scand.* 71: 140–150.

Blom, P.C.S (1989). Post-exercise glucose uptake and glycogen synthesis in human muscle during oral or IV glucose intake. *Eur. J. Appl. Physiol.* 59: 327–333.

Blom, P.C.S., A.T. Hostmark, O. Vaage, K.R. Kardel, and S. Maehlum (1987a). Effect of different post-exercise sugar diets on the rate of muscle glycogen synthesis. *Med. Sci. Sports Exerc.* 19: 491–496.

Blom, P.C.S. D.L. Costill, and N.K. Vollestad (1987b). Exhaustive running: inappropriate stimulus of muscle glycogen supercompensation. *Med. Sci. Sports Exerc.* 19: 398–403.

Bonen, A., B.W. Ness, A.N. Belcastro, and R.L. Kirby (1985). Mild exercise impedes glycogen repletion in muscle. *J. Appl. Physiol.* 58: 1622–1629.

Bonen, A., S.A. Malcolm, R.D. Kilgour, K.P. MacIntyre, and A.N. Belcastro (1981). Glucose ingestion before and during intense exercise. *J. Appl. Physiol.* 50: 766–771.

Bourey, R.E., A.R. Coggan, W.M. Kohrt, J.P. Kirwan, D.S. King, and J.O. Holloszy (1990). Effect of exercise on glucose disposal: response to a maximal insulin stimulus. *J. Appl. Physiol.* 69:1689–1694.

Brewer, J., C. Williams, and A. Patton (1988). The influence of high carbohydrate diets on endurance running performance. *Eur. J. Apppl. Physiol.* 57: 698–706.

Brooke, J.D., and L.F. Green (1974). The effect of a high carbohydrate diet on recovery following prolonged work to exhaustion. *Ergonomics* 17: 489–497.

Brotherhood, J.R. Nutrition and sports performance (1984). *Sports Medicine* 1: 350–389.

Burke, L.M., and R.S.D. Read (1987). Diet patterns of elite Australian male triathletes. *Physician and Sportsmedicine* 15: 140–155.

Costill, D.L., D.D. Pascoe, W.J. Fink, R.A. Robergs, and S.I. Barr (1990). Impaired muscle glycogen resynthesis after eccentric exercise. *J. Appl. Physiol.* 69: 46–50.

Costill, D.L., D.R. Pearson, and W.J. Fink (1988). Impaired muscle glycogen storage after muscle biopsy. *J. Appl. Physiol.* 64: 2245–2248.

Costill, D.L., W.M. Sherman, W.J. Fink, C. Maresh, M. Witten, and J.M. Miller (1981). The role of dietary carbohydrates in muscle glycogen resynthesis after strenuous running. *Am. J. Clin. Nutr.* 34: 1831–1836.

Costill, D.L., and J.M. Miller (1980). Nutrition for endurance sport: Carbohydrate and fluid balance. *Int. J. Sports Med.* 1: 2–14.

Costill, D.L., E.F. Coyle, G. Dalsky, W. Evans, W. Fink, and D. Hoopes (1977). Effects of elevated plasma FFA and insulin on muscle glycogen useage during exercise. *J. Appl. Physiol.* 43: 695–699.

Coyle, E.F., A.R. Coggan, M.K. Hemmert, and J.L. Ivy (1986). Muscle glycogen utilization during prolonged strenuous exercise when fed carbohydrate. *J. Appl. Physiol.* 61: 165–172.

Coyle, E.F., A.R. Coggan, M.K. Hemmert, R.C. Lowe, and T.J. Walters (1985). Substrate useage during prolonged exercise following a preexercise meal. *J. Appl. Physiol.* 59: 429–433.

Coyle, E.F., and A.R. Coggan (1984). Effectiveness of carbohydrate feeding in delaying fatigue during prolonged exercise. *Sports Medicine* 1: 446–458.

Coyle, E.F., J.M. Hagberg, B.F. Hurley, W.H. Martin, III, A.A. Ehsani, and J.O. Holloszy (1983). Carbohydrate feeding during prolonged strenuous exercise can delay fatigue. *J. Appl. Physiol.* 55: 230–235.

Deuster, P.A., S.B. Kyle, P.B. Moser, R.A. Vigersky, A. Singh, and E.B. Schoomaker (1986). Nutritional intakes and status of highly trained amenorrheic and eumenorrheic women runners. *Fertility & Sterility* 46: 636–643.

Devlin, J.T., J. Calles-Escandon, and E.S. Horton (1986). Effects of preexercise snack feeding on endurance cycle exercise. *J. Appl. Physiol.* 60: 980–985.

Ferrannini, E., O. Bjorkman, G.A. Reichard, Jr., A. Pilo, M. Olsson, J. Wahren, and R.A. DeFronzo (1985). The disposal of an oral glucose load in healthy subjects: a quantitative study. *Diabetes* 34: 580–588.

Fielding, R.A., D.L. Costill, W.J. Fink, D.S. King, J.E. Kovaleski, and J.P. Kirwan (1987). Effects of pre-exercise carbohydrate feedings on muscle glycogen use during exercise in well-trained runners. *Eur. J. Appl. Physiol.* 56: 225–229.

Flynn, M.G., T.J. Michaud, J. Rodriguez-Zayas, C.P. Lambert, J.B. Boone, and R.W. Moleski (1989). Effects of 4- and 8-h preexercise feedings on substrate use and performance. *J. Appl. Physiol.* 67: 2066–2071.

Foster, C., D.L. Costill, and W.J. Fink (1979). Effects of preexercise feedings on endurance performance. *Med. Sci. Sports Exerc.* 11: 1–5.

Gleeson, M., P.L. Greenhaff, and R.J. Maughan (1988). Influence of a 24 h fast on high intensity cycle exercise performance in man. *Eur. J. Appl. Physiol.* 57: 653–659.

Gleeson, M., R.J. Maughan, and P.L. Greenhaff (1986). Comparison of the effects of preexercise feedings of glucose, glycerol and placebo on endurance and fuel homeostasis in man. *Eur. J. Appl. Physiol.* 55: 645–653.

Gollnick, P.D., P.D. Pernow, B. Essen, E. Jansson, and B. Saltin (1981). Availability of glycogen and FFA for substrate utilization in leg muscle of man during exercise. *Clin. Physiol.* 1: 27–42.

Hargreaves, M., D.L. Costill, W.J. Fink, D.S. King, and R.A. Fielding (1987). Effect of pre-exercise carbohydrate feedings on endurance cycling performance. *Med. Sci. Sports Exerc.* 19: 33–36.

Heinz, F (1972). Metabolism of fructose in the liver. *Acta Med. Scand.* (suppl.) 542: 27–33.

Hikida, R.S., R.S. Staron, F.C. Hagerman, W.M. Sherman, and D.L. Costill (1983). Muscle fiber necrosis associated with human marathon runners. *J. Neurol. Sci.* 59:185–203.

Hultman, E (1978). Liver as a glucose supplying source during rest and exercise with special reference to diet. In: J. Parizkova and V.A. Rogozkin (eds.). *Nutrition, Physical Fitness and Health.* Baltimore: University Park Press, pp. 9–30.

Ivy, J.L., A.L. Katz, C.L. Cutler, W.M. Sherman, and E.F. Coyle (1988a). Muscle glycogen synthesis after exercise: effect of time of carbohydrate ingestion. *J. Appl. Physiol.* 64:1480–1485.

Ivy, J.L., M.C. Lee, J.T. Broznick, Jr., and M.J. Reed (1988b). Muscle glycogen storage after different amounts of carbohydrate ingestion. *J. Appl. Physiol.* 65: 2018–2023.

Jandrain, B., G. Krzentowski, F. Pirnay, F. Mosora, M. Lacroix, A. Luyckx, and P. Lefebvre (1984). Metabolic availability of glucose ingested 3 h before prolonged exercise in humans. *J. Appl. Physiol.* 56: 1314–1319.

Johnson, A., P. Collins, I. Higgins, D. Harrington, J. Connolly, C. Dolphin, M. McCreery, L. Brady, and M. O'Brien (1985). Psychological, nutritional, and physical status of Olympic road cyclists. *Brit. J. Sports Med.* 19: 11–14.

Keizer, H.A., H. Kuipers, G. van Kranenburg, and P. Geurten (1987). Influence of liquid and solid meals on muscle glycogen resynthesis, plasma fuel hormone response, and maximal physical working capacity. *Int. J. Sports Med.* 8: 99–104.

Keller K., and R. Schwarzkopf (1984). Preexercise snacks may decrease exercise performance. *Physician and Sportsmedicine* 12: 89–91.

Kiens, B., A.B. Raben, A-K Valeus, and E.A. Richter (1990). Benefit of dietary simple carbohydrates on the early postexercise muscle glycogen repletion in male athletes. *Med. Sci. Sports Exerc.* 22:S88, abstract.

Kochan, R.G., D.R. Lamb, S.A. Lutz, C.V. Perrill, E.M. Reimann, and K.K. Schlender (1979). Glycogen synthase activation in human skeletal muscle: effects of diet and exercise. *Am. J. Physiol.* 236: E660–E666.

Koivisto, V., M. Harkonen. S.-L. Karonen, P.H. Groop, R. Elovainio, E. Ferrannini, L. Sacca, and R.A. Defronzo (1985). Glycogen depletion during prolonged exercise: influence of glucose, fructose or placebo. *J. Appl. Physiol.* 58: 731–737.

Koivisto, V., S.-L. Karonen, and E.O. Nikkila (1981). Carbohydrate ingestion before exercise: comparison of glucose, fructose, and sweet placebo. *J. Appl. Physiol.* 51: 783–787.

Krzentowski, G., F. Pirnay, A.S. Luyckx, N. Pallikarakis, M. Lacroix, F. Mosora, and P.J. Lefebvre (1982). Metabolic adaptations in post-exercise recovery. *Clin. Physiol.* 2: 277–288.

Kuipers, H., H.A. Keizer, F.T.J. Verstappen, and D.L. Costill (1985). Influence of prostaglandin-inhibiting drug on muscle soreness after eccentric exercise. *Int. J. Sports Med.* 6: 336–349.

Lamb, D.R., T.S. Baur, G.R. Brodowicz, C.S. Blair, and D.L. Corrigan (1986). Consumption of carbohydrates, electrolytes, and acid buffers on brief, high intensity exercise performance. *Activities Report of the R&D Associates* 38: 44–52.

Levine, L., W.J. Evans, B.S. Cadarette, E.C. Fisher, and B.A. Bullen (1983). Fructose and glucose ingestion and muscle glycogen use during submaximal exercise. *J. Appl. Physiol.* 55: 1767–1771.

Loy, S.F., R.K. Conlee, W.W. Winder, A.G. Nelson, D.A. Arnall, and A.G. Fisher (1986). Effects of 24-hour fast on cycling endurance time at two different intensities. *J. Appl. Physiol.* 61: 654–659.

MacDougall, G.R. Ward, D.G. Sale, and J.R. Sutton (1977). Muscle glycogen repletion after high-intensity intermittent exercise. *J. Appl. Physiol.* 42: 129–132.

Maehlum, S., P. Felig, and J. Wahren (1978). Splanchnic glucose and muscle glycogen metabolism after glucose feeding during postexercise recovery. *Am. J. Physiol.* 235: E255-E260.

McMurray, R.G., J.R. Wilson, and B.S. Kitchell (1983). The effects of glucose and fructose on high intensity endurance performance. *Res. Q. Exerc. and Sport* 54: 156–162.

Neufer, P.D., D.L. Costill, M.G. Flynn, J.P Kirwan, J.B. Mitchell, and J. Houmard (1987). Improvements in exercise performance: effects of carbohydrate feedings and diet. *J. Appl. Physiol.* 62: 983–988.

Nilson, L.H., and E. Hultman (1974). Liver and muscle glycogen in man after glucose and fructose infusion. *Scand. J. Clin. Lab. Invest.* 33: 5–10.

Okano, G., H. Takeda, I. Morita, M. Katoh, Z. Mu, and S. Miyake (1988). Effects of preexercise fructose ingestion on endurance performance in man. *Med. Sci. Sports Exerc.* 20: 105–109.

O'Reilly, K.P., M.J. Warhol, R.A. Fielding, W.R. Frontera, C.N. Meredith, and W.J. Evans (1987). Eccentric exercise-induced muscle damage impairs muscle glycogen repletion. *J. Appl. Physiol.* 63: 252–256.

Peden, C., W.M. Sherman, L. D'Aquisto, and D.A. Wright (1989). 1 h preexercise carbohydrate meals enhance performance. *Med. Sci. Sports. Exerc.* 21: S59, abstract.

Peters, A.J., R.H. Dressendorfer, J. Rimar, and C.L. Keen (1986). Diets of endurance runners competing in a 20-day road race. *Physician and Sportsmedicine* 14: 63–70.

Piehl, K (1974). Time course for refilling of glycogen stores in human muscle fibers following exercise-induced glycogen depletion. *Acta Physiol. Scand.* 90: 297–302.

Piehl, K., S. Adolfsson, and K. Nazar (1974). Glycogen storage and glycogen synthase activity in trained and untrained muscle of man. *Acta Physiol. Scand.* 90: 779–788.

Ravussin, L., P. Pahus, A. Dorner, M.J. Arnaud, and E. Jequier (1979). Substrate utilization during prolonged exercise preceded by ingestion of 13C-glucose in glycogen depleted and control subjects. *Pflugers Arch.* 382: 197–202.

Reed, M.J., J.T. Broznick, Jr., M.C. Lee, and J.L. Ivy (1989). Muscle glycogen storage postexercise: effect of mode of carbohydrate administration. *Med. Sci. Sports Exerc.* 66: 720–726.

Roedde, S., J.D. MacDougall, J.R. Sutton, and H.J. Green (1986). Supercompensation of muscle glycogen in trained and untrained subjects. *Can. J. Appl. Sport Sci.* 11: 42–46.

Saltin, B., and J. Karlsson (1971). Muscle glycogen utilization during work of different intensities. In: B. Pernow and B. Saltin (eds.) *Muscle Metabolism during Exercise*, New York: Plenum Press, pp. 289–300.

Sherman, W.M., G. Brodowicz, D.A. Wright, W.K. Allen, J. Simonsen, and A. Dernbach (1989). Effects of 4 h preexercise carbohydrate feedings on cycling performance. *Med. Sci. Sports Exerc.* 21:598–604.

Sherman, W.M. and D.A. Wright (1989). Preevent Nutrition for Prolonged Exercise. In: A. C.

Grandjean and J. Storlie (eds.) *Ross Symposium on the Theory and Practice of Athletic Nutrition.* Columbus: Ross Laboratories, pp. 30–46.

Sherman, W.M. and D.R. Lamb (1988). Nutrition and prolonged exercise. In: D.R. Lamb and R. Murray (eds.) *Perspectives in Exercise Science and Sports Medicine: vol 1. Prolonged Exercise.* Indianapolis: Benchmark, pp. 213–280.

Sherman, W.M., L.E. Armstrong, T.M. Murray, F.C. Hagerman, D.L. Costill, R.C. Staron, and J.L. Ivy (1984). Effect of a 42.2-km footrace and subsequent rest or exercise on muscular strength and work capacity. *J. Appl. Physiol.* 57: 1668–1673.

Sherman, W.M., D.L. Costill, W.J. Fink, F.C. Hagerman, L.E. Armstrong, and T.F. Murray (1983). Effect of a 42.2-km footrace and subsequent rest or exercise on muscle glycogen and enzymes. *J. Appl. Physiol.* 55: 1219–1224.

Sherman, W.M., D.L. Costill, W.J. Fink, and J.M. Miller (1981). The effect of exercise and diet manipulation on muscle glycogen and its subsequent use during performance. *Int. J. Sports Med.* 2: 114–118.

Simonsen, J.C., W.M. Sherman, D.R. Lamb, A.A. Dernbach, J.A. Doyle, and R. Strauss (1991). Dietary carbohydrate, muscle gycogen, and power output during rowing training. *J. App. Physiol.* 70(4): 000–000. (In press.)

Vollestad, N.K., P.C.S. Blom, and O. Gronnerod (1989). Resynthesis of glycogen in different muscle fibre types after prolonged exhaustive exercise in man. *Acta Physiol. Scand.* 137: 15–21.

Wright, D.A., and W.M. Sherman (1989). Carbohydrate feedings 3 h before and during exercise improve cycling performance. *Med. Sci. Sports Exerc.* 21: S58, abstract.

Young, K., and C.T.M. Davies (1984). Effect of diet on human muscle weakness following prolonged exercise. *Eur. J. Appl. Physiol.* 53: 81–85.

DISCUSSION

COSTILL: There is no question that if you give subjects a pre-competition or pre-exercise feeding 2–3 h ahead of time, they will certainly perform better; but if you give it to them 30 min beforehand, some individuals will develop an exertional hypoglycemia. Furthermore, in one of the early studies we did, we showed that exercise performance time is decreased with such feedings. Therefore, the optimal time frame for pre-exercise feedings should be clarified.

SHERMAN: There are about four studies that show a performance enhancing effect of pre-exercise carbohydrate feedings provided from 1–4 h before exercise when individuals were fed between 5 g/kg body weight 4 h before and 1–2 g/kg body weight 1 h before. Although some individuals in these studies had initial exertional hypoglycemia, they were able to exercise through that reduction in blood glucose. These individuals have to identify themselves and avoid this dietary manipulation if they are indeed sensitive to exertional hypoglycemia. I don't want to belittle the fact that exertional hypoglycemia exists, but our experience is that this response is not very common in most subjects.

COSTILL: In most of the studies where attempts were made to identify people who tended to be sensitive to that condition, feedings were given 30–45 min beforehand, so the subjects were hitting the exercise at a time when their insulins were very high. In the same individuals, an hour later, insulin may be quite normal.

SHERMAN: In all of our studies, which included more than 30 subjects, insulin concentrations were at least 1.7—fold higher at the

start of exercise and remained higher throughout most of the exercise, but no one experienced serious reductions in blood glucose.
COSTILL: How many went below 2.5 mM?
SHERMAN: No subjects reached clinically hypoglycemic levels, but they did have at least a 1 mM drop in glucose during the first 15 min of exercise. It has been suggested that there are some individuals who are sensitive to such a modest drop, so we have to be aware that preexercise feedings could adversely affect this small proportion of athletes.
COGGAN: Hypoglycemia is often used to vaguely describe central nervous system symptoms, but it also simply means a lowering of blood glucose. We might be better off to characterize hypoglycemia as a reduction of glucose and neuroglucopenia as the onset of symptoms. We also have to realize that there may be adverse effects long before a person shows symptoms, as has been shown with insulin-induced neuroglycopenia. Therefore, simply because a person doesn't report an increase in perceived exertion doesn't mean that the preexercise feeding didn't have an effect upon motor function. We need objective measurements of presymptomatic effects of hypoglycemia.
SHERMAN: To my knowledge, in studies where subjects had a lowering of blood glucose, it has never been shown that these subjects stopped as the result of hypoglycemia. That does not mean they did not have some hypoglycemic effects, but there is no solid evidence that any such effects led to premature exhaustion.
COGGAN: You left out the classic studies of Boje in 1936 and Christensen and Hansen in 1939, in which hypoglycemic responses were very clearly shown; I think that is where the idea first became established.
SHERMAN: You're right. Those early studies did show some individuals who apparently suffered adverse hypoglycemic effects.
KNUTTGEN: Most of the available data are from studies of marathon runners, and laboratory subjects exercising on cycle ergometers and treadmills. I would like you to comment on the implications of pre- and postexercise carbohydrate feedings for athletes who compete in a the wide variety of sports activities that we have on both the secondary school and university level.
SHERMAN: I think the recommendations about preexercise carbohydrate feedings apply to athletes who participate in sports events that are limited in any way by the body's carbohydrate reserves. The important thing is to identify those sports and the conditions under which these recommendations would apply.
COYLE: Blood glucose concentration is the balance between glucose introduction to the circulation from the liver versus glucose

removal by muscles and other tissues. Our lab recently showed that most of the usual decline in blood glucose during exercise at 70% $\dot{V}O_2$max 4 h after a carbohydrate meal could be prevented by asking the subject to increase his exercise intensity. This presumably is a stimulus to increase liver glucose output. I am not sure if there is any practical value to this observation, but perhaps at the least we need to recommend to Ethan Nadel that as soon as he feels hypoglycemic attack coming on, he should pick up the pace.

NADEL: Easier said than done!

SHERMAN: Although preexercise feedings have demonstrated ergogenic effects, the studies haven't examined the mechanism whereby the feedings work. It has been suggested that feedings delay the decline in the rate of carbohydrate oxidation, similar to what Ed Coyle and others have noted for carbohydrate feedings during exercise. Turnover studies and other techniques need to be applied to these dietary manipulations.

HEIGENHAUSER: Are different types of carbohydrates such as fructose, glucose, and sucrose equally effective? Is there any advantage or disadvantage to using more complex forms?

SHERMAN: With respect to preexercise carbohydrate feedings, studies by Evans et al. with fructose ingestion suggested there is a 30% sparing of muscle glycogen during a fixed exercise task. They didn't study performance, but they implied that if muscle glycogen is spared, performance should be enhanced. But that glycogen sparing observation of Evans et al. has not been replicated in studies at Ball State and other places; I don't know of any study that shows fructose to be more beneficial to performance than other sugars.

The postexercise feeding studies demonstrate generally that with fructose the rate of muscle glycogen synthesis tends to be lower than with glucose or sucrose, probably as the result of more of the fructose being taken up and delivered to the liver to stimulate liver glycogen synthesis.

HEIGENHAUSER: What are the effects of recovery carbohydrate feedings on liver glycogen?

SHERMAN: That is an important question, but in the absence of data from liver biopsies, we need to come up with a marker for liver glycogen turnover to answer it.

GISOLFI: You indicated that muscle glycogen can be restored within 24 h after exhaustive exercise. If glycogen starts from a supercompensated state, can it be totally replenished to that state within 24 h?

SHERMAN: The results from the marathon work that we did and some work that Per Blom has published suggest that it is very difficult to resynthesize in 24 h to a supercompensated level, but I don't think there are direct studies to answer how much time is required.

GISOLFI: Within that 24 h period, does it make any difference what form of carbohydrate you are consuming?

SHERMAN: I don't know of a study that has directly addressed that question.

HEIGENHAUSER: Are there any differences in the characteristics of glycogen supercompensation between elite athletes and average well-conditioned subjects?

SHERMAN: The only paper that I know of that addresses that is the Roedde paper, and their results suggest that the capacity to supercompensate is fairly similar between trained and untrained individuals. I find that surprising in light of the fact that the both the sensitivity to activation of glycogen synthase by its activators and total glycogen synthase activity are less in untrained people.

BUTTERFIELD: The rate of consumption of dietary carbohydrate that you suggest should be started immediately after exercise works out to be something like 5000 kcal over a 24 h period. I assume that you don't advise athletes to eat at that rate for the whole day? Such high carbohydrate feedings can result in elevated blood triglyceride levels, and it is nearly impossible to force that much carbohydrate down in a few hours. If the athlete tries to eat this much carbohydrate as normal solid foods, the high fiber content of these foods usually results in very high volumes of food, gastrointestinal distress, and a loss of some trace minerals in the feces. People have difficulty eating enough carbohydrate at high energy demands to cover their energy needs.

SHERMAN: I agree that it is difficult to have individuals consume that amount of carbohydrate from solid food sources. All of our studies used rapidly absorbable glucose or glucose polymer supplement solutions. We have had very few problems with compliance or acceptability of our feeding schedules in the subjects that we have used. For preexercise feedings or just daily carbohydrate intake, we can quite easily feed subjects 10 g/kg per day, which in these athletes ends up being about 70%-85% of their energy from carbohydrates. We give them meals which have about 50–60% carbohydrate and supplement their caloric intake with a carbohydrate beverage. In studies where we have looked at blood lipids, we found absolutely no effect of carbohydrate feedings on cholesterol profiles or triglyceridemia. It appears that the exercise training on a daily basis to some extent counters the triglyceridemia that the carbohydrate intake sometimes causes.

NADEL: Is the muscle biopsy the right tool for studying changes in muscle glycogen?

SHERMAN: A lot of people are looking for an alternative method to assess muscle glycogen without doing a biopsy, and there are some nuclear magnetic resonance spectroscopy procedures that may soon take the place of biopsies. Costill's group suggested that an earlier biopsy could have some effect on glycogen measurements in a subsequent biopsy if the biopsies were taken within 7 d of each other. They found an adverse effect on glycogen when a second biopsy was taken within 1 cm proximal or medial to or within 3 cm distal to the initial site. That is why I make the recommendation that repeated biopsies should be taken from alternate legs if possible and that when biopsies have to come from the same leg within a 5–7 d period, the subsequent biopsy sites should be at least 5 cm away from the first site. In the more than 400 biopsies we have done in the last 2 y, we have found no problem with the effect of the previous biopsy when the subsequent biopsy was taken 5 cm proximal or distal to the first site.

SPRIET: What is the ability of the muscle to use fructose with respect to glucose?

SHERMAN: Fructose kinase activity is low in the muscle compared to the liver, and the muscle glycogen synthesis rate for fructose is a lot lower than that for glucose or sucrose.

CONLEE: The liver captures most of the fructose coming out of the gut; therefore, very little gets into the systemic circulation. Fructose in the liver doesn't turn over very quickly to glucose to get into the system either; fructose is a poor source for both liver and muscle glycogen.

HICKSON: What are the critical diet controls that must be included in an experiment to answer this question of ergogenicity for preexercise carbohydrate feedings "once and for all?"

SHERMAN: Most studies controlled the diet during the 3–5 d before the experimental manipulation by either having people follow a recalled diet from a similar protocol during the weeks before or by carefully supervising the feeding of those subjects. Some studies also have incorporated a familiarization trial in which the subjects go through the entire experimental procedure before they are randomized into the experimental treatments. The studies of exercise at moderate intensities have produced both indeterminate and positive results. I think most of those were pretty well designed. The studies of high intensity exercise are the earlier studies, and the controls on those were not quite as rigid.

HICKSON: If individuals are supercompensated to start with, is the high carbohydrate preexercise meal necessary? What if you gave a very low carbohydrate or carbohydrate-free meal within several hours before the start of the event to an athlete who was already supercompensated?

SHERMAN: Most of these subjects that have been studied were fasted for 10 h and then fed 1–4 h before exercise. At Ohio State, we try to manipulate their diet and exercise so that they come into the study with muscle glycogen between 130 and 150 mmol/kg, which is not supercompensated. There is one study reported in which glycogen levels did not affect the oxidation of a preexercise carbohydrate feeding.

CLARKSON: Do you think that during the days after muscle-damaging exercise, when considerable muscle repair takes place, it is possible for the muscle to shift its energy expenditure away from glycogen resynthesis to the repair of contractile elements? If so, there may be no defect in glycogen synthesis but rather a useful shift of energy to the repair process.

SHERMAN: I think that is a very reasonable hypothesis. The animal studies that have damaged muscle with blunt objects and looked at the effects of insulin on stimulation of glucose uptake, protein synthesis, and protein degradation are consistent with your hypothesis. Of course, this has not yet been proved in humans following eccentric exercise.

COYLE: Do you think that some of the beneficial effects of preexercise feeding, in addition to providing extra substrate, are the results of an insulin effect? The studies that have shown improved performance have also shown a high rate of carbohydrate oxidation. Do you think that is one of the mechanisms by which preexercise feedings improve performance, that is, allowing for a marked elevation blood glucose utilization and, therefore, increased carbohydrate oxidation?

SHERMAN: I think that is a reasonable hypothesis. The studies that would have to be done to test that would be studies where the glucose was elevated but insulin secretion was depressed. Those studies would probably be done more invasively than what has been done.

COGGAN: We have glucose turnover data with ^{13}C glucose in one subject given a preexercise meal about 2 h before exercise at 60% $\dot{V}O_2max$, and he showed the classic pattern of an early drop in blood glucose and then a gradual glucose recovery. But the glucose turnover rates were greatly accelerated early in exercise. The rate of disappearance was elevated, which is consistent with the increase in R values and the increase in glycogen utilization.

SHERMAN: Bjorkman found increased muscle glucose uptake with preexercise feedings; this is consistent with the insulin effect.

MURRAY: The studies that are done on postexercise carbohydrate feedings show that sucrose does a pretty good job compared to glucose, yet sucrose has on a weight by weight basis one-half the amount of glucose. Do you have an idea why that might be?

SHERMAN: No.

COYLE: I think Kuipers postulated that the muscle and liver are in competition for the substrate, and when sucrose is fed, the liver will prefer the fructose, leaving the glucose more available to muscles. His conclusion was that muscle is not deprived of glucose when sucrose is fed.

DOHM: There is a lot of evidence that most ingested glucose does not go to the liver for direct glycogen synthesis but, in fact, goes to some of the other tissues to be converted to three-carbon compounds before entering the liver. Fructose, on the other hand, would go to the liver and be synthesized to glycogen right away, so there could be a real benefit to using fructose if you want to replete glycogen in the liver. Maybe that is part of the explanation of why sucrose is effective. With sucrose you are generating liver glycogen, which is beneficial during the exercise period.

COGGAN: What is the distribution of the carbohydrate that is ingested following exercise? I know that rat studies have suggested that the liver loses out in this competition and the muscle glycogen synthesis takes preference. Most of the studies of fasted, rested subjects show that muscle sees only about 50% of the orally ingested carbohydrate; half of that ends up in muscle glycogen, and the remainder is oxidized. We have a very poor handle on where the carbohydrate goes, even in people who have not exercised. When you start throwing exercise into the equation, it becomes even a bigger question. This has a lot of relevance not only for erogenics and recovery from exercise, but also for understanding how exercise affects oral glucose tolerance. We know that the insulin response is less, but where is the carbohydrate going?

SHERMAN: It's an important question, but I don't know the answer.

GREGG: We have a huge number of athletes who train twice a day. Obviously, they don't have 24 h between their workouts to replenish muscle glycogen. What do we recommend to these athletes?

SHERMAN: They should consume as much carbohydrate as possible to keep carbohydrate stores elevated. They should also probably decrease the frequency of their training, according to work from Costill's lab.

KREIDER: Regarding the postexercise feedings and the observation that glycogen resynthesis requires 24 h, the ultra-endurance cyclist rides 5–6 h/d and expends huge amounts of energy, often without total energy replacement from one day to the next. Yet these cyclists are still able to perform well for many days and weeks. How do you think they can make these adjustment to inadequate energy intake?

SHERMAN: I think that particular example is an extreme of adaptability in humans. There is a possibility that these very highly trained athletes adapt to more efficient utilization of ingested carbohydrate or more efficient storage of muscle glycogen. Also, their muscles have adapted to a greater utilization of fats.

KREIDER: Is there any evidence that training the athlete to eat frequently during performance enables the athlete to somehow store glycogen more efficiently?

SHERMAN: I don't know of any such evidence.

2

Carbohydrate-Electrolyte Solutions During Prolonged Exercise

RON MAUGHAN, PH.D.

INTRODUCTION

The physiological and biochemical responses to exercise have been extensively studied by scientists interested in the nature of the fatigue process. A more empirical approach has been adopted by athletes with a view to delaying the onset of fatigue and improving exercise performance. While both these methods have clearly established that the most effective way to improve performance is by a systematic training program, it is equally apparent that nutritional factors can exert a significant effect. It is now well recognized that

35

this applies as much to nutrients consumed during the exercise period itself as to the training and pre-competition diet.

More than 20 years ago, it was possible for Roger Bannister (1967), with his experience as an athlete and a scientist, to say in a review of the medical aspects of competitive athletics that the dangers of marathon running were "hypoglycaemia, salt depletion and dehydration" with the clear implication that provision of glucose, salt, and water could effectively avoid these problems. Almost 20 years later, however, Williams (1985) reviewed the available literature and concluded that, in most situations, water was as effective a replacement fluid for the athlete as a glucose-electrolyte solution. Much has happened in the last few years to increase our understanding of this area, and the current consensus would appear to be that performance can be improved by the ingestion of correctly formulated carbohydrate-electrolyte solutions during exercise. The evidence on which this is based will be examined here.

SUBSTRATE PROVISION

In the early years of this century, it was established that both fat and carbohydrate (CHO) could serve as metabolic fuels (Zuntz, 1911). In these studies, Zuntz was able to show from respiratory exchange ratio (R) measurements in exercising human subjects that, if the subjects were fed a high-fat diet prior to exercise, low-intensity work could be performed with little contribution from CHO to oxidative metabolism. These results were not immediately accepted, however, as earlier studies on isolated muscle had indicated that fat was not metabolised by muscle. It was not until the work of Krogh and Lindhard (1920) that the controversy was finally resolved. In a series of careful experiments, they confirmed that both fat and CHO oxidation contributed to energy production in resting and exercising subjects, and that the relative contributions of these two substrates were influenced by the preceding diet.

The importance of the body's CHO stores was indicated by the results of Levine et al. (1924), who studied competitors in the 1923 Boston marathon race, held over a distance of 42.2 km (26.2 miles). A marked fall in blood glucose concentration occurred during the race in the majority of the runners studied; three of the 12 competitors studied had blood glucose levels of less than 2.8 mmol/L (50 mg/dL) after the race. The physical condition of these subjects after the race was described as "very poor." Consumption of a high-CHO diet prior to the following year's race, in combination with sugar ingestion during the race, was effective in preventing these problems and led to an improved performance (Gordon et al., 1925).

In 1928, Bock et al. reported that the contribution of CHO to metabolism was dependent on the workload, being greater at high workloads than at low workloads. In 1936, Boje showed that feeding carbohydrate solutions could restore exercise capacity in exhausted individuals. Shortly after this, Christensen and Hansen (1939) demonstrated the critical role of CHO in the performance of prolonged exercise. They found that the time for which work could be maintained was greater after a high-CHO diet than after a normal mixed diet, whereas endurance was decreased if a high-fat diet was consumed prior to the exercise test. Ingestion of a large amount (200 g) of glucose at the point of exhaustion enabled a further hour of work to be performed, confirming the earlier result of Boje (1936).

These studies, carried out more than half a century ago, clearly established the importance of CHO availability during exercise. Furthermore, they pointed out that CHO feeding prior to or during exercise could improve exercise performance. In all of the early experiments, estimates of carbohydrate oxidation were based on measurements of the R value. Although some of these measurements were carried out with a degree of precision that is unlikely to be matched by modern analytical techniques, they were able to provide no information on the source of the endogenous substrates oxidized by the working muscles. Equally, the measurement of concentrations of substrates and metabolites in peripheral blood could not identify the substrate source.

New techniques were needed, and these became available and came into general use in the 1960s. The most important of these were the introduction of the percutaneous needle biopsy technique, the use of isotopic tracers, and the application to man of the measurement of arterio-venous differences across muscle.

In 1966, Bergstrom and Hultman performed an ingenious experiment which showed that, during one-leg exercise on a cycle ergometer, the glycogen content of the working muscles fell to very low levels at exhaustion, whereas that of the resting leg remained normal; refeeding resulted in glycogen supercompensation only in the exercised leg. Experiments into the time course of glycogen disappearance during prolonged heavy exercise showed that a progressive utilization of muscle glycogen took place and that exhaustion occurred when the muscle glycogen had almost totally disappeared (Hermansen et al., 1967). Subsequently, it was shown that the pattern of glycogen depletion is muscle fiber specific; in high intensity exercise, depletion of glycogen is most marked in Type 2 fibers, but in prolonged exercise at lower intensities depletion occurs first in the Type 1 fibers, and the Type 2 fibers lose their glycogen only in the later stages of exercise.

It was also found that feeding diets containing different amounts of carbohydrate after exercise influenced the rate of glycogen resynthesis and allowed the muscle glycogen content to be manipulated. When muscle glycogen was low at the beginning of exercise, endurance capacity was restricted and a shift towards fat metabolism was evident; if exercise began with unusually high muscle glycogen, both the rate of CHO utilization and the endurance capacity were increased (Ahlborg et al., 1967). When the working muscles have exhausted their glycogen store, even exercise of moderately heavy intensity (70% of maximum oxygen uptake—$\dot{V}O_2max$) cannot be sustained, although low intensity work can be carried out (Hultman, 1967). These studies, which demonstrated the crucial role played by the muscle glycogen stores and focused attention on preexercise nutritional strategies aimed at maximizing the muscle glycogen content prior to exercise, have been reviewed in Chapter 1.

The muscle is able to use blood glucose in addition to the local glycogen store as a carbohydrate source. Blood glucose is derived from the liver, with glycogenolysis and gluconeogenesis both contributing. The percutaneous needle biopsy technique permitted measurements of changes in the liver glycogen content in response to exercise (Hultman & Nilsson, 1971; Nilsson et al., 1973). The effect of heavy exercise on the liver glycogen content was similar to that on muscle glycogen; there was a progressive decrease to very low levels at exhaustion. Unlike muscle, however, the liver glycogen was rapidly depleted by fasting, even in the absence of exercise.

Carbohydrate ingested during exercise will enter the blood glucose pool if it is absorbed from the gastrointestinal tract; if this exogenous glucose can substitute for the body's limited endogenous glycogen stores, then exercise capacity should be increased in situations where liver or muscle glycogen availability limits endurance. Several studies have shown that the ingestion of glucose during exercise will maintain or raise the circulating glucose concentration (Costill et al., 1973; Pirnay et al., 1982; Erickson et al., 1987). Substitution of glucose polymers for glucose does not alter this response (Ivy et al., 1979; Coyle et al., 1983, 1986; Maughan et al., 1987; Coggan & Coyle, 1988; Hargreaves & Briggs, 1988); similar effects are seen with the feeding of sucrose (Sasaki et al., 1987) or mixtures of sugars (Murray et al., 1987; Mitchell et al., 1988; Carter & Gisolfi, 1989).

There is some evidence that this increased supply of substrate will result in a decreased rate of muscle glycogen utilization during exercise if the carbohydrate is administered orally (Erickson et al., 1987; Hargreaves et al., 1984) or by intravenous infusion (Bergstrom & Hultman, 1967; Galbo et al., 1977; Bagby et al., 1978). It should be noted, however, that Bergstrom and Hultman reported that this effect was small and that muscle glycogen utilization continued at a high rate even when the blood glucose level was elevated to over 20 mmol/L, well beyond the concentration observed after oral administration of glucose; furthermore, the results of Galbo et al. involved only four subjects and appear not to have reached statistical significance, and the experiment of Bagby et al. was carried out in rats.

In contrast to these results, some studies have shown no effect of carbohydrate feeding during exercise on the rate of muscle glycogen utilization (Fielding et al., 1985; Coyle et al., 1986; Hargreaves & Briggs, 1988; Noakes et al., 1988b). Coyle et al. (1986) found that oral administration of large amounts of glucose polymer had no effect on the rate of muscle glycogen utilization during 3 h of exercise; however, these glucose feedings allowed an additional hour of exercise to be performed with a high rate of CHO oxidation, very little of which was derived from muscle glycogen, which had fallen to a low level by this time. It was not clear in these studies why the subjects became fatigued, nor how the CHO feedings were able to extend the exercise period. Flynn et al. (1987) found that CHO feeding during exercise had no effect on the rate of muscle glycogen breakdown when the glycogen was elevated prior to exercise by a CHO-loading procedure. These conflicting results may be explained by a differential effect of exogenous glucose depending on the muscle glycogen content.

Many sports involve periods of high-intensity exercise interspersed with rest or low-intensity exercise. Kuipers et al. (1987) measured glycogen resynthesis rates during rest or low-intensity cycling (40% $\dot{V}O_2max$) following intermittent exercise to exhaustion; during the 3 h recovery period, subjects drank 2 L of a 25% solution of a glucose polymer-fructose mixture. In the resting trial, glycogen resynthesis was observed in all muscle fiber types, but during exercise, glycogen repletion was observed only in the Type 2 fibers. This suggests that when large amounts of CHO are given orally during low-intensity exercise, glycogen resynthesis can occur in inactive muscle fibers; it also suggests that measurement of the glycogen content of whole muscle extracts may not reflect the fiber-specific pattern of glycogen metabolism.

The use of isotopic tracers has allowed estimates to be made of the extent to which ingested substrates are oxidized during exercise. Pirnay et al. (1977) showed that when a dose of 100 g of glucose was given orally as a concentrated (1389 mmol/L; 25%) solution during treadmill walking at 50% $\dot{V}O_2max$, the carbon tracer was detected in expired air within 15 min after ingestion. After 1–2 h, oxidation of the ingested glucose accounted for 55% of total CHO oxidation. The same authors later showed that the rate of exogenous glucose oxidation was directly proportional to workload up to about 50% $\dot{V}O_2$max, and tended to level off at higher work intensities; the relative contribution to total energy production was not influenced by the work intensity in the range of 22–64% $\dot{V}O_2$max (Pirnay et al., 1982). They also showed that glucose, taken in a 25% solution at a rate of 50 g every 30 min during low-intensity (45% $\dot{V}O_2$max) treadmill exercise could account for 85–90% of total glucose oxidation towards the end of a prolonged walk (Pallikarakis et al., 1986).

In contrast to these results, however, Costill et al. (1973) found that when a smaller amount (31.8 g) of glucose was given in a more dilute (589 mmol/L; 10.6%) solution during running or cycling at 60–72% $\dot{V}O_2$max, the rate of oxidation of the ingested glucose was 6.5-fold higher than at rest, but accounted for only about 5% of total CHO oxidation. They later found similar results using cycling exercise at 50% $\dot{V}O_2$max (Van Handel et al., 1980). The reason for the different results obtained by these two groups of investigators is not clear, but may be at least partly a function of the amount of glucose given, because the amount of an oral glucose load which is oxidized increases as the total glucose load increases (Mosora et al., 1981).

Support for the suggestion that ingested CHO can make a significant contribution to oxidative energy supply during exercise came from the results of Massicotte et al. (1986), who gave ^{13}C-labelled glucose or fructose as 389 mmol/L (7%) solutions at intervals during 3 h of cycling exercise at 50% $\dot{V}O_2$max. The ingested glucose accounted for 38% of the total CHO oxidized; during the second half of the exercise period this figure was 56%. More of the ingested glucose (75%) than of the fructose (56%) was oxidized during the exercise period; glucose ingestion, however, resulted in higher plasma insulin levels during exercise, leading to a lower rate of fat oxidation. This effect of insulin on substrate oxidation is probably related to the inhibition of fatty acid mobilization from adipose tissue rather than a stimulation of glucose uptake by the active muscles. The sparing of endogenous CHO stores, compared with the control trial when water only was given, was thus the same for glucose and fructose ingestion, and is in contrast to some of the reports described above. This sparing effect was observed during the second, but not the first, half of the exercise period. The same authors have more recently confirmed the greater availability of ingested glucose compared with fructose, and have also shown that there is no difference in the oxidation rates of ingested glucose and glucose polymers (Massicotte et al., 1989). Another recent study, however, indicated that fructose given orally during treadmill exercise at 50% VO₂max is oxidized to approximately the same extent as glucose (Slama et al., 1989).

The possibility that ingestion of carbohydrates and other substrates during exercise may have metabolic effects other than simply sparing endogenous energy stores has largely been ignored. Ingestion of carbohydrate at rest may stimulate the uptake of plasma tryptophan by the brain as a result of an insulin-mediated fall in the circulating concentration of branched chain amino acids, which compete with tryptophan for uptake; tryptophan availability is the limiting step in the synthesis within the brain of the neurotransmitter 5-hydroxytryptamine, which is known to influence mood and the perception of pain (Wurtman, 1983). Prolonged exercise can also cause a rise in the plasma free tryptophan levels and a fall in circulating branched-chain amino acids that compete with tryptophan for uptake by the brain (Blomstrand et al., 1988). The effect of exercise on the plasma concentration of branched-chain amino acids is also known to be modified by nutritional status (Gleeson & Maughan, 1987). The experiments remain to be done, but it does seem possible that at least a part of the effect of CHO ingestion on exercise performance might be mediated by effects on brain neurotransmitters.

The effects of CHO ingestion during exercise on endurance capacity and exercise performance will be considered later.

WATER AND ELECTROLYTE PROVISION

Fluid loss during exercise is linked to the need to maintain the body's core temperature within narrow limits. Of the available chemical energy of foods, only 20–25% is converted to useful work in the body, the remainder being lost as heat. At rest the rate of energy turnover is low; oxygen consumption of a 70 kg man at rest is about 250 mL/min, corresponding to a heat production of about 4 kJ/min (1 kcal/min). Heat is exchanged with the environment by the physical processes of conduction, convection, and radiation. The body will gain or lose by these mechanisms depending on the relative temperatures of the skin and the environment. Heat can also be lost by evaporation, which depends on the difference in water vapor pressure between the skin and the surrounding air. The regulation of body temperature at rest is normally achieved by behavioral mechanisms which involve the adjustment of the amount of clothing worn or of the environmental temperature.

During exercise, the rate of heat production is increased; a 70 kg runner completing a marathon race in a time of 2.5 h requires an oxygen consumption of about 4 L/min to be sustained through-out the race (Maughan & Leiper, 1983). At this pace, the rate of heat production would be about 80 kJ/min (20 kcal/min). If no heat exchange with the environment was to take place, this would cause body temperature to rise by about 1° C every 3 min. A rise of body temperature by as little as 5° C from the normal resting range of 37–38° C can lead to collapse and even death. This point would be reached after only 15 min of running, but measurements made on marathon runners have shown that body temperature does not normally rise by more than 2–3° C, even in the fastest runners (Pugh et al., 1967; Maughan, 1985). After the initial phase during which body temperature rises, the additional heat produced during marathon running is not stored in the body but is dissipated at a rate equal to the rate of production.

At high rates of heat production, the major avenue of heat loss is usually by evaporation of sweat secreted onto the skin surface. Exceptions to this are exercise in water which is below skin temperature, or in very cold environments. When the ambient temperature exceeds that of the skin, heat will be gained from the environment by radiation and convection, conduction being generally insignificant; evaporation is then the only mechanism by which heat can be lost. Evaporation of 1 L of water from the skin surface will result in the loss of 2.4 MJ (580 kcal) of heat energy. If the 2.5 h marathon runner can produce sweat at a rate of 2 L/h, and if all of this evaporates, this will remove about 80 kJ of heat energy from the body per minute, and the sweating mechanism will prevent any rise in body temperature, assuming no sources of heat gain other than metabolism and no other avenues of heat loss.

A disadvantage of high sweat rates is that a significant proportion of the fluid secreted onto the skin surface may not evaporate, but simply drip from the skin, increasing the water loss from the body without promoting heat loss. The maximum evaporative capacity will depend on the ambient water vapor pressure; when this is high, the potential for heat loss by evaporation will be limited. High humidity may therefore pose more of a threat to the athlete than does a high ambient temperature.

The rate of sweat secretion depends mainly on the rate of heat production by the body and the ambient temperature. In an event such as a marathon race, the faster runners sweat at a higher rate than do the slower runners because their rate of energy expenditure is higher (Figure 2–1), but they are active for a shorter period of time. Neither the total sweat loss during the race nor postrace rectal temperature is related to the finishing time (Maughan, 1985).

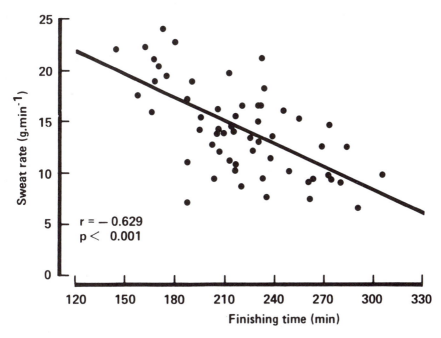

FIGURE 2-1. *The calculated mean sweating rate during a marathon race is closely related to finishing time. These results were obtained from 59 male runners taking part in the same race. In spite of the strong statistical relationship, there is a large variation between individuals running at the same speed. Reproduced from Maughan (1985).*

It is a common observation that there is a large variation between individuals in the rate of sweat production, even when they are exercising under the same conditions and at the same intensity. Marathon runners in the same race finishing with the same time and with the same fluid intake may lose from as little as 1% to as much as 6% of body weight during the race and yet finish the race with the same body temperature (Maughan, 1985). The reasons for this large inter-individual variability in sweat production are not apparent, and the implications are generally ignored. Differences between individuals in the energy cost of running are generally relatively small, and differences in the rate of heat production cannot therefore account for the observed differences in sweating rate. If the rate of heat production is the same, and the heat storage (increment in body temperature) is also the same, then the rate of heat loss must also be equal. This leads us to the apparently contradictory conclusion that the rate of evaporative heat loss must be independent of the sweating rate. For the individual who is sweating profusely it is certainly true that a large part of the sweat drips from the skin without evaporating.

During a race at high ambient temperatures, marathon runners may lose as much as 8% of body weight, corresponding to about 13% of total body water (Costill, 1972). Sweat losses of up to 7 L have been reported during an 85 km ski race lasting about 7 h (Saltin, 1964). We have observed one individual whose body weight consistently decreased by 2.0–2.5 kg during 45 min of exercise at 60% $\dot{V}O_2max$ in the heat (35° C).

The water lost during sweating is derived in varying proportions from the plasma, the extravascular extracellular space, and the intracellular water. Water accounts for about 60% of body mass in men and about 50% in women, the fraction depending primarily on body fat content. About 70% of total body water is intracellular. Plasma accounts for about 4–5% of total body weight, corresponding to 8–9% of total body water. In the first 10–15 min of exercise, there is generally a marked (5–15%) reduction in plasma volume, this fall being proportional to the exercise intensity and greater in cycling than in running exercise (Senay et al., 1980). This response is by no means consistent, however, and depends on a number of factors, including the exercise mode, the ambient temperature, and the degree of heat acclimation of the subjects (Harrison, 1985).

The initial response to exercise represents a redistribution of body water in response to an increased capillary filtration pressure in the working muscles and an increased tissue osmolality rather than a net water loss from the body. In the later stages of exercise, this process is reversed; the loss of hypotonic fluid as sweat results in an increased osmolality of the extracellular fluid and a consequent shift of fluid from the intracellular space. Costill and Fink (1974) found that plasma volume was reduced by 12% within 10 min of the onset of exercise at 60–75% $\dot{V}O_2max$; a further 110 min of exercise resulted in body weight being decreased by 4% with only a further 4% reduction in plasma volume; similar results were obtained by Francis (1979). In prolonged exercise at moderate intensity, a hemodilution may be observed at the end of exercise, even though there has been an initial hemoconcentration (Harrison, 1985).

The ambient temperature also appears to influence the distribution of body water losses. Kozlowski and Saltin (1964) found that a greater proportion of the total body water loss was derived from intracellular water when 3 h of exercise was performed at an ambient temperature of 18° C, than when the same degree of dehydration was induced by exercise at 38° C, although exercise time in the heat was only about 30 min less. In subjects cycling in the heat (40° C), Costill et al. (1976a) found that intracellular water accounted for only 30% of the total water loss after about 1.5 h of exercise, when the subjects were dehydrated by 2% of body weight, but for 50% of total water loss when they were dehydrated by 4% or 6%.

It is widely quoted that exercise performance is impaired when an individual is dehydrated by as little as 2% of body weight, representing a loss of about 3.3% of total body water. The studies on which this is based have been reviewed by Herbert (1983). The decrease in plasma volume that accompanies dehydration may be of particular importance in influencing work capacity; blood flow to the muscles must be maintained at a high level to supply oxygen and substrates, but a high blood flow to the skin is also necessary to convect heat to the body surface where it can be dissipated (Nadel, 1980). When the ambient temperature is high and blood volume has been decreased by sweat loss during prolonged exercise, there may be difficulty in meeting the requirement for a high blood flow to both these tissues. In this situation, skin blood flow is likely to be compromised, allowing central venous pressure and muscle blood flow to be maintained but reducing heat loss and causing body temperature to rise (Rowell, 1986). Fortney et al. (1984) observed a 32% reduction in forearm skin blood flow after dehydration corresponding to 3% of body weight. Such a decrease in peripheral blood flow would reduce the transfer of heat from the working muscles to the body surface.

With moderate dehydration, the cardiac output is generally well maintained during submaximal work, a reduction in stroke volume being compensated for by an increased heart rate, but rectal temperatures are elevated in dehydration in proportion to the degree of water deficit (Gisolfi & Copping, 1974). If some degree of dehydration is present at the onset of exercise, the effects of fluid loss during exercise are likely to be more pronounced, and thermoregulation will be impaired (Horowitz and Nadel, 1984). Even in subjects who are well hydrated prior to exercise, endurance times in the heat are often much less than at more moderate temperatures, although the pattern of substrate utilization appears not to be greatly different. In some situations, dehydration may therefore be more important than substrate depletion in causing fatigue during prolonged exercise. This idea is supported by the observation that intravenous saline infusion during exercise at 84% $\dot{V}O_2$max can reduce the decrease in plasma volume which occurs, and results in a lower rectal temperature and lower heart rate during exercise compared with a control test (Deschamps et al., 1989). In this study there was no difference in endurance time between the two test conditions, but neither dehydration nor hyperthermia would be expected to limit performance in exercise at this intensity as the duration is necessarily short (about 21 min). Large increases in treadmill running time (from 68 to 94 min, P < 0.01) in the heat have been reported to occur in rats when the plasma volume was expanded prior to exercise (Francesconi et al., 1989).

As well as causing dehydration, the loss of large volumes of sweat will lead to a loss of electrolytes from the body. The extent of the electrolyte loss depends on sweat volume and composition. Sweat is frequently described as an ultrafiltrate of plasma, and the concentrations of the major ionic components of sweat and plasma are shown in Table 2–1. The total osmolality of sweat is considerably lower than that of plasma, largely due to the relatively low concentrations of sodium and chloride, but the sweat content of some electrolytes, particularly potassium and magnesium, is relatively high. The very wide range reported in sweat composition probably reflects not only biological variability but also difficulties associated with the collection of sweat for analysis. The major problems are evaporative loss, incomplete collection, and contamination with skin cells. It has been reported that the sweat rate increases and the electrolyte content decreases as a consequence of heat acclimation (Leithead & Lind, 1964). Costill (1977) found that the sodium and chloride concentrations in sweat increased as the sweat rate increased, but Verde et al. (1982) reported that the concentration of these ions was independent of sweat rate. The potassium content of sweat appears to be unaffected by sweat rate, and the magnesium content is unchanged or decreases slightly.

Because sweat is hypotonic with respect to body fluids, the effect of prolonged sweating is to increase the plasma osmolality, which may have a significant effect on the ability to maintain body temperature. A direct relationship between plasma osmolality and body temperature has been demonstrated during exercise (Greenleaf et al., 1974; Harrison et al., 1978). Hyperosmolality of plasma, induced

TABLE 2-1. *Concentrations of the major electrolytes present in sweat, plasma, and intracellular (muscle) water in man. The values for sweat are derived from data reported in the literature (Costill, 1977; Costill et al., 1981; Verde et al., 1982). Plasma values are laboratory reference ranges for normal resting individuals. Values for intracellular concentrations are from Pitts (1959).*

| Electrolyte | Electrolyte Concentrations in Body Fluids (mEq/L) | | |
	Plasma	Sweat	Intracellular
Sodium	137–144	40–80	10
Potassium	3.5–4.9	4–8	148
Calcium	4.4–5.2	3–4	0–2
Magnesium	1.5–2.1	1–4	30–40
Chloride	100–108	30–70	2

prior to exercise, has been shown to result in a decreased thermo-regulatory effector response; the threshold for sweating is elevated and the cutaneous vasodilator response is reduced (Fortney et al., 1984). In short term (30 min) exercise, however, the cardiovascular and thermoregulatory response appears to be independent of changes in osmolality induced during the exercise period (Fortney et al., 1988).

The changes in the concentration of individual electrolytes are more variable, but an increase in the plasma sodium and chloride concentrations is generally observed in response to both running and cycling exercise. Exceptions to this are rare and occur only when excessively large volumes of drinks low in electrolytes are consumed over long time periods. These situations are discussed further below.

The plasma potassium concentration has been reported to remain constant after marathon running (Meytes et al., 1969; Whiting et al., 1984), although others have reported small increases, irrespective of whether drinks containing large amounts of potassium (Kavanagh & Shephard, 1975) or no electrolytes (Costill et al., 1976b; Cohen & Zimmerman, 1978) were given. Much of the inconsistency in the literature relating to changes in the circulating potassium concentration can be explained by the variable time taken to obtain blood samples after exercise under field conditions; the plasma potassium concentration rapidly returns to normal in the post-exercise period (Stansbie et al., 1982). The potassium concentration of extracellular fluid (4–5 mmol/L) is small relative to the intracellular concentration (150–160 mmol/L), and release of potassium from liver, muscle, and red blood cells will tend to elevate plasma potassium levels during exercise in spite of the losses in sweat.

The plasma magnesium concentration is unchanged after 60 min of moderate intensity cycling exercise (Joborn et al., 1985), but Rose et al. (1970) observed a 20% fall in the serum magnesium concentration after a marathon race and attributed this to a loss in sweat. A fall of similar magnitude was reported by Cohen and Zimmerman (1978). A larger fall in the serum magnesium concentration has been observed during exercise in the heat than at neutral temperatures (Beller et al., 1972), supporting the idea that losses in sweat are responsible. There are, however, reports that the fall in plasma magnesium concentration that occurs during prolonged exercise is a consequence of redistribution, with uptake of magnesium by red blood cells (Refsum et al., 1973), active muscle (Costill, 1977), or adipose tissue (Lijnen et al., 1988). The plasma content of potassium and magnesium represents only a small fraction of the whole body stores; Costill and Miller (1980) estimated that only about 1% of the body stores of these electrolytes was lost when individuals were dehydrated by 5.8% of body weight.

Numerous studies have shown that the physiological response to exercise can be modified if fluids are given orally during the exercise period. In many of these trials, plain water has been shown to enhance performance, whereas others have shown added benefits if sugars, electrolytes, and other components are present in solution. Because of the role of sugars and sodium in promoting water uptake in the small intestine, it is sometimes difficult to separate the effects of water replacement from those of substrate and electrolyte replacement when CHO-electrolyte solutions are ingested. In practice it is difficult to administer large amounts of CHO during exercise without also giving a significant amount of water. The effects of fluid ingestion on exercise performance are described below.

EFFECTS ON PERFORMANCE

Laboratory Studies—Cycling

Laboratory investigations into the ergogenic effects of the administration of CHO-electrolyte drinks during exercise have usually relied upon changes in physiological function during submaximal exercise or on the exercise time to exhaustion at a fixed work rate as a measure of performance. While this is a perfectly valid approach in itself, it must be appreciated that there are difficulties in extrapolating results obtained in this way to a race situation where the workload is likely to fluctuate with variations in the pace, weather conditions, and topography, and where tactical considerations and motivational factors are involved. To take account of some of these factors, some recent investigations have used exercise tests involving intermittent exercise, simulated races, or prolonged exercise followed by a sprint finish. Because different exercise tests and different solutions and rates of administration have been used in these various studies, comparisons between studies are difficult. Some studies have included a trial where no fluids were given, whereas others have compared the effects of test solutions with trials where plain water or flavored placebo drinks were given. These studies have been the subject of a number of extensive reviews which have concentrated on the effects of administration of CHO, electrolytes, and water on exercise performance (Coyle & Coggan, 1984; Lamb & Brodowicz, 1986; Murray, 1987).

Even where the exercise model used is similar, different results have been obtained. Of nine seemingly well controlled trials where continuous cycling exercise for 2 h or more was performed, six showed improvements in exercise performance (Björkman et al., 1984; Brooke et al., 1975; Coggan & Coyle, 1988, 1989; Coyle et al., 1983, 1986), and three showed no significant effect of administration of CHO-containing drinks (Felig et al., 1982; Flynn et al., 1987; Ivy et al., 1979). In none of these studies was performance adversely affected. In only one of these experiments did the drink used contain added electrolytes (Brooke et al., 1975). In two of the trials, exercise was performed on an isokinetic ergometer, and performance was measured as the total work output achieved in a 2 h period; neither of these trials showed a significant increase in total work output as a result of CHO ingestion (Flynn et al., 1987; Ivy et al., 1979). In one study, exercise consisted of alternate 15 min periods at 60% and 85% $\dot{V}O_2$max (Coggan and Coyle, 1988).

Variations in the total volume of fluids consumed could not explain differences between trials. In the trials showing a positive effect, intake varied from approximately 0.4 to 2.7 L; where no effect was seen, fluid intake was 0.2 to 2.2 L. Trials showing positive effects generally involved administration of relatively large amounts of substrate. Total CHO intake was 90 g or less in two of the trials where no effect was seen; the third trial investigated the effects of two different doses, 114 and 212 g. In studies where positive effects were seen, intake was in the range 120–410 g except for one study where intake appeared to be approximately 935 g over a period of 214 min. There was, perhaps, a tendency for the duration of the exercise task to be greater in those trials where a positive effect was observed. In exercise of shorter duration (70–90 min), endurance time was increased by ingestion (100 mL every 10 min) of an isotonic glucose-electrolyte solution, containing 40 g/L glucose, but not by ingestion of large amounts (360 g/L) of glucose polymer or fructose solutions (Maughan et al., 1989). The fructose solution caused severe gastrointestinal distress in a number of subjects.

Davis et al. (1988a) exercised subjects for approximately 2 h in a warm environment (27° C) at 75% $\dot{V}O_2$max; 275 mL of fluid, consisting of a 6% or 2.5% CHO-electrolyte drink or a flavored placebo, was given every 20 min during exercise. After a 30 min rest, subjects completed 2,700 pedal revolutions on the cycle ergometer as fast as possible. Performance time for the trial where the 6% CHO-electrolyte solution was given (31.3 min) was better than on the placebo trial (34.3 min), but the 2.5% solution (31.9 min) was not significantly better than the placebo.

Several studies have employed an experimental model consisting of prolonged intermittent exercise followed by a brief high intensity sprint, and again the results are not altogether consistent. Mitchell et al. (1988) showed that, compared with a trial where water was given, performance of a sprint lasting 12 min was enhanced if solutions containing 50, 60, or 75 g/L of various sugars were given at a rate of 8.5 mL/kg every hour during the prolonged exercise period; performance was not related to the amount of substrate given (58–87 g). Murray et al. (1987), however, found that performance of a sprint ride lasting about 6 min was not improved when 39 g of glucose polymer was given in a volume of 780 mL, but that improvements were seen when 47 g of a glucose-sucrose mixture with added electrolytes or 55 g of a glucose polymer-fructose mixture, again with added electrolytes, was given. In another study, Murray et al. (1989a) showed that sprint performance was reduced when fructose (76 g in 1.27 L) was given, compared with trials where glucose or sucrose were given at the same rate; no placebo or control trial was included in this study. The same authors (Murray et al., 1989b) found improvements in a sprint lasting about 14 min when a 6% sucrose solution (42 g in 692 mL) was given, but not when 8% or 10% sucrose solutions were given. Concentrated (12%) glucose-electrolyte drinks have also been reported to cause gastrointestinal distress during prolonged intermittent exercise (Davis et al., 1988b). In that same study, a 6% glucose-electrolyte beverage also failed to improve exercise performance relative to a flavored placebo. Kingwell et al. (1989) also failed to find differences in performance of a 5 min sprint test when 1.6 L of a 10% glucose polymer solution or an equal volume of placebo solution was given during the 160 min intermittent exercise period which preceded the sprint.

Laboratory Studies—Treadmill Exercise

As with studies during cycling exercise, many different exercise models have been used to investigate the effects of the administration of CHO-electrolyte solutions during walking and running. Again, conflicting results have been obtained. Sasaki et al. (1987) found that running time at 80% $\dot{V}O_2$max was increased, compared with a placebo trial, by ingestion of 90 g of sucrose in a volume of 500 mL. Macaraeg (1983) reported an increased endurance time during running at 85% of maximum heart rate when a 7% CHO-electrolyte solution was given, providing 84 g of CHO in a volume of 1.2 L, compared with either a trial without fluids or a trial with water only. In contrast to these results, however, Fruth and Gisolfi (1983) gave subjects a placebo or 150 g of glucose or fructose as a 10% solution during treadmill running at 70% $\dot{V}O_2$max; running time on the fructose trial was less than on the other two runs, but there was no difference in running time between the glucose and placebo trials. Riley et al. (1988) also found no difference in running time when a 7% CHO-electrolyte solution was given compared with a placebo trial; in this study subjects fasted for 21 h before exercise tests, and the first drink was given 20 min before exercise. In a study of very prolonged walking, Ivy et al. (1983) reported an increased walking time (299 min) when 120 g of glucose polymer was given in a volume of 1.5 L compared with a placebo trial (268 min).

Williams et al. (1988, 1990) have used an experimental model in which the subject is able to adjust the treadmill speed while running; the subject can then be encouraged either to cover the maximum distance possible in a fixed time or to complete a fixed distance in the fastest time possible. They showed that ingestion of 1 L of a glucose polymer-sucrose (50 g/L) solution did not increase the total distance covered in a 2 h run, but that the running speed was greater over the last 30 min of exercise when CHO was given compared with a placebo trial (Williams et al., 1988). They observed a similar effect when a CHO solution (70 g of glucose-glucose polymer, or 70 g of fructose-glucose polymer) or water was given in a 30 km treadmill time trial (Williams et al., 1990). The running speed decreased (from 4.14 to 3.75 m/s) over the last 10 km of the water trial, but was maintained in the other two runs. There was no significant difference between the three trials in the time taken to cover the total distance, although there was a tendency for performance to be better in the glucose (124.8 min) and fructose (125.9 min) trials than in the run where water only was given (129.3 min).

Field Studies

There are many practical difficulties associated with the conduct of field trials to assess the efficacy of ergogenic aids, which accounts for the fact that few well controlled studies of the effects of administration of glucose-electrolyte solutions have been carried out in this way. The main problem is with the design of an adequately controlled trial. Where a cross-over design is used, this is likely to be confounded by changes in the environmental conditions between trials, and the use of parallel control and test groups raises the difficulty of matching the groups. Many of the early studies purporting to show beneficial effects of ingestion of CHO-containing solutions on performance in events such as cycling, canoeing, and soccer were so poorly designed that the results are of no value.

In a study reported by Wells et al. (1985), experienced marathon runners completed a 20 mile (32 km) run on three separate occasions; water, a CHO-electrolyte solution, or a caffeine solution was given before and during the run. No effects of the different drinks on heart rate, rectal temperature, body weight loss, or decrease in plasma volume were observed. Again, however, the experimental design was poor, as environmental conditions varied greatly between trial days, and subjects were allowed to consume water in addition to the test beverages.

Studies where matched groups of competitors consumed 1.4 L of either water or a glucose-electrolyte solution during a marathon race (Maughan & Whiting, 1985) or 1.4 L of different CHO-containing drinks during marathon and ultramarathon races (Noakes et al., 1988) have shown no differences between the groups in finishing time. In the study of Maughan and Whiting (1985), subjects were matched on the basis of their anticipated finishing times. Mean finishing time for the runners (n = 43) drinking the CHO-electrolyte solution was 220 ± 40 min compared with a predicted finishing time of 220 ± 35 min; for the group drinking water (n = 47) actual finishing time was 217 ± 32 min and predicted time was 212 ± 32 min. Twenty four runners (60%) in the CHO-electrolyte group ran faster than expected, compared with 19 (40%) in the water group, suggesting that there may have been a benefit obtained from drinking the CHO-electrolyte solution.

Leatt (1986) gave 1 L of a 7% glucose polymer solution or a flavoured placebo to soccer players during a practice game. During the match, the group who had been given CHO utilized 31% less glycogen than the placebo group. No measure of performance of the two groups was made, but it was proposed that a beneficial effect would be experienced in the later stages of the game by the players taking the glucose polymer.

Summary of Effects on Performance

The time for which exercise at intensities of about 70–85% $\dot{V}O_2max$ can be sustained is generally improved by the ingestion of CHO-containing drinks during exercise. If prolonged strenuous exercise is followed by a high intensity sprint test, performance in the sprint is also generally improved if CHO-containing drinks are taken during the prolonged exercise. There are few reported adverse effects of CHO-electrolyte solutions on exercise performance, except where large doses of fructose are given, although concentrated (12% or more) glucose solutions may also cause problems. The CHO content of drinks used has been in the form of glucose, fructose, sucrose, short chain glucose polymers, or combinations of these. Different CHO sources seem to be equally effective, with the exception of fructose which, given alone, may cause gastrointestinal distress; given in combination with glucose or sucrose, however, fructose seems to be effective and acceptable.

FORMULATION OF FLUID REPLENISHMENT

The fate of ingested fluids depends on the rate at which they are emptied from the stomach and on the rate of absorption in the small intestine, and these factors must be taken into account in the formulation of drinks. Of these two processes, it is likely that gastric emptying limits the availability of ingested fluids; if the rate of fluid delivery from the stomach was to exceed the absorptive capacity of the intestine and large bowel for a significant period of time, diarrhea would ensue. Although this condition is by no means unknown during exercise, it does not normally occur in most individuals.

Control of Gastric Emptying

Some exchange of water does occur in the stomach, but it is not clear whether there is net absorption; no significant absorption of nutrients, other than alcohol to a limited extent, takes place in the stomach (Karel, 1948). The gastric emptying rate regulates the rate at which ingested food and fluids are delivered to the site of absorption in the small intestine and the extent to which these are modified by the gastric solutions. Many factors have been shown to influence the rate of gastric emptying of liquids, and some of these are listed in Table 2-2. Most of this information is derived from studies on resting individuals; the effects of exercise will be discussed later, but these appear not to materially alter the effects of fluid composition on gastric emptying.

A more important limitation to the usefulness of many studies in the literature is a consequence of the methodology used; most have relied on gastric aspiration techniques in which the stomach contents are recovered at a fixed time interval after fluid ingestion. This method assumes a linear rate of emptying. If repeated sampling techniques are used, however, it is observed that emptying follows an exponential time course (Rehrer et al., 1989a); use of scintigraphic techniques to assess emptying rates confirms these obser-

TABLE 2-2. *Factors reported to influence gastric emptying rate in humans.*

Osmolality	Fatty acid chain length
Energy density	Presence of particulate matter
pH	Exercise intensity
Volume	Hormonal environment
Temperature	Stress
Acclimation	Environmental temperature
Fear	Time of day
Anger	Phase of menstrual cycle

vations (Leiper & Maughan, 1988). The interpretation of the results is therefore strongly influenced by the time at which measurements are made. Where sampling at a single time point has been used, different investigators have chosen different intervals in the range 10–60 min between drink ingestion and sampling, making comparisons between drinks and between studies difficult. The exponential nature of the emptying curve also indicates the crucial importance of the volume of the stomach contents in controlling the rate of emptying. As fluid is emptied and the stomach volume falls, so the rate of emptying is decreased.

Accepting these problems, however, and considering only the effects of the composition of ingested fluids, the most important observations with respect to their fate are that emptying is slowed if solutions are markedly hypertonic with respect to the osmolality of body fluids (Hunt & Pathak, 1960), by increasing acidity (Hunt & Knox, 1969) and by increasing energy density (Hunt & Stubbs, 1975). It seems well established that the emptying rate of CHO solutions is slowed relative to isotonic saline solutions (M^CHugh & Moran, 1979; Brener et al., 1983), although Barker et al. (1974) found no difference in the emptying rates of isosmotic solutions of glucose and potassium chloride. The emptying rate is also highly dependent on the volume of the stomach contents as mentioned above, and maintaining a large fluid volume in the stomach will promote emptying.

The effect of increasing glucose concentration on the time course of emptying is shown in Figure 2–2; the emptying rate is slowed in proportion to the glucose content and slows as the volume of fluid remaining in the stomach decreases. From these results, it appears that even a 5% glucose solution will delay gastric emptying. Some previous reports have indicated that the rate of gastric emptying is decreased if the CHO content of the drink exceeds 2.5% (Costill & Saltin, 1974; Foster et al., 1980), but more recent studies have shown that emptying of solutions containing up to 10% glucose or glucose polymer is not delayed relative to water (Owen et al., 1986; Rehrer et al., 1989a). At least part of this apparent discrepancy is probably the result of the design of these studies. If a fixed volume of two different glucose solutions, one dilute and one concentrated, is given, the initial emptying rate for the dilute solution will be more rapid; as the volume falls, so the emptying rate is reduced, but this effect will be less marked for the more concentrated solution. It is also apparent from Figure 2–2 that, although increasing the glucose content of the ingested fluid does slow the rate at which fluid leaves the stomach, it results in a faster delivery of glucose, in agreement with the results of Hunt et al. (1985). The non-linear nature of the

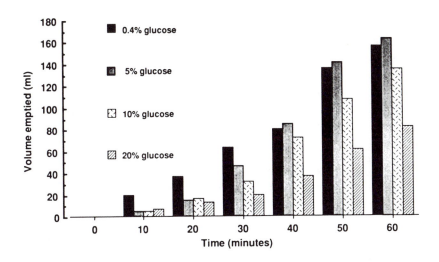

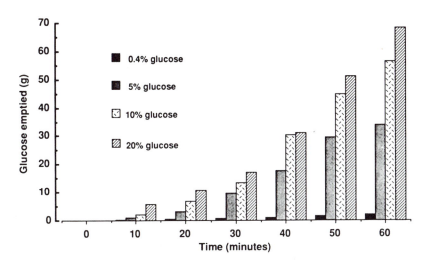

FIGURE 2-2. *Effects of glucose concentration on the rate of gastric emptying.*
Upper panel. *Volume of solution emptied after ingestion of 200 mL of flavored water (0.4% glucose) or solutions containing 5%, 10% or 20% glucose.*
Lower panel. *Amount of glucose emptied from the stomach when these solutions are consumed. Reproduced from Maughan and Leiper (1990).*

time course of emptying makes it difficult to accept that the rate of energy delivery to the intestine is constant as has been proposed by Brener et al. (1983).

Ahlborg and Felig (1976) gave 200 g of glucose as a 30% solution during exercise at 30% of $\dot{V}O_2$max and showed a rapid elevation of blood glucose concentration and an increased glucose oxidation, indicating that the ingested solution had been emptied and absorbed. In many of the studies where addition of tracers to ingested glucose solutions has shown that the ingested glucose is readily available for oxidation during exercise, concentrated (25%) solutions of glucose without added electrolytes have been used and appeared to be well tolerated (e.g., Pirnay et al., 1977, 1982; Pallikarakis et al., 1986). The same investigators have also shown that 86–98% of a glucose load (50 g) ingested during walking at 45% $\dot{V}O_2$max was oxidized within 4 h and that the amount oxidized was not significantly different if the glucose was added to volumes of 200, 400, or 600 mL of water (Jandrain et al., 1989).

Substitution of glucose polymers for free glucose may help to promote the emptying of glucose-electrolyte solutions from the stomach by reducing the osmolality of the solution while maintaining the total glucose content, although the studies reported in the literature are by no means in agreement. In an early report, Hunt (1960), found no major differences in the emptying rates of solutions containing isoenergetic amounts of monomeric glucose or starch. Foster et al. (1980), however, reported that substituting glucose oligomers 3–4 units in length resulted in a rate of emptying approximately one third faster compared with a solution of free glucose which had the same energy density when a 5% solution was used, but no difference in emptying rates between free glucose and polymers for 10, 20, and 40% solutions. These results are in marked contrast to those reported recently by Sole and Noakes (1989); they found that a 15% glucose polymer solution emptied faster than a 15% solution of free glucose, although 5% and 10% solutions of free glucose and polymer appeared to be emptied at the same rates. In another recent study, Naveri et al. (1989) found that the emptying rates of electrolyte solutions with 3% CHO added in the form of glucose or a polymer were the same. Owen et al. (1986) also found no difference in the rate of emptying of 10% solutions of glucose or glucose polymer, in spite of the higher osmolality of the free glucose solution. Even dilute polymer solutions are generally emptied more slowly than plain water, but Seiple et al. (1983) did report that a 7% glucose polymer solution with an osmolality of 216 mosmol/kg was emptied as fast as water; however, the first sampling point in this study was at 30 min, by which time at least 90% of total volume had emptied for all the solutions studied. In none of the above studies was the emptying rate of polymer solutions slower than that of free glucose solutions with the same energy density, and the polymer solutions were generally emptied faster even when the differences were not statistically significant.

The temperature of ingested drinks may also have an influence on the rate of emptying. Costill and Saltin (1974) gave subjects 400 mL of a dilute glucose solution at temperatures ranging from 5–35° C; the volume emptied in the first 15 min after ingestion was approximately twice as great for the solution at 5° C as for the solution at 35° C. More recent reports, however, have cast some doubt on the importance of temperature in affecting emptying of liquids. Sun et al. (1988) gave isosmotic orange juice at different temperatures, and found that the initial emptying rate for cold (4° C) drinks was slower than for drinks given at body temperature (37° C); the emptying rate of warm (50° C) drinks was intermediate to and statistically indistinguishable from the other two drinks. McArthur and Feldman (1989) have also recently shown that the emptying rates for coffee drinks given at 4, 37, or 58° C were not different.

Other factors, such as pH, may have a minor role to play in the control of gastric emptying. Interestingly, in view of the introduction of carbonated sports drinks, there is some evidence that emptying is hastened if drinks are carbonated (Lolli et al., 1952).

In summary, gastric emptying of liquids is regulated by many factors, of which the most important are the osmolality and the energy density. Increasing the carbohydrate content of drinks will delay emptying. Substitution of glucose polymers for free glucose appears to slightly increase the rate of delivery of fluid and substrate to the small intestine. The factors regulating gastric emptying have been the subject of extensive reviews (Murray, 1987; Brouns et al., 1987).

Regulation of Intestinal Transport

Because of the practical difficulties involved, there have been few attempts to measure intestinal absorption during exercise. These measurements require the presence of a multi-lumen perfusion set in the proximal small intestine; apart from the obvious discomfort to the subject, valid results are obtained only when a steady state is achieved. This can require a perfusion period of two hours or more, limiting the application during exercise (Leiper & Maughan, 1988). As with gastric emptying therefore, most of our information comes from studies of resting individuals.

Absorption of glucose in the small intestine is an active process linked to the transport of sodium, and is therefore dependent on the concentrations of glucose and sodium in the lumen. The absorption of water, however, is a purely passive process, and follows the osmotic gradients set up by the uptake of solutes by the intestinal mucosa. The uptake of water is influenced by the luminal concentrations of glucose, sodium, and other actively transported solutes, and by the pH and the osmolality of the luminal contents.

Glucose-electrolyte solutions that are moderately hypotonic with respect to plasma seem to promote the fastest rates of water transport, with the optimum osmolality being in the range of 200–250 mosmol/kg (Wapnir & Lifshitz, 1985; Leiper & Maughan, 1986). The presence of very high glucose concentrations does not lead to increased glucose uptake and results in an increased osmotic load. When hypertonic solutions are perfused through the gut, net secretion of water into the lumen occurs; this will not only exacerbate the effects of dehydration (Figures 2-3, 2-4), but will also increase the risk of gastrointestinal discomfort by increasing the volume of fluid in the gut. Other sugars can be substituted for glucose, and an increased uptake of glucose has been demonstrated when glucose oligomers with a chain length of 5–9 glucose units have been used in the rat (Daum et al., 1978) or 3–6 glucose units in man (Jones

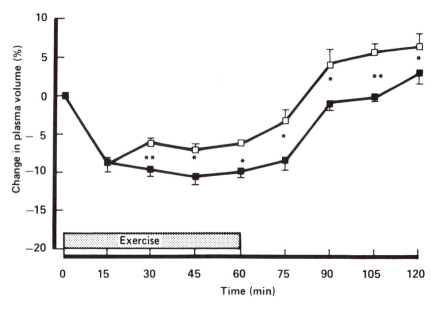

FIGURE 2-3. *Plasma volume changes during and after 60 min of cycle exercise at 68% of $\dot{V}O_2max$. On one trial (□) an isotonic (310 mosmol/kg) glucose-electrolyte solution was given at a rate of 100 mL every 10 min; on the other trial (■) a hypertonic (630 mosmol/kg) glucose polymer solution was given at the same rate. Values are Mean and SE (n = 6); significant differences between trials are indicated as follows : * P < 0.05, ** P < 0.01. Reproduced from Maughan et al (1987).*

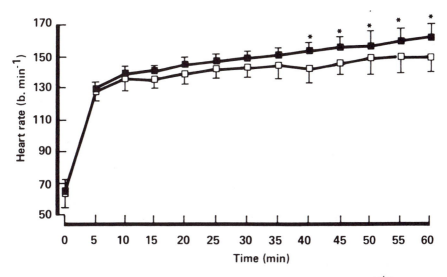

FIGURE 2-4. *Heart rate before and during 60 min of cycle exercise at 68% of $\dot{V}O_2max$. On one trial (□) an isotonic (310 mosmol/kg) glucose-electrolyte solution was given at a rate of 100 mL every 10 min; on the other trial (■) a hypertonic (630 mosmol/kg) glucose polymer solution was given at the same rate. Towards the end of exercise, heart rate was significantly higher on the trial where the hypertonic solution was given; this response helps maintain cardiac output in spite of the lower plasma volume (Figure 2-3). Values are Mean and SE (n = 6); significant differences between trials are indicated as follows : * P < 0.05. Reproduced from Maughan et al (1987).*

et al., 1983; 1987); these short chain polymers are rapidly hydrolysed by the actions of pancreatic α-amylase and a group of enzymes located on the enterocyte brush border (Kenny and Maroux, 1982). Sucrose has been shown to be as effective as glucose in promoting glucose and water uptake (Spiller et al., 1982); this can be accounted for by the rapid intestinal hydrolysis of sucrose to glucose and fructose with subsequent uptake of the liberated monosaccharides (Gray & Ingelfinger 1966), although there is some evidence that absorption of sucrose as such can take place in the intestine (Chain et al., 1960). Wheeler and Banwell (1986), however, found that substituting an equivalent amount of sucrose for a part of the glucose polymer content of a CHO-electrolyte solution resulted in a reduced rate of water uptake; since they appear not to have measured sugar uptake, the mechanism responsible for this is not apparent. Contrary to most other reports, these authors also found no difference in water uptake when plain water or CHO-electrolyte solutions were perfused.

The absorption of fructose by the intestine is not an active process in man, and it does not compete with glucose for uptake; its absorption appears to be stimulated by glucose and independent of the luminal sodium content (Rumessen & Gudmand-Hoyer, 1986). Fructose is less rapidly absorbed than glucose, the transport rate being about two thirds that of glucose at the same concentration, and stimulates less sodium and water absorption (Fordtran, 1975). The ingestion of large amounts of fructose is to be avoided as it commonly results in disturbances of gastrointestinal function, with vomiting and diarrhea.

The major benefit derived from the addition of electrolytes to drinks consumed during exercise is their stimulation of glucose and water uptake. The most important addition, therefore, is sodium which is co-transported with glucose; addition of other cations serves no useful purpose, as far as is presently known, and will result in an increased osmolality. Many of the currently available sports drinks, however, contain small but significant amounts of divalent cations, particularly calcium and magnesium. Perfusion studies have established that the optimum sodium concentration, from the point of view of the stimulation of glucose uptake, is in the range of 60–120 mmol/L; when the luminal sodium concentration is less than 70–90 mmol/L, there will be a net flux of sodium from mucosa to lumen. This is much higher than the sodium content generally found in sports drinks, but glucose-electrolyte solutions used for oral rehydration in the treatment of diarrhea-induced dehydration commonly use such high concentrations (Table 2-3).

It is possible that studies in which a short segment of the proximal intestine is perfused may give misleading results with respect to the optimum sodium concentration. If the solution present in the intestinal lumen has a low sodium content, sodium ions will be secreted into the lumen until they are present in sufficient concentra-

TABLE 2-3. *Carbohydrate and electrolyte content of two commonly used sports drinks, a soft drink, the World Health Organization recommended oral rehydration solution (WHO-ORS), and a commercially-available hypotonic oral rehydration solution (Dioralyte). Most of the solutions contain some additional electrolytes, including bicarbonate, citrate, and phosphate. The composition of Coca Cola appears to vary widely between different countries.*

Beverage	Carbohydrate (g/L)	Na^+ (mM)	K^+ (mM)	Cl^- (mM)	Osmolality (mosmol/L)
Isostar	73	24	4	12	296
Gatorade	62	23	3	14	349
Coca Cola	105	3	0	1	650
WHO-ORS	20	90	20	80	331
Dioralyte	16	60	20	60	240

tion to stimulate glucose uptake. Thus it is possible to achieve net uptake of water and glucose in the presence of net secretion of sodium. When the whole gut is available, sodium secreted into the proximal region of the intestine in response to low luminal sodium concentrations will eventually reach an equilibrium level and will be reabsorbed by more distal regions of the gut. It is not at present clear whether the delay introduced by the need for sodium secretion before absorption can take place will significantly retard the delivery of glucose and water to the circulation. However, in one study where a glucose load (87 g) was given in combination with either NaCl or an equimolar amount of mannitol, the plasma glucose level was significantly higher between 45–105 min after ingestion when NaCl was given (Ferrannini et al., 1982). Although not conclusive, this does imply that the presence of sodium will increase the availability of ingested glucose. The choice of anion does not appear to be of critical importance, and chloride is normally used in combination with bicarbonate, citrate, and sometimes phosphate, all of which serve as acidity regulators. Chloride uptake occurs by diffusion down the electrochemical gradient established by active sodium uptake; as well as maintaining electrical neutrality, this adds to the osmotic gradient driving water uptake.

An alternative method to examine the fate of ingested fluids involves measurement of the rate of accumulation in body water of an isotopic tracer for water added to the drink. Davis et al. (1987) found that accumulation in plasma and saliva of deuterium (^{2}H) added to drinks was slower for concentrated (15% and 40%) glucose solutions than for hypotonic saline or dilute CHO-electrolyte solutions, in accordance with the known gastric emptying and intestinal absorption characteristics of these solutions. More recently, the same authors measured the rate of plasma ^{2}H accumulation after ingestion of water, a 6% glucose polymer solution, and glucose-fructose mixtures at concentrations of 6%, 8%, and 10%; all solutions contained a ^{2}H$_2$O tracer and also low (20 mmol/L) concentrations of sodium (Davis et al. 1990). The rate of tracer accumulation in the plasma was the same for all drinks, suggesting that the availability of ingested fluids is not impaired if the carbohydrate content is in the form of a glucose-fructose mixture and does not exceed 10%. In a comparison of the rates of blood ^{2}H accumulation after ingestion of water or a dilute glucose-electrolyte solution containing a ^{2}H$_2$O tracer, the rate of tracer accumulation was found to be higher for the glucose-electrolyte solution than for plain water, supporting the suggestion that these beverages will promote the absorption of water (Leiper and Maughan, 1988). In all studies where the appearance of tracers for water uptake has been followed, a rapid accumulation of tracer has been observed, suggesting that ingested fluids are readily available.

Effects of Exercise on Gastric Emptying and Intestinal Absorption

Relatively few measurements of gastric emptying, and even fewer of intestinal transport, have been made during exercise. Costill and Saltin (1974) showed that 15 min of cycling exercise had no effect on gastric emptying of a dilute glucose-electrolyte solution until a work intensity of about 70% $\dot{V}O_2$max was reached; at 80–90% $\dot{V}O_2$max, the emptying rate was only about 50% of the resting rate. In a rather poorly controlled study, Ramsbottom and Hunt (1974) found that 20 min of "severe exercise" (100W!) reduced the emptying rate of a 278 mmol/L (5%) glucose solution in 4 of 6 subjects. During intermittent cycling exercise at 74% of $\dot{V}O_2$max, gastrointestinal transit time, estimated by breath hydrogen analysis, was not different from rest, and was not different when concentrated glucose (1000 mmol/L) or flavoured dilute (150 mmol/L) solutions were given (Segal et al., 1985). Mitchell et al. (1989) found that prolonged (105 min) cycling at 70% $\dot{V}O_2$max did not affect the rate of emptying of a 6% CHO (4% glucose polymer, 2% sucrose) solution compared with rest; their subjects drank approximately 620 mL/h and the calculated emptying rate was close to 600 mL/h. Similar results were obtained during intermittent exercise (Mitchell et al., 1988). Emptying rates in excess of 1 L/h, corresponding to over 90% of the ingested volume, can be achieved during prolonged (3 h) exercise at 60% $\dot{V}O_2$max in the heat (Ryan et al., 1989). Using a double sampling gastric aspiration technique that allowed the time course of emptying to be measured, Rehrer et al. (1989a) reported that exercise at 50% or 70% $\dot{V}O_2$max had no significant effect on the emptying rate of sweetened water or CHO-electrolyte solutions, although there was a trend towards a decreased emptying rate of the CHO-electrolyte solutions, but not of water, with increasing exercise intensity. They also showed that gastric emptying and gastric secretion were not different between trained and untrained individuals.

When a dilute glucose-electrolyte solution labeled with ^2H_2O is given at rest or during exercise, the rate of accumulation of deuterium in the plasma decreases during exercise in proportion to the exercise intensity, and the time to peak plasma deuterium concentration increases with increasing exercise intensities in the range 40–

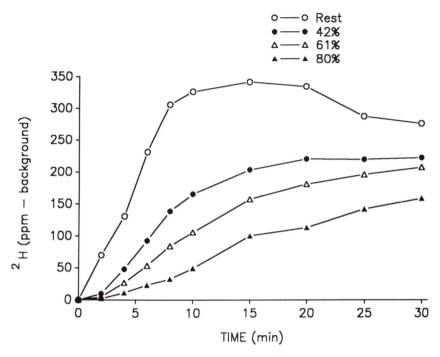

FIGURE 2-5. *Accumulation in the plasma of deuterium (^{2}H) after ingestion of 200 mL of a dilute glucose-electrolyte solution containing trace amounts of deuterium oxide. Results were obtained from six subjects at rest and during exercise at 42%, 61%, and 80% of VO$_2$max. Reproduced from Maughan et al (1990).*

80% V̇O$_2$max (Figure 2-5). These results imply a decreased availability of ingested fluids during exercise (Maughan et al., 1990). It has been suggested, however, that the use of tracer techniques in this way may not give a valid measure of net water flux in the small intestine (Gisolfi et al., 1990).

The above studies all involved cycling exercise, but earlier, poorly controlled investigations had established that gastric emptying is delayed during running (Campbell et al., 1928). In 1967, Fordtran and Saltin reported that the rate of emptying of a concentrated glucose-electrolyte solution (740 mmol/L [13.3%] glucose; 52 mmol/L NaCl) was not changed during 1 h of treadmill running at 70% V̇O$_2$max compared with rest; emptying of plain water was much faster and was slightly delayed by exercise. Costill et al. (1970) found no differences in the gastric emptying rates of water and a dilute glucose-electrolyte solution during 2 h of treadmill running at

70% $\dot{V}O_2$max in highly trained runners. Owen et al. (1986) found no difference in emptying rates of solutions containing 10% glucose (586 mosmol/kg) or 10% glucose polymers (194 mosmol/kg) compared with sweetened water during 2 h of treadmill running in the heat (35° C) at 65% $\dot{V}O_2$max; emptying of the glucose solution, but not of the others was retarded relative to sweetened water ingested at a lower (25° C) ambient temperature. In contrast to these results, Neufer et al. (1986) found that 15 min of running at 50 or 70% $\dot{V}O_2$max increased the rates of emptying of water and of carbohydrate-containing solutions relative to rest. Later, Neufer et al. (1989a) confirmed these results for walking and running at 28–65% $\dot{V}O_2$max, but found a decreased emptying rate at 75% $\dot{V}O_2$max compared with rest. The same authors also reported that exercise in the heat (49° C) or after dehydration reduced gastric emptying compared with exercise at a neutral temperature (Neufer et al., 1989b). Sole and Noakes (1989) have reported that gastric emptying of water, but not of a 10% glucose polymer solution, is delayed during 30 min of treadmill running at 75% $\dot{V}O_2$max; this result is the opposite of that obtained by Rehrer et al. (1989a) during cycling.

As with the resting studies described above, some of the variability between these exercise studies is probably an effect of differences in sampling times. In some of the exercise studies also, the experimental protocol required the subjects to ingest several different test beverages sequentially during a single session. The effects of the presence of previous drinks in the small intestine cannot be excluded as a source of error (Rehrer et al., 1989a). The effects of exercise on gastric emptying have been reviewed and summarised by Brouns et al. (1987).

There have been few studies on the effects of exercise on intestinal absorption, largely due to the practical problems associated with perfusing the small intestine in exercising individuals. Using this technique, Fordtran and Saltin (1967) found no effect of treadmill exercise at 70% $\dot{V}O_2$max on intestinal absorption of glucose, water, or electrolytes from a glucose-electrolyte solution. More recently, Barclay and Turnberg (1988) reported large reductions in water and electrolyte absorption when an electrolyte solution containing no carbohydrate was perfused during low intensity cycling exercise. The workload was poorly controlled in this study and was varied to achieve a heart rate 40–50% above the resting rate.

The mechanisms by which exercise might influence the function of the gastrointestinal tract are thought to be related to the increased circulating catecholamine level and reduced perfusion of the splanchnic vascular bed during strenuous exercise; this has been reviewed by Murray (1987).

Formulation of Sports Drinks

In most situations the primary aim of fluids ingested during prolonged exercise is to provide both substrate for the working muscles and water to offset the effects of dehydration. The supply of electrolytes to replace losses in sweat is not usually a priority during the exercise period. Many of the studies quoted above show that endurance capacity can be increased if fluids are taken during exercise, particularly when the ambient temperature is high. Although plain water can be effective in this respect, the addition of sugars, electrolytes, and possibly other components can give added benefits. Addition of electrolytes can also have negative effects if their concentration is high.

The commercial products that are available represent a variety of different approaches to the problem of finding the optimal solution for the provision of substrate and the maintenance of fluid and electrolyte balance. Table 2–3 shows the composition of two currently available sports drinks which have very similar formulations; for comparison, the composition of a popular soft drink and of two solutions intended for oral rehydration in patients with diarrhea-induced dehydration are also shown.

Several important points should be borne in mind when planning fluid replacement strategies. First, there is a need to take account of individual circumstances, including the duration and intensity of the exercise and the environmental conditions, and to make some allowance for the differences among individuals. In prolonged exercise (up to about 3–4 h) at high ambient temperatures, there is a need to minimize the decrease in plasma volume and the increase in plasma osmolality which normally occur, so replacement of water losses is a primary requirement. Replacement of the electrolytes lost in sweat during exercise is not a priority for the overwhelming majority of participants in sports events; the primary purpose of adding sodium to fluids ingested during exercise should be perceived as its stimulatory effect on glucose and water absorption. A second role played by sodium is in the maintenance of extracellular volume. As the main osmotically active component of extracellular fluid, sodium is important in the distribution of water between the intracellular and extracellular compartments (Nose et al., 1988). When sweat losses are high and are replaced by plain water, extracellular osmolality will fall, resulting in a shift of water into the intracellular space. However, several studies have indicated that addition of sodium chloride to ingested fluids is not beneficial in terms of improving exercise performance (see Noakes et al., 1985). In the cold, fluid replacement has a lower priority, and increasing the CHO content of drinks will provide more fuel for the muscles.

PRACTICAL CONSIDERATIONS

Frequency and Volume of Drinks

In many sporting situations the volume of fluids that can be consumed during the event is limited by the rules of the competition. In other events, drinks are more or less freely available, and the volume taken will be limited by the capacity of the individual to assimilate the ingested fluid and to tolerate the presence of unabsorbed fluid in the gut. The large loss of plasma volume that occurs within the first 10–15 min of exercise is a consequence of shifts between body water compartments and is not influenced by the ingestion of fluids (Maughan et al., 1987). Rapid infusion of isotonic saline can reduce this initial decrease in plasma volume (from 14% to 5%) but does not abolish it (Deschamps et al., 1989). In more prolonged exercise, the water loss will depend on the exercise intensity and on the ambient temperature and humidity; there is also a large inter-individual variability in sweating rates. All these factors will influence the need to replace fluids.

The first obstacle to fluid absorption is gastric emptying. The maximum rate of gastric emptying that can be achieved will depend on the regulatory factors described above. Because the emptying rate is so dependent on the volume in the stomach, the time period over which measurements are made is also of critical importance; low rates of emptying are generally reported when long sampling periods are used. Neufer et al. (1986) found emptying rates for water of about 20 mL/min during 15 min of treadmill running at 50–70% $\dot{V}O_2$max when 400 mL of fluid was ingested; emptying rates for CHO-containing solutions were lower (approximately 12–16 mL/min). Rehrer et al. (1989a) reported much higher initial emptying rates of water and of a CHO-electrolyte solution; over the first 10 min after ingestion of a volume of about 600 mL (8 mL/kg), about 37 mL/min (2.2 L/h) were emptied. The emptying rate decreased rapidly as the volume remaining in the stomach decreased but was not affected by exercise. These results suggest that when a high rate of gastric emptying is required and where the presence of a large volume in the stomach does not cause discomfort, the volume of liquid in the stomach should be kept high (about 600 mL) by frequent ingestion of small volumes.

The capacity of the small intestine for absorption will not normally limit CHO or water uptake when CHO-electrolyte solutions are taken orally, but ingestion of large volumes of isotonic saline in the fasted individual will result in diarrhea.

In laboratory studies, large volumes of fluid are often consumed by subjects during exercise, and volumes in excess of 1 L/h appear to be well tolerated during running and cycling if given in frequent small volumes. In contrast to the laboratory situation, the amounts of fluids consumed during competition in sport are generally small. The total fluid intake of elite marathon runners is often less than 200 mL in an event lasting more than 2 h (Costill et al., 1970; Brouns et al., 1987). Rehrer et al. (1989b) reported mean fluid intakes of 109 mL in a 25 km race and 577 mL in a marathon. When required to do so, marathon runners can, however, tolerate larger volumes (at least 1.4 L) without apparent problems (Maughan, 1985). Magazanik et al. (1974) reported a mean fluid intake of 1.5 L (range 0.57–2.57) in six runners during a marathon race.

Where the finishing times of runners vary greatly, the rates of fluid intake may be more relevant than the total intake. Noakes et al. (1988a) measured fluid intakes of 0.45–0.62 L/h in a total of 109 runners competing in a number of marathon and 56 km races; finishing times ranged from 2 h 16 min to 5 h 38 min, and there was a tendency for the slower runners to have the greatest water intake. Costill et al. (1970), however, gave marathon runners 100 mL of water every 5 min for the first 100 min of a 2 h treadmill run at 70% $\dot{V}O_2$max; the subjects complained of gastrointestinal discomfort in the later stages of exercise, by which time a volume of 2 L had been consumed, and they were unable to continue drinking. In contrast, cyclists commonly have much higher intakes and can achieve intakes of up to 1 L/h over prolonged periods during simulated competition (Brouns et al., 1989). Fluid intakes in excess of 10 L/d have been reported for competitors in the Tour de France cycle race (Saris et al., 1989). Large volumes of fluid appear to be better tolerated in cycling than in running, perhaps due to the more pronounced movement of the abdominal contents during running. There is generally little difference in gastric emptying rates between these two exercise modes when the work intensity is the same (Rehrer et al., 1990), although Neufer et al. (1986) found that emptying was faster during running than during cycling at 70% $\dot{V}O_2$max.

It appears from these results that it should be possible to achieve fluid intakes considerably in excess of those normally taken by athletes. There are many reports of athletes, particularly runners, suffering from varying degrees of gastrointestinal distress during training and competition. These surveys have been reviewed by Moses (1990). These symptoms, however, seem not to be influenced by the amount or composition of fluids consumed (Brouns et al., 1987). In a study carried out by Ahlborg and Felig (1976), subjects were able to ingest 200 g of glucose as a 30% solution over a period of 5–10 min during low intensity (30% $\dot{V}O_2$max) bicycle exercise without any reported problems.

Relatively little attention has been paid to the role of beverage palatability in influencing the volume of fluid that is tolerable during exercise. It is well known that voluntary fluid intake during prolonged exercise is generally less than the deficit incurred (Pitts et al., 1944), and efforts to promote adequate fluid intake must take account of the subjective perception of taste. Costill et al. (1975) reported that the volume of fluid consumed during exercise in the heat was greater when a CHO-electrolyte solution was available than when plain water was provided. Hubbard et al. (1984) found that the temperature as well as the taste of drinks influenced the volume consumed during walking in the heat, with cool (15° C) drinks being preferred to warm (40° C) ones.

Water Overload and Hyponatraemia

It has often been reported that the fluid intakes of participants in endurance events are low, and it is recognized that this may lead to dehydration and heat illness in prolonged exercise when the ambient temperature is high. Accordingly, the advice given to participants in endurance events is that they should ensure a high fluid intake to minimize the effects of dehydration and that drinks should contain low levels of glucose and electrolytes so as not to delay gastric emptying (American College of Sports Medicine, 1984). In accordance with these recommendations, most CHO-electrolyte drinks intended for consumption during prolonged exercise also have a low electrolyte content, with sodium and chloride concentrations typically in the range of 10–20 mmol/L (Table 2-3). While this might represent a reasonable strategy for providing substrates and water (although it can be argued that a higher sodium concentration would enhance water uptake and that a higher carbohydrate content would increase substrate provision), these recommendations may not be appropriate in all circumstances.

Physicians dealing with individuals in distress at the end of long distance races have become accustomed to dealing with hyperthermia associated with dehydration and hypernatraemia, but it has become clear that a small number of individuals at the end of very prolonged events may be suffering from hyponatraemia in conjunction with either hyperhydration (Noakes et al., 1985, 1990; Frizell et al., 1986; Saltin & Costill, 1988) or dehydration (Hiller, 1989).

All the reported cases have been associated with ultramarathon or prolonged triathlon events; most of the cases have occurred in events lasting in excess of 8 h, and there are few reports of cases where the exercise duration is less than 4 h. Noakes et al. (1985) reported four cases of exercise-induced hyponatraemia; race times were between 7 and 10 h, and postrace serum sodium concentrations were between 115 and 125 mmol/L. Estimated fluid intakes were between 6 and 12 L, and consisted of water or drinks containing low levels of electrolytes; estimated total sodium chloride intake during the race was 20–40 mmol. Frizell et al. (1986) reported even more astonishing fluid intakes of 20–24 L of fluids (an intake of almost 2.5 L/h) with a mean sodium content of only 5–10 mmol/L in two runners who collapsed after an ultramarathon run and who were found to be hyponatraemic (serum sodium concentration 118–123 mmol/L). Hyponatraemia as a consequence of ingestion of large volumes of fluids with a low sodium content has also been recognized in resting individuals. Flear et al. (1981) reported the case of a man who drank 9 L of beer, with a sodium content of 1.5 mmol/L, in the space of 20 min; plasma sodium fell from 143 mmol/L before to 127 mmol/L after drinking, but the man appeared unaffected. In these cases, there is clearly a replacement of water in excess of losses with inadequate electrolyte replacement. In competitors in the Hawaii Ironman Triathlon who have been found to be hyponatraemic, however, dehydration has also been reported to be present (Hiller, 1989). Fellmann et al. (1988) reported a small but statistically significant fall in serum sodium concentration, from 141 to 137 mmol/L, in runners who completed a 24-h run, but food and fluid intakes were neither controlled nor measured.

These reports are interesting and indicate that some supplementation with sodium chloride may be required in extremely prolonged events where large sweat losses can be expected and where it is possible to consume large volumes of fluid. This should not, however, divert attention away from the fact that electrolyte replacement during exercise is not a priority for most participants in most sporting events, although it is certainly helpful after the event to restore body water and electrolyte content.

SUMMARY

The available evidence supports the idea that ingestion of CHO-electrolyte solutions during prolonged exercise can improve performance. Ingestion of CHO-containing beverages during prolonged exercise will maintain the blood glucose level and increase the contribution of CHO to oxidative metabolism; when these solutions are taken, heart rate and rectal temperature will generally be lower, and plasma volume will be better maintained than when no fluids are given. There is, however, no agreement on the optimum formulation nor on the frequency or volume of drinking that is most appropriate. In practice, the ideal solution will depend on a number of factors, including the duration and intensity of the exercise, the environmental conditions, and the characteristics of the individual. Based on what is known regarding the regulation of gastric emptying and intestinal absorption of ingested fluids, a solution of glucose, sucrose, or maltodextrins containing about 5–10% carbohydrate and added sodium chloride (20–50 mmol/L) taken at a rate of 100–200 mL every 15–20 min might appear best. Practical experience, however, indicates that most individuals can tolerate solutions with a higher carbohydrate content, and these might be preferable where high sweat losses are not anticipated and where the major requirement is for substrate provision. In some circumstances, e.g., exercise at low intensity in hot environments, it is likely that dehydration rather than carbohydrate depletion will limit performance. In such conditions, the carbohydrate concentration should be reduced to less than 5% and the sodium concentration increased to 50 mmol/L or even higher. Under all circumstances, the variation between individuals is large, and the optimum strategy can only be established by subjective experience.

BIBLIOGRAPHY

Ahlborg, G., and P. Felig (1976). Influence of glucose ingestion on fuel-hormone response during prolonged exercise. *J. Appl. Physiol.* 41: 683–688.
Ahlborg, B., J. Bergstrom, J. Brohult, L.-G. Ekelund, E. Hultman, and G. Maschio (1967). Human muscle glycogen content and capacity for prolonged exercise after different diets. *Forsvarsmedicin.* 3: 85–99.
American College of Sports Medicine (1984). Prevention of thermal injuries during distance running. *Phys. Sportsmed.* 12: 43–51.
Bagby, G.J., H.J. Green, S. Katsuta, and P.D. Gollnick (1978). Glycogen depletion in exercising rats infused with glucose, lactate, or pyruvate. *J. Appl. Physiol.* 45: 425–429.
Bannister, R.G. (1967). Medical aspects of competitive athletics. *Trans. Med. Soc. Lond.* 83: 145–147.
Barclay, G.R., and L.A. Turnberg (1988). Effect of moderate exercise on salt and water transport in the human jejunum. *Gut* 29: 816–820.
Barker, G.R., G.M. Cochrane, G.A. Corbett, J.N. Hunt, and S.K. Roberts (1974). Actions of glucose and potassium chloride on osmoreceptors slowing gastric emptying. *J. Physiol.* 237: 183–186.
Beller, G.A., J.T. Maher, L.H. Hartley, D.E. Bass, and W.E.C. Wacker (1972). Serum Mg and K concentrations during exercise in thermoneutral and hot conditions. *Physiologist* 15: 94.
Bergstrom, J., and E. Hultman (1966). Muscle glycogen synthesis after exercise: an enhancing factor localised to the muscle cells in man. *Nature* 210: 309–310.
Bergstrom, J., and E. Hultman (1967). A study of the glycogen metabolism during exercise in man. *Scand. J. Clin. Lab. Invest.* 19: 218–228.
Björkman, O., K. Sahlin, L. Hagenfeldt, and J. Wahren (1984). Influence of glucose and fructose ingestion on the capacity for long-term exercise in well-trained men. *Clin. Physiol.* 4: 483–494.
Blomstrand, E., F. Celsing, and E.A. Newsholme (1988). Changes in plasma concentrations of aromatic and branched-chain amino acids during sustained exercise in man and their possible role in fatigue. *Acta. Physiol. Scand.* 133: 115–121.
Bock, A.V., C. Vancaulaert, D.B. Dill, A. Folling, and L. Hurxthal (1928). Studies in muscular activity, IV. *J. Physiol.* 66: 162–174.
Boje, O. (1936). Der Blutzucker während und nach körperlicher Arbeit. *Skand. Arch. Physiol.* 74 Suppl 10: 1–48.
Brener, W., T.R. Hendrix, and P.R. M^{C}Hugh (1983). Regulation of the gastric emptying of glucose. *Gastroenterology* 85: 76–82.
Brooke, J.D., G.J. Davies, and L.F. Green (1975). The effects of normal and glucose syrup work diets on the performance of racing cyclists. *J. Sports Med.* 15: 257–265.

Brouns, F., W.H.M. Saris, and N.J. Rehrer (1987). Abdominal complaints and gastrointestinal function during long-lasting exercise. *Int. J. Sports Med.* 8: 175–189.

Brouns, F., W.H.M. Saris, J. Stroeken, E. Beckers, R. Thijssen, N.J. Rehrer, and F. ten Hoor (1989). Eating, drinking, and cycling. A controlled Tour de France simulation study, part 1. *Int. J. Sports Med.* 10 Suppl 1: S32–S40.

Campbell J.M.H., G.O. Mitchell, and A.T.W. Powell (1928). The influence of exercise on digestion. *Guy's Hospital Reports* 78: 279–293.

Carter, J.E., and C.V. Gisolfi (1989). Fluid replacement during and after exercise in the heat. *Med. Sci. Sports Exerc.* 21: 532–539.

Chain, E.B., K.R.L. Mansford, and F. Pocchiari (1960). The absorption of sucrose, maltose and higher oligosaccharides from the isolated rat small intestine. *J. Physiol.* 154: 39–51.

Christensen, E.H., and O. Hansen (1939). Zur methodik der Respiratorischen Quotient-Bestimmungen in Ruhe und bei Arbeit. *Skand. Arch. Physiol.* 81: 137–189.

Coggan, A.R., and E.F. Coyle (1988). Effect of carbohydrate feedings during high-intensity exercise. *J. Appl. Physiol.* 65: 1703–1709.

Coggan, A.R., and E.F. Coyle (1989). Metabolism and performance following carbohydrate ingestion late in exercise. *Med. Sci. Sports Exerc.* 21: 59–65.

Cohen, I, and AL Zimmerman (1978). Changes in serum electrolyte levels during marathon running. *S. Afr. Med. J.* 53: 449–453.

Costill, D.L. (1972). Physiology of marathon running. *J. Am. Med. Assoc.* 221: 1024–1029.

Costill, D.L. (1977). Sweating: its composition and effects on body fluids. *Ann. NY Acad. Sci.* 301: 160–174.

Costill, D.L., and W.J. Fink (1974). Plasma volume changes following exercise and thermal dehydration *J. Appl. Physiol.* 37: 521–525.

Costill, D.L., and J.M. Miller (1980). Nutrition for endurance sport. *Int. J. Sports Med.* 1: 2–14.

Costill, D.L., and B. Saltin (1974). Factors limiting gastric emptying during rest and exercise. *J. Appl. Physiol.* 37: 679–683.

Costill, D.L., W.F. Kammer, and A. Fisher (1970). Fluid ingestion during distance running. *Arch. Environ. Health* 21: 520–525.

Costill, D.L., A. Bennett, G. Branam, and D. Eddy (1973). Glucose ingestion at rest and during prolonged exercise. *J. Appl. Physiol.* 34: 764–769.

Costill, D.L., R. Cote, E. Miller, T. Miller, and S. Wynder (1975). Water and electrolyte replacement during repeated days of work in the heat. *Aviat. Space Environ. Med.* 46: 795–800.

Costill, D.L., R. Cote, and W. Fink (1976a). Muscle water and electrolytes following varied levels of dehydration in man. *J. Appl. Physiol.* 40: 6–11.

Costill, D.L., G. Branam, W. Fink, and R. Nelson (1976b). Exercise induced sodium conservation: changes in plasma renin and aldosterone. *Med. Sci. Sports Exerc.* 8: 209–213.

Costill, D.L., R. Cote, W.J. Fink, and P. Van Handel (1981). Muscle water and electrolyte distribution during prolonged exercise. *Int. J. Sports Med.* 2: 130–134.

Coyle, E.F., and A.R. Coggan (1984). Effectiveness of carbohydrate feeding in delaying fatigue during prolonged exercise. *Sports Med.* 1: 446–458.

Coyle, E.F., J.M. Hagberg, B.F. Hurley, W.H. Martin, A.H. Ehsani, and J.O. Holloszy (1983). Carbohydrate feeding during prolonged strenuous exercise can delay fatigue. *J. Appl. Physiol.* 55: 230–235.

Coyle, E.F., A.R. Coggan, M.K. Hemmert, and J.L. Ivy (1986). Muscle glycogen utilisation during prolonged strenuous exercise when fed carbohydrate. *J. Appl. Physiol.* 61: 165–172.

Daum, F., M.I. Cohen, H. McNamara, and L. Finberg (1978). Intestinal osmolality and carbohydrate absorption in rats treated with polymerized glucose. *Pediat. Res.* 12: 24–26.

Davis, J.M., D.R. Lamb, W.A. Burgess, and W.P. Bartoli (1987). Accumulation of deuterium oxide in body fluids after ingestion of D_2O-labeled beverages. *J. Appl. Physiol.* 63: 2060–2066.

Davis, J.M., D.R. Lamb, R.R. Pate, C.A. Slentz, W.A. Burgess, and W.P. Bartoli (1988a). Carbohydrate-electrolyte drinks: effects on endurance cycling in the heat. *Am. J. Clin. Nutr.* 48: 1023–1030.

Davis, J.M., W.A. Burgess, C.A. Slentz, W.P. Bartoli, and R.R. Pate (1988b). Effects of ingesting 6% and 12% glucose/electrolyte beverages during prolonged intermittent cycling in the heat. *Eur. J. Appl. Physiol.* 57: 563–569.

Davis, J.M., W.A. Burgess, C.A. Slentz, and W.P. Bartoli (1990). Fluid availability of sports drinks differing in carbohydrate type and concentration. *Am. J. Clin. Nutr.* 51: 1054–1057.

Deschamps, A., R.D. Levy, M.G. Cosio, E.B. Marliss, and S. Magder (1989). Effect of saline infusion on body temperature and endurance during heavy exercise. *J. Appl. Physiol.* 66: 2799–2804.

Erickson, M.A., R.J. Schwartzkopf, and R.D. M^CKenzie (1987). Effects of caffeine, fructose, and glucose ingestion on muscle glycogen utilisation during exercise. *Med. Sci. Sports Exerc.* 19: 579–583.

Felig, P., A. Cherif, A. Minigawa, and J. Wahren (1982). Hypoglycaemia during prolonged exercise in normal men. *New Engl. J. Med.* 306: 895–900.

Fellmann, N., M. Sagnol, M. Bedu, G. Falgairette, E. Van Praagh, G. Gaillard, P. Jouanel, and J. Coudert (1988). Enzymatic and hormonal responses following a 24 h endurance run and a 10 h triathlon race. *Eur. J. Appl. Physiol.* 57: 545–553.

Ferrannini, E., E. Barrett, S. Bevilacqua, J. Dupre, and R.A. Defronzo (1982). Sodium elevates the plasma glucose response to glucose ingestion in man. *J. Clin. Endocrinol. Metab.* 54: 455–458.

Fielding, R.A., D.L. Costill, W.J. Fink, D.S. King, M. Hargreaves, and J.E. Kovaleski (1985). Effect of carbohydrate feeding frequencies on muscle glycogen use during exercise. *Med. Sci. Sports Exerc.* 17: 472–476.

Flear, C.T.G., C.V. Gill, and J. Burn (1981). Beer drinking and hyponatraemia. *Lancet* 2: 477.

Flynn, M.G., D.L. Costill, J.A. Hawley, W.J. Fink, P.D. Neufer, R.A. Fielding, and M.D. Sleeper (1987). Influence of selected carbohydrate drinks on cycling performance and glycogen use. *Med. Sci. Sports Exerc.* 19: 37–40.

Fordtran, J.S. (1975). Stimulation of active and passive sodium absorption by sugars in the human jejunum. *J. Clin. Invest.* 55: 728–737.

Fordtran, J.S., and B. Saltin (1967). Gastric emptying and intestinal absorption during prolonged severe exercise. *J. Appl. Physiol.* 23: 331–335.

Fortney, S.M., C.B. Wenger, J.R. Bove, and E.R. Nadel (1984). Effect of hyperosmolality on control of blood flow and sweating. *J. Appl. Physiol.* 57: 1688–1695.

Fortney, S.M., N.B. Vroman, W.S. Beckett, S. Permutt, and N.D. LaFrance (1988). Effect of exercise hemoconcentration and hyperosmolality on exercise responses. *J. Appl. Physiol.* 65: 519–524.

Foster, C., D.L. Costill, and W.J. Fink (1980). Gastric emptying characteristics of glucose and glucose polymers. *Res. Quart.* 51: 299–305.

Francesconi, R.P., M. Bosselaers, C. Matthew, and R.W. Hubbard (1989). Plasma volume expansion in rats: effects on thermoregulation and exercise. *J. Appl. Physiol.* 66: 1749–1755.

Francis, K.T. (1979). Effect of water and electrolyte replacement during exercise in the heat on biochemical indices of stress and performance. *Aviat. Space Environ. Med.* 50: 115–119.

Frizell, R.T., G.H. Lang, D.C. Lowance, and S.R. Lathan (1986). Hyponatraemia and ultramarathon running. *J. Am. Med. Assoc.* 255: 772–774.

Fruth, J.M., and C.V. Gisolfi (1983). Effects of carbohydrate consumption on endurance performance: fructose versus glucose. In: Fox EL (Ed) *Nutrient utilisation during exercise.* Ross Laboratories, Columbus pp 68–75.

Galbo, H., N.J. Christensen, and J.J. Holst (1977). Glucose-induced decrease in glucagon and epinephrine responses to exercise in man. *J. Appl. Physiol.* 42: 525–530.

Gisolfi, C.V. and J.R. Copping (1974). Thermal effects of prolonged treadmill exercise in the heat. *Med. Sci. Sports* 6: 108–113.

Gisolfi, C.V., R.W. Summers, H.P. Schedl, T.L. Bleiler, and R.A. Oppliger (1990). Human intestinal water absorption: direct vs. indirect measurements. *Am. J. Physiol.* 258: G216-G222.

Gleeson, M., and R.J. Maughan (1987). The effect of nutritional status on circulating concentrations of amino acids and urea during prolonged strenuous exercise in man. *J. Physiol.* 390: 251P.

Gordon, B., L.A. Cohn, S.A. Levine, M. Matton, W.D.M. Scriver, and W.B. Whiting (1925). Sugar content of the blood in runners following a marathon race. *J. Am. Med. Assoc.* 185: 508–509.

Gray, G.M., and F.J. Ingelfinger (1966). Intestinal absorption of sucrose in man: interrelation of hydrolysis and monosaccharide product absorption. *J. Clin. Invest.* 45: 388–398.

Greenleaf, J.E., B.L. Castle, and D.H. Card (1974). Blood electrolytes and temperature regulation during exercise in man. *Acta. Physiol. Pol.* 25: 397–410.

Hargreaves, M., and C.A. Briggs (1988). Effect of carbohydrate ingestion on exercise metabolism. *J. Appl. Physiol.* 65: 1553–1555.

Hargreaves, M., D.L. Costill, A. Coggan, W.J. Fink, and I. Nishibata (1984). Effect of carbohydrate feedings on muscle glycogen utilisation and exercise performance. *Med. Sci. Sports Exerc.* 16: 219–222.

Harrison, M.H. (1985). Effects of thermal stress and exercise on blood volume in humans. *Physiol. Rev.* 65: 149–209.

Harrison, M.H., R.J. Edwards, and P.A. Fennessy (1978). Intravascular volume and tonicity as factors in the regulation of body temperature. *J. Appl. Physiol.* 44: 69–75.

Herbert, W.G. (1983). Water and electrolytes. In: Williams MH (Ed) *Ergogenic Aids in Sport.* Human Kinetics, Champaign pp56–98.

Hermansen, L., E. Hultman, and B. Saltin (1967). Muscle glycogen during prolonged severe exercise. *Acta. Physiol. Scand.* 71: 129–139.

Hiller, W.D.B. (1989). Dehydration and hyponatraemia during triathlons. *Med. Sci. Sports Exerc.* 21: S219-S221.

Horowitz, M., and E.R. Nadel (1984). Effect of plasma volume on thermoregulation in the dog. *Pflüg. Arch.* 400: 211–213.

Hubbard, R.W., B.L. Sandick, W.T. Matthews, R.P. Francesconi, and J.B. Sampson (1984). Voluntary dehydration and alliesthesia for water. *J. Appl. Physiol.* 57: 868–875.

Hultman, E. (1967). Studies on muscle metabolism of glycogen and active phosphate in man with special reference to exercise and diet. *Scand. J. Clin. Lab. Invest.* 19 Suppl 94: 11–63.

Hultman, E., and L.H. Nilsson (1971). Liver glycogen in man. Effect of different diets and muscular exercise. *Adv. Exp. Biol. Med.* 11: 143–151.

Hunt, J.N. (1960). The site of receptors slowing gastric emptying in response to starch in test meals. *J. Physiol.* 154: 270–276.

Hunt, J.N., and M.T. Knox (1969). The slowing of gastric emptying by nine acids. *J. Physiol.* 201: 161–179.

Hunt, J.N., and J.D. Pathak (1960). The osmotic effect of some simple molecules and ions on gastric emptying. *J. Physiol.* 154: 254–269.

Hunt, J.N., and D.F. Stubbs (1975). The volume and energy content of meals as determinants of gastric emptying. *J. Physiol.* 245: 209–225.

Hunt, J.N., J.L. Smith, and C.L. Jiang (1985). Effect of meal volume and energy density on the gastric emptying rate of carbohydrates. *Gastroenterology* 89: 1326–1330.

Ivy, J., D.L. Costill, W.J. Fink, and R.W. Lower (1979). Influence of caffeine and carbohydrate feedings on endurance performance. *Med. Sci. Sports* 11: 6–11.

Ivy, J.L., W. Miller, V. Dover, L.G. Goodyear, W.M. Sherman, S. Farrell, and H. Williams (1983). Endurance improved by ingestion of a glucose polymer supplement. *Med. Sci. Sports Exerc.* 15: 466–471.

Jandrain, B.J., F. Pirnay, M. Lacroix, F. Mosora, A.J. Scheen, and P.J. Lefebvre (1989). Effect of osmolality on availability of glucose ingested during prolonged exercise in humans. *J. Appl. Physiol.* 67: 76–82.

Joborn, H., G. Åkerström, and S. Ljunghall (1985). Effects of exogenous catecholamines and exercise on plasma magnesium concentrations. *Clin. Endocrinol.* 23: 219–226.

Jones, B.J.M., B.E. Brown, J.S. Loran, D. Edgerton, and J.F. Kennedy (1983). Glucose absorption from starch hydrolysates in the human jejunum. *Gut* 24: 1152–1160.

Jones, B.J.M., B.E. Higgins, and D.B.A. Silk (1987). Glucose absorption from maltotriose and glucose oligomers in the human jejunum. *Clin. Sci.* 72: 409–414.

Karel, L. (1948). Gastric Absorption. *Physiol. Rev.* 28: 433–450.

Kavanagh, T., and R.J. Shephard (1975). Maintenance of hydration in "post-coronary" marathon runners. *Br. J. Sports Med.* 9: 130–135.

Kenny, A.J., and S. Maroux (1982). Topology of microvillar membrane hydrolases of kidney and intestine. *Physiol. Rev.* 62: 91–128.

Kingwell, B., M.J. MᶜKenna, E.R. Sandstrom, M. Hargreaves (1989). Effect of glucose polymer ingestion on energy and fluid balance during exercise. *J. Sports Sci.* 7: 3–8.

Kozlowski, S., and B. Saltin (1964). Effect of sweat loss on body fluids. *J. Appl. Physiol.* 19: 1119–1124.

Krogh, A. and J. Lindhard (1920). The relative value of fat and carbohydrate as sources of muscular energy. *Biochem. J.* 14: 293–360.

Kuipers, H., H.A. Keizer, F. Brouns, and W.H.M. Saris (1987). Carbohydrate feeding and glycogen synthesis during exercise in man. *Pflüg. Arch.* 410: 652–656.

Lamb, D.R., and G.R. Brodowicz (1986). Optimal use of fluids of varying formulations to minimize exercise-induced disturbances in homeostasis. *Sports Med.* 3: 247–274.

Leatt, P. (1986). The effect of glucose polymer ingestion on skeletal muscle glycogen depletion during soccer match-play and its resynthesis following a match. (Unpublished M Sc Thesis, University of Toronto, Toronto, Ontario, Canada.).

Leiper, J.B., and R.J. Maughan (1986). The effect of luminal tonicity on water absorption from a segment of the intact human jejunum. *J. Physiol.* 378: 95P.

Leiper, J.B., and R.J. Maughan (1988). Experimental models for the investigation of water and solute transport in man: implications for oral rehydration solutions. *Drugs* 36 Suppl 4: 65–79.

Leithead, C.S., and A.R. Lind (1964). *Heat stress and heat disorders.* Casell, London..

Levine, S.A., B. Gordon, and C.L. Derick (1924). Some changes in the chemical constituents of the blood following a marathon race. *J. Am. Med. Assoc.* 82: 1778–1779.

Lijnen, P., P. Hespel, R. Fagard, R. Lysens, E. Vanden Eynde, and A. Amery (1988). Erythrocyte, plasma and urinary magnesium in men before and after a marathon. *Eur. J. Appl. Physiol.* 58: 252–256.

Lolli, G., L.A. Greenberg, and D. Lester (1952). The influence of carbonated water on gastric emptying. *New Engl. J. Med.* 246: 490–492.

McArthur, K.E., and M. Feldman (1989). Gastric acid secretion, gastrin release, and gastric temperature in humans as affected by liquid meal temperature. *Am. J. Clin. Nutr.* 49: 51–54.

MᶜHugh, P.R., and T.H. Moran (1979). Calories and gastric emptying: a regulatory capacity with implications for feeding. *Am. J. Physiol.* 236: R254–260.

Macaraeg, P.V.J. (1983). Influence of carbohydrate electrolyte ingestion on running endurance. In: Fox EL (Ed) *Nutrient utilisation during exercise.* Ross Laboratories, Columbus pp 91–96.

Magazanik, A., Y. Shapiro, D. Meytes, and I. Meytes (1974). Enzyme blood levels and water balance during a marathon race. *J. Appl. Physiol.* 36: 214–217.

Massicotte, D., F. Péronnet, C. Allah, C. Hillaire-Marcel, M. Ledoux, and G. Brisson (1986). Metabolic response to [^{13}C]glucose and [^{13}C]fructose ingestion during exercise. *J. Appl. Physiol.* 61: 1180–1184.

Massicotte, D., F. Péronnet, G. Brisson, K. Bakkouch, and C. Hilaire-Marcel (1989). Oxidation of a glucose polymer during exercise: comparison with glucose and fructose. *J. Appl. Physiol.* 66: 179–183.

Maughan, R.J. (1985). Thermoregulation and fluid balance in marathon competition at low ambient temperature. *Int. J. Sports Med.* 6: 15–19.

Maughan, R.J., and J.B. Leiper (1983). Aerobic capacity and fractional utilisation of aerobic capacity in elite and non-elite male and female marathon runners. *Eur. J. Appl. Physiol.* 52: 80–87.

Maughan, R.J., and J.B. Leiper (1990). Studies in human models. *Clinical Therapeutics* 12, Suppl. A: 63–72.

Maughan, R.J., and P.H. Whiting (1985). Factors influencing plasma glucose concentration during marathon running. In:Dotson CO, JH Humphrey (Eds) *Exercise Physiology.* Volume 1, New York: AMS Press.

Maughan, R.J., C.E. Fenn, M. Gleeson, and J.B. Leiper (1987). Metabolic and circulatory responses to the ingestion of glucose polymer andglucose/electrolyte solutions during exercise in man. *Eur. J. Appl. Physiol.* 56: 356–362.

Maughan, R.J., C.E. Fenn, and J.B. Leiper (1989). Effects of fluid, electrolyte and substrate ingestion on endurance capacity. *Eur. J. Appl. Physiol.* 58: 481–486.

Maughan, R.J., J.B. Leiper, and B.A. McGaw (1990). Effects of exercise intensity on absorption of ingested fluids in man. *Exp. Physiol.* 75: 419–421.

Meytes, I., Y. Shapira, A. Magazanik, D. Meytes, and U. Seligsohn (1969). Physiological and biochemical changes during a marathon race. *Int. J. Biometeorol.* 13: 317.

Mitchell, J.B., D.L. Costill, J.A. Houmard, M.G. Flynn, W.J. Fink, and J.D. Beltz (1988). Effects of carbohydrate ingestion on gastric emptying and exercise performance. *Med. Sci. Sports Ex.* 20: 110–115.

Mitchell, J.B., D.L. Costill, J.A. Houmard, W.J. Fink, R.A. Robergs, and J.A. Davis (1989). Gastric emptying: influence of prolonged exercise and carbohydrate concentration. *Med. Sci. Sports Exerc.* 21: 269–274.

Moses, F.M. (1990). The effect of exercise on the gastrointestinal tract. *Sports Med.* 9: 159–172.

Mosora, F., M. Lacroix, A. Luckyx, N. Pallikarakis, F. Pirnay, G. Krzentowski, and P. Lefebvre (1981). Glucose oxidation in relation to the size of the oral glucose loading dose. *Metabolism* 30: 1143–1149.

Murray, R. (1987). The effects of consuming carbohydrate-electrolyte beverages on gastric emptying and fluid absorption during and following exercise. *Sports Med.* 4: 322–351.

Murray, R., D.E. Eddy, T.W. Murray, J.G. Seifert, G.L. Paul, and G.A. Halaby (1987). The effect of fluid and carbohydrate feedings during intermittent cycling exercise. *Med. Sci. Sports Exerc.* 19: 597–604.

Murray, R., G.L. Paul, J.G. Seifert, D.E. Eddy, and G.A. Halaby (1989a). The effects of glucose, fructose, and sucrose ingestion during exercise. *Med. Sci. Sports Exerc.* 21: 275–282.

Murray, R., J.G. Seifert, D.E. Eddy, G.L. Paul, and G.A. Halaby (1989b). Carbohydrate feeding and exercise: effect of beverage carbohydrate content. *Eur. J. Appl. Physiol.* 59: 152–158.

Nadel, E.R. (1980). Circulatory and thermal regulations during exercise. *Fed. Proc.* 39: 1491–1497.

Naveri, H., H. Tikkanen, A.-L. Kairento, and M. Harkonen (1989). Gastric emptying and serum insulin levels after intake of glucose-polymer solutions. *Eur. J. Appl. Physiol.* 58: 661–665.

Neufer, P.D., D.L. Costill, W.J. Fink, J.P. Kirwan, R.A. Fielding, and M.G. Flynn (1986). Effect of exercise and carbohydrate composition on gastric emptying. *Med. Sci. Sports Exerc.* 18: 658–662.

Neufer, P.D., A.J. Young, and M.N. Sawka (1989a). Gastric emptying during walking and running: effects of varied exercise intensity. *Eur. J. Appl. Physiol.* 58: 440–445.

Neufer, P.D., A.J. Young, and M.N. Sawka (1989b). Gastric emptying during exercise: effect of heat stress and hypohydration. *Eur. J. Appl. Physiol.* 58: 433–439.

Nilsson, L.H., P. Furst, and E. Hultman (1973). Carbohydrate metabolism of the liver in normal man under varying dietary conditions. *Scand. J. Clin. Lab. Invest.* 32: 331–337.

Noakes, T.D., N. Goodwin, B.L. Rayner, T. Branken, and R.K.N. Taylor (1985). Water intoxication: a possible complication during endurance exercise. *Med. Sci. Sports Exerc.* 17: 370–375.

Noakes, T.D., B.A. Adams, K.H. Myburgh, C. Greeff, T. Lotz, and M. Nathan (1988a). The danger of an inadequate water intake during prolonged exercise. A novel concept re-visited. *Eur. J. Appl. Physiol.* 57: 210–219.

Noakes, T.D., E.V. Lambert, M.I. Lambert, P.S. M^{C}Arthur, K.H. Myburgh, and A.J.S. Benade (1988b). Carbohydrate ingestion and muscle glycogen depletion during marathon and ultra-marathon racing. *Eur. J. Appl. Physiol.* 57: 482–489.

Noakes, T.D., R.J. Norman, R.H. Buck, J. Godlonton, K. Stevenson, and D. Pittaway (1990). The incidence of hyponatremia during prolonged ultraendurance exercise. *Med. Sci. Sports Exerc.* 22: 165–170.

Nose, H., G.W. Mack, H. Lhi, and E.R. Nadel (1988). Role of osmolarity and plasma volume during dehydration in humans. *J. Appl. Physiol.* 65: 325–331.

Owen, M.D., K.C. Kregel, P.T. Wall, and C.V. Gisolfi (1986). Effects of ingesting carbohydrate beverages during exercise in the heat. *Med. Sci. Sports Exerc.* 18: 568–575.

Pallikarakis, N., B. Jandrain, F. Pirnay, F. Mosora, M. Lacroix, A.S. Luyckx, and P.J. Lefebvre (1986). Remarkable metabolic availability of oral glucose during long-duration exercise in humans. *J. Appl. Physiol.* 60: 1035–1042.

Pirnay, F., M. Lacroix, F. Mosora, A. Luyckx, and P. Lefebvre (1977). Glucose oxidation during prolonged exercise evaluated with naturally labeled [^{13}C]glucose. *J. Appl. Physiol.* 43: 258–261.

Pirnay, F., J.M. Crielaard, N. Pallikarakis, M. Lacroix, F. Mosora, G. Krzentowski, A.S. Luyckx, and P.J. Lefebvre (1982). Fate of exogenous glucose during exercise of different intensities in humans. *J. Appl. Physiol.* 53: 1620–1624.

Pitts, G.L., R.E. Johnson, and C.F. Consolazio (1944). Work in the heat as affected by intake of water, salt and glucose. *Am. J. Physiol.* 142: 253–259.

Pitts, R.F. (1959). *The Physiological Basis of Diuretic Therapy.* CC Thomas, Springfield.

Pugh, L.G.C.E., J.L. Corbett, and R.H. Johnson (1967). Rectal temperatures, weight losses, and sweat rates in marathon running. *J. Appl. Physiol.* 23: 347–352.

Ramsbottom, N., J.N. Hunt (1974). Effect of exercise on gastric emptying and gastric secretion. *Digestion* 10: 1–8.

Refsum, H.E., H.D. Meen, and S.B. Stromme (1973). Whole blood, serum and erythrocyte magnesium concentrations after repeated heavy exercise of long duration. *Scand. J. Clin. Lab. Invest.* 32: 123–127.

Rehrer, N.J., E. Beckers, F. Brouns, F. Ten Hoor, and W.H.M. Saris (1989a). Exercise and training effects on gastric emptying of carbohydrate beverages. *Med. Sci. Sports Exerc.* 21: 540–549.

Rehrer, N.J., G.M.E. Janssen, F. Brouns, and W.H.M. Saris (1989b). Fluid intake and gastrointestinal problems in runners competing in a 25-km race and a marathon. *Int. J. Sports Med.* 10 Suppl 1: S22-S25.

Rehrer, N.J., F. Brouns, E. Beckers, F. Ten Hoor, and W.H.M. Saris (1990). Gastric emptying with repeated drinking during running and bicycling. *Int. J. Sports Med.* 11:238–243.

Riley, M.L., R.G. Israel, D. Holbert, E.B. Tapscott, and G.L. Dohm (1988). Effect of carbohydrate ingestion on exercise endurance and metabolism after a 1-day fast. *Int. J. Sports Med.* 9: 320–324.

Rose, L.I., D.R. Carroll, S.L. Lowe, E.W. Peterson, and K.H. Cooper (1970). Serum electrolyte changes after marathon running. *J. Appl. Physiol.* 29: 449–451.

Rowell, L.B. (1986). *Human Circulation.* Oxford University Press, New York.

Rumessen, J.J., E. Gudmand-Hoyer (1986). Absorption capacity of fructose in healthy adults. Comparison with sucrose and its component monosaccharides. *Gut* 27: 1161–1168.

Ryan, A.J., T.L. Bleiler, J.E. Carter, and C.V. Gisolfi (1989). Gastric emptying during prolonged exercise in the heat. *Med. Sci. Sports Exerc.* 21: 51–58.

Saltin, B. (1964). Aerobic work capacity and circulation at exercise in man. *Acta. Physiol. Scand.* 62 Suppl 230: 1–52.

Saltin, B., and D.L. Costill (1988). Fluid and electrolyte balance during prolonged exercise. In: Horton ES, RL Terjung (Eds), *Exercise, Nutrition, and Energy Metabolism.* New York: Macmillan, pp 150–158.

Saris, W.H.M., M.A. van Erp-Baart, F. Brouns, K.R. Westerterp, and F. ten Hoor (1989). Study on food intake and energy expenditure during extreme sustained exercise: the Tour de France. *Int. J. Sports Med.* 10 Suppl 1: S26-S31.

Sasaki, H., J. Maeda, S. Usui, and T. Ishiko (1987). Effect of sucrose and caffeine ingestion on performance of prolonged strenuous running. *Int. J. Sports Med.* 8: 261–265.

Segal, K., A. Nyman, J.G. Kral, P. Bjorntorp, D.P. Kotler, and F.X. Pi-Sunyer (1985). Effects of glucose ingestion on submaximal intermittent exercise. *Med. Sci. Sports Exerc.* 17: 205.

Seiple, R.S., V.M. Vivian, E.L. Fox, and R.L. Bartels (1983). Gastric-emptying characteristics of two glucose polymer-electrolyte solutions. *Med. Sci. Sports Exerc.* 15: 366–399.

Senay, L.C., G. Rogers, and P. Jooste (1980). Changes in blood plasma during progressive treadmill and cycle exercise. *J. Appl. Physiol* 49: 59–65.

Slama, G., J. Boillot, I. Hellal, D. Darmaun, S.W. Rizkalla, E. Orveon-Frija, M.F. Dore, G.

Guille, J. Fretault, and J. Coursaget (1989). Fructose is as good a fuel as glucose for exercise in normal subjects. *Diabete Metab (Paris)* 15: 105–106.
Sole, C.C., and T.D. Noakes (1989). Faster gastric emptying for glucose-polymer and fructose solutions than for glucose in humans. *Eur. J. Appl. Physiol.* 58: 605–612.
Spiller, R.C., B.J.M. Jones, B.E. Brown, and D.B.A. Silk (1982). Enhancement of carbohydrate absorption by the addition of sucrose to enteric diets. *J. Parent Ent. Nutr.* 6: 321.
Stansbie, D., K. Tomlinson, J.M. Potman, and E.G. Walters (1982). Hypothermia, hypokalaemia and marathon running. *Lancet* 2: 1336.
Sun, W.M., L.A. Houghton, N.W. Read, D.G. Grundy, and A.G. Johnson (1988). Effect of meal temperature on gastric emptying of liquids in man. *Gut* 29: 302–305.
Van Handel, P.J., W.J. Fink, G. Branam, and D.L. Costill (1980). Fate of ^{14}C glucose ingested during prolonged exercise. *Int. J. Sports Med.* 1: 127–131.
Verde, T., R.J. Shephard, P. Corey, and R. Moore (1982). Sweat composition in exercise and in heat. *J. Appl. Physiol.* 53: 1540–1545.
Wapnir, R.A., and F. Lifshitz (1985). Osmolality and solute concentration—their relationship with oral rehydration solution effectiveness: an experimental assessment. *Pediatr. Res.* 19: 894–898.
Wells, C.L., T.A. Schrader, J.R. Stern, and G.S. Krahenbuhl (1985). Physiological responses to a 20-mile run under three fluid replacement treatments. *Med. Sci. Sports Exerc.* 17: 364–369.
Whiting, P.H., R.J. Maughan, and J.D.B. Miller (1984). Dehydration and serum biochemical changes in runners. *Eur. J. Appl. Physiol.* 52: 183–187.
Wheeler, K.B., and J.G. Banwell (1986). Intestinal water and electrolyte flux of glucose-polymer electrolyte solutions. *Med. Sci. Sports Exerc.* 18: 436–439.
Williams, C., M.G. Nute, and M.P. Walker (1988). Influence of carbohydrate supplementation on running performance. *Proc. Nutr. Soc.*.
Williams, C., M.G. Nute, L. Broadbank, and S. Vinall (1990). Influence of fluid intake on endurance running performance: a comparison between water, glucose and fructose solutions. *Eur. J. Appl. Physiol.* 60: 112–119.
Williams, M.H. (1985). *Nutritional aspects of human physical and athletic performance.* CC Thomas, Springfield..
Wurtman, R., (1983). Behavioural effects of nutrients. *Lancet* 1: 1145–1147.
Zuntz, N. (1911). Bebrachtungen über die Beziehungen zwischen Nährstoffen und Leishingen des Körpers. *Oppenheimers Handbuch der Biochemie* 4: 826–821.

DISCUSSION

GISOLFI: You indicate that if athletes want to avoid dehydration, they should consume a fluid replacement beverage that has less than 5% carbohydrate, and if athletes are interested in replacing electrolytes, they should consider a solution that has 50–100 mEq/L of sodium. What is the justification for those recommendations?.

MAUGHAN: I don't think there is much doubt that if the rate of intestinal water uptake is to be maximized, a hypotonic solution with an osmolality between 210 and 250 is required. If we are going to limit ourselves to a hypotonic solution, we can only put in a limited amount of sodium and glucose, and we have to put something in to balance the sodium, i.e., usually chloride. From the intestinal perfusion studies that I have seen, we get the best water uptake with something akin to the formulation I've suggested. The problem with that conclusion is that we are looking at only a part of the gut in these studies. We can probably get by with a slightly lower sodium concentration. If we put in a much lower sodium solution, we will see sodium accumulation in the small intestine with subsequent potential water reabsorption trouble. I don't think we know whether that sodium accumulation is going to impair water uptake or not, but my suspicion is that it will.

GISOLFI: We have done two studies on how much sodium should be put in an oral rehydration solution. If we double the amount of sodium from 25 mEq/L to 50 mEq/L, we see no difference in water absorption. Furthermore, if we compare a 6% carbohydrate solution with no electrolytes to a 6% carbohydrate solution with 20 mEq/L sodium, there is no difference in water absorption. This suggests that it is the carbohydrate content that is most important in terms of generating fluid absorption, presumably because the gut is contributing the necessary sodium. That doesn't mean that we shouldn't have sodium in an oral rehydration solution, but I challenge the statement that the most important reason for having sodium in the oral rehydration beverage is to stimulate water absorption. I think sodium is terribly important in helping to maintain plasma volume.

MAUGHAN: I'm familiar with those studies of yours, but there are other studies in the literature showing increased water uptake with higher sodium concentrations; this is in direct disagreement with your results. Similar experimental models are giving contradictory results.

GISOLFI: It depends on the technique being used. A double lumen tube as opposed to a triple lumen tube is going to give very different results. I think the studies that you are quoting used double lumen tubes.

MAUGHAN: Even some of the triple lumen experiments showed increased water uptake with increased sodium. I know you don't agree entirely with that. The thing that worries me about putting in large amounts of sodium to maintain plasma volume is that in most of these exercise situations, we see an increase in the plasma sodium concentration anyway. If there were a decrease in plasma sodium, we would want to put some sodium in, but we see an increase in plasma sodium in most situations. Hyponatremia occurs in a very small number of people. Do we really want to add sodium to a drink to maintain plasma sodium when plasma sodium is already higher than baseline? I don't see why. What function will the extra sodium have? We are trying to make recommendations for all situations in the space of two or three sentences, and we can't do it. We have to consider individuals. We have to consider different modes, different durations, and different intensities of exercise. We have to consider different climatic conditions and different fluid losses. But we always end up with trying to make a few generalizations that are so general they become meaningless. To cover all the bases, we should say to people: You should drink between 50 and 300 mL of fluid every 5–25 min during exercise; the sodium concentration should be anything from 0–100 mM; and the glucose should be anywhere from 0–20%. Such guidelines become useless. We have to look at an individual and ask what we are going to do for that individual in that situation.

NADEL: While I agree with you that we need to customize our ideas somewhat, we can still generalize because these are physiological and physical events that are occurring.

MAUGHAN: The danger comes when people take that generalization and apply it to themselves individually. That is what the coach and the athlete do. They take the generalization and apply it without considering the individual situation.

NADEL: I think we have enough information among us to generate a mathematical model for predicting water, sodium, and carbohydrate requirements for most circumstances. We could then develop a three dimensional graph or nomogram in which we can plug in variables such as environmental temperature, exercise intensity, exercise duration, state of training of the athlete, the type of event, and so forth.

MAUGHAN: I think that is effectively what we are asking individual athletes to do. We are asking them to take a generalization and to fit it to their own situations.

NADEL: I'm going a step beyond that. I'm saying that we have the knowledge to do it for more than any one individual. We have the knowledge to do it for different groups and different communities.

SAWKA: I am less optimistic than Ethan Nadel about our ability to develop a useful model for fluid replenishment. We have used a number of different models for sweating, and an important part of that is just simple metabolic rate. I have examined the literature and the results over the years from our lab and from Costill's lab for running at different speeds and different grades, and what really impressed me was the big differences in the metabolic rates required for different subjects to run at a given grade and speed. They are so diverse that you get very gross differences for given environmental conditions. I think we can give good advice on glucose and sodium concentrations, but the proper volume for fluid replacement is really an individual factor.

MAUGHAN: I think producing the equation would be very difficult, especially because there is so much variability. If we look at the variation between subjects in gastric emptying or the variation between subjects in intestinal absorption, we are going to have a very difficult equation. It is not necessarily impossible, but very difficult. I just wonder if for the individual it is easier to do it by trial and error.

NADEL: On another issue, you have a graph where you have wildly differing sweating rates for runners in a marathon. That is reasonable, given the fact that people may be different sizes, they produce different amounts of energy, and so forth. But you say that you made a comparison of two people exactly the same size running at exactly the same speed, and one of them lost 1 L of sweat and the other 6 L in the same conditions. Given the law of conservation of energy, how can that be explained? For example, if one person is not sweating in a given environment where the heat production is the same as his neighbor, the heat loss by radiation and convection is similar, and skin temperatures are somewhat similar, how is it that the poorly sweating person doesn't store heat at the rate of 1° C every 3–5 min? I just don't think those data are reasonable.

MAUGHAN: We see big differences between individuals. The runner who is sweating 6 L in the marathon isn't evaporating most of that sweat; it is dripping from the skin. Some people in the lab and in sports sweat much more than they should. The textbooks tell us that when the skin is wet, sweat secretion should be decreased, but with these particular runners it is not. These very profuse sweaters lose large amounts of fluid that isn't effective in cooling.

NADEL: The amount of water that can be lost by dripping is not tremendous. I don't think it could account for that difference.

Do you agree that during recovery it is important to have electrolytes in the replacement drink? Without the sodium coming back into the body, the fluid can't really stay in the body to any great extent.

MAUGHAN: I agree entirely. In recovery, you need the sodium there to retain the water. If you don't get the sodium in, you don't retain the water. But during exercise you retain the water whether you put the sodium in or not.

NADEL: Because the urine flow is reduced?

MAUGHAN: Yes.

NADEL: That is a good point and requires investigation. We have recently done a study showing that consumption of a solution containing cations during exercise attenuates the loss of plasma volume that occurs with a placebo.

I totally agree that palatability is very important. Sodium concentrations higher than about 30 or 40 mEq/L are unpalatable, and palatability changes between resting conditions and exercising conditions. The taste intensity of salt is markedly decreased during exercise. This was surprising to me. Further, that decrease in salt taste perception is related to the plasma sodium concentration. I think it is a very important point, but I don't claim to understand it.

MAUGHAN: Yes, the taste for salt does change with dehydration. I think body temperature also probably plays a role here.

A few years ago we did a study of a marathon. We studied 190 people and weighed them all before and after the race. Half the people got water to drink, and the other half got a glucose/electrolyte solution containing 90 mM sodium. They got 200 mL every 6 km. The runners had agreed beforehand that they would drink the entire 200 mL every time. Those who drank the salty drink said it was very unpleasant for the first couple of feeding stations, but towards the end, they began to enjoy it. So, their tastes had changed. People prefer the saltier fluid in the latter stages of exercise. Certainly most athletes don't give "sports drinks" proper taste trials. They drink them sitting at rest. If we want to see how we are going to respond to them during exercise, we should consume them during exercise.

WILMORE: The issue of palatability certainly influences voluntary fluid consumption, which is the bottom line in athletics. Is there much of a data base available on the influence of palatability on voluntary fluid consumption?

MAUGHAN: Roger Hubbard and others have shown that if you give people pleasant tasting fluids at a reasonable temperature, they will drink greater volumes; palatability is crucially important. It sometimes works the other way as well. If you give athletes something that doesn't taste too good, they think it must be good for them.

EICHNER: I'd like to make a clinical point on hyponatremia and exercise duration. I have seen hyponatremia after a 10 km race. The runner was a physician and a heavy sweater. It was a hot day, and he ran about 40 min and then worked in the medical tent for about 90 min, drinking copious amounts of water until he got a headache and mild confusion. He walked across the street into his own emergency room, where his plasma sodium concentration was recorded at 125 mEq/L. After infusion of a liter of saline, he was fine. Apparently, hyponatremia can happen after shorter exercise than we think.

I have a question about gender differences in palatability. I have heard, for instance, that caffeine added to cola makes it taste better to men but not women. Are there gender differences in palatability?

MAUGHAN: I don't know anything about that.

MURRAY: We have done a lot of that type of work at Quaker, and we haven't seen any gender specific differences. There is, however, definitely a link between palatability and the volume people will consume. The whole beverage industry is based on that concept, and it applies during exercise. If a formulated beverage tastes good when people are hot and sweaty and thirsty, they will drink more of it during exercise than beverages that do not taste good under those conditions.

HEIGENHAUSER: One of the areas that needs to be addressed is athletic events in which the exercise is done in very short intervals with a lot of rest in between, such as in North American Football. There are lots of problems with thermoregulation in such sports because when the players are resting, heat dissipation is impeded by the protective gear they wear. Are there any differences in the electrolyte requirements for these types of athletes and those individuals who run marathons or do bicycling?

MAUGHAN: I don't see why there should be. I think one of the problems in the past has been that these individuals haven't appreciated the need to replace fluids. Soccer players certainly tend not to take fluids on board. Traditionally, at half time they suck an orange. Even when they are playing in 27° C temperatures, they don't drink fluids. That is beginning to change. They are beginning to appreciate that their performance can be improved with fluids. But I certainly haven't seen any data. These athletic team sports can be extremely difficult to study. We tend to go for something simple like running or cycling or swimming.

LOMBARDO: We noticed in American football players that running backs and others who lose little weight are the most likely players to get heat cramps. We think that heat cramps may be more of an electrolyte problem than a fluid problem. A lineman will lose 20 pounds during practice or in a game, but it's the back who loses only 1 pound who shows up with heat cramps.

COYLE: I am still a little confused about the recommendation for the high sodium concentration you are recommending in rehydration solutions. You are suggesting a sodium concentration between 50 and 100 mM. Are you recommending that there be such a high concentration in the drink consumed during exercise? This seemed to be contrary to your premise that the body is becoming hypernatremic and should not be loaded with more sodium. Are you suggesting that these high sodium concentrations be included in drinks consumed during exercise?

MAUGHAN: Yes. I don't think there is necessarily such a big difference between sodium requirements during exercise and those after exercise. Drinks containing sodium concentrations at 50 to 100 mM are still substantially below the sodium concentration in plasma, and are not so different from the sodium concentration being lost in sweat. The evidence from the intestinal transport studies is that 50–100 mM sodium is going to maximize water uptake. I know that Carl Gisolfi thinks that water transport will be maximized at sodium concentrations lower than that, but our feeling is that 500–100 mM is the concentration range that should be maintained.

COYLE: That is going to be hypertonic to sweat in many athletes because sweat sodium concentration is usually 40 to 60 mM.

COSTILL: I agree with Ed Coyle. I think you are proposing sodium values that would be more concentrated than those in the sweat of many athletes. Admittedly, there are some individuals who would have sodium concentrations in their sweat in the higher range, but I think you are going to the extreme with your recommendation. You ought to be giving them a more dilute, rather than a higher concentration of sodium.

MAUGHAN: According to the literature, there is a wide range for sodium values in sweat.

COSTILL: In well trained people, sodium concentration in sweat is pretty low.

MAUGHAN: But looking at the values in the literature from moderately trained to untrained people, sweat sodium tends to be in that 50–100 mM concentration range.

COSTILL: But you are not bringing the plasma sodium down with drinks that are concentrated in sodium.

MAUGHAN: Plasma sodium rises only slightly during exercise. We are not talking about large increases in circulating sodium.

HEIGENHAUSER: When you talk about sodium concentrations, are they observed during the activity or after the activity? If you are looking at the changes during exercise, some of those changes have occurred due to movement of fluid between the various fluid compartments. If you try to maintain sodium levels during exercise at concentrations seen during rest, then you are going to run into problems. I don't know if anybody has considered that when making comparisons in electrolytes.

NADEL: I think George is right. At the beginning of exercise, fluid is pushed out of the vascular compartment, and the sodium concentration in the blood tends to become elevated. The value of that elevated sodium concentration is that it tends to draw fluid back from other compartments and ultimately from the intracellular fluid compartment. The second part of this issue is consideration of the total body sodium. As we sweat and lose water, we are also losing some sodium. In our studies, the range of sodium concentrations in sweat was 20–100 mM, with the average about 55 mM. This was in a cross-sectional group. One relatively fit subject had 20 mEq/L sodium in his sweat, and the mean was around 55 mEq/L, much as you showed. But the point is that sodium is being lost, and if the body is to recover after exercise and replenish lost water, then it seems to me inevitable that sodium should be ingested to aid in the absorption of water from the gut and to help hold water in the body fluids. The elevated sodium concentration in body fluids will help maintain the osmotic drive for drinking, and that is something that we often overlook. If the plasma sodium concentration is too dilute, in most conditions that completely removes the osmotic drive for drinking, and people will voluntarily stop drinking.

HEIGENHAUSER: Following short-term work, e.g., four bouts of exercise with 4 min rest in between, renal function shuts down dramatically for a period of 24 h after the exercise period. I don't know what happens during long-term activity, but is there any sort of beverage that can be used to bring renal function back? Howie Green has some data that showing that untrained individuals who exercise very severely will retain a lot of fluid during the time that the kidney is shut down. Why? Is there any drink that you can take to overcome this sort of thing?

MAUGHAN: Presumably, if you consume enough of a hypertonic, low sodium solution, you will overcome this type of problem and stimulate urine production.

HEIGENHAUSER: They even gave diuretics to these individuals, and they could not overcome the renal hypofunction.

MAUGHAN: If we take individuals who aren't used to exercise and exercise them hard, whether it is short term and high intensity or prolonged, we see a marked elevation in body water for 24–72 h after exercise, which is associated with the decreased urine excretion. But in most situations, fluid intake should overcome that problem.

HEIGENHAUSER: Howie has even taken his subjects out and bought them a lot of beer after exercise, which should stimulate urine output, but it does not.

SPRIET: Is it true that there really isn't very much information about fluid replenishment for exercise at intensities above 70% $\dot{V}O_2$max? Some well-trained athletes can sustain a work rate of 80 or 85% $\dot{V}O_2$max for a couple of hours.

MAUGHAN: I certainly haven't seen much in the literature on heavy exercise sustained for long periods, probably because there are very few subjects able to do that. Yes, if you get some highly trained individuals, they can sustain 80% $\dot{V}O_2$max or better for long periods. I would assume that the response won't be very different from those reported for subjects at 70–75% $\dot{V}O_2$max. I think it is the duration that is critically important. If they can sustain that exercise intensity for 2 h, I think the physiologic response would be similar, as long as the intensity is at least 65% $\dot{V}O_2$max.

SPRIET: I guess my puzzlement comes from the fact that few studies really simulate athletic situations as closely as I expected.

MAUGHAN: You really can't do good field studies in this area because conditions change. You can't do a good double-blind experiment. Clyde Williams' group has made a good effort to simulate racing on a treadmill. They set the speed initially at 70 to 75% $\dot{V}O_2$max. The subjects had a hand-held control and could adjust the speed as it suited them; that is a lot closer to the race situation. In that situation the results showed that if people take plain water, they tend to slow down over the last 10 km. If they take either a glucose/fructose solution or a sucrose/glucose solution, they tend to maintain speed over the last 10 km. But there was no difference in running speed in the early stages. I don't think we will get much closer to our modeling of this situation.

GISOLFI: I would like to come back to the sodium issue one more time. It's been clearly shown that you don't need to add very much sodium to an oral rehydration solution in order to produce an intraluminal sodium concentration in the intestine of 80 to 90 mEq/L to optimally stimulate water absorption. Could we not maximize water absorption with considerably less than 50–100 mM sodium in the oral rehydration solution, especially when we take into consideration the influence of palatability of that oral solution on voluntary fluid consumption?

MAUGHAN: I think this is where we need to start looking at models other than the simple intestinal perfusion model, which tends to be confusing. Hopefully, we can start to use some of the isotopic tracer models to answer some of these questions. Even though it provides only an index, perhaps the simple deuterium uptake model will help us see how quickly we are getting fluid uptake into the blood under different situations. This model seems to take into account both gastric emptying and intestinal absorption.

COGGAN: One of the problems with all tracers is the underlying assumption that the tracer and the tracee are treated identically by the body, but whenever you have a two-way exchange going on, that isn't necessarily true. The tracer will diffuse down its concentration gradient at the same time the tracee is going the other direction. Therefore, there will be major problems with interpretation of tracer data.

MAUGHAN: I appreciate some of the problems—probably not all of them.

COYLE: What is the limiting factor in fluid replenishment—gastric emptying or intestinal absorption? Isn't the intestinal absorption rate much more rapid than the rate of gastric emptying?

MAUGHAN: By and large, you are right. However, in some situations when we give individuals large volumes of fluid, they can be emptied faster than they are absorbed, and those individuals have diarrhea. If we fast an individual and give him water at a rate of 1.5–2.0 L/h, he will produce a fairly spectacular diarrhea because he can't absorb that water fast enough. Strongly hypertonic solutions can also be emptied from the stomach faster than they are absorbed by the intestine because of fluid secretion into the gut. So, in some situations, we will see intestinal transport unable to cope with the rate of gastric emptying. We see that during races. Many runners have to stop during races because of abdominal cramps or diarrhea. Furthermore, there is an enormous variation in gastric emptying rates reported in the literature, with some studies showing between 5 and 10 mL/min and others showing 40 mL/min for similar solutions. But in most situations, I agree that intestinal absorption rate is unlikely to be a limiting factor in fluid replenishment.

3

Amino Acids and High Protein Diets

GAIL BUTTERFIELD, PH.D., R.D., FACSM

INTRODUCTION

The amino acids that constitute protein may be considered as potential ergogenic aids for two reasons. First, amino acids may be used as substrate for energy transformations, a well-documented function, but one for which no exercise performance evaluation has been made. Second, they may be used to form body protein, particularly muscle, and thus serve to maintain or augment the tissue responsible for sport and exercise performance. Without *adequate* protein intake over sustained periods of time, performance eventually suffers markedly.

The controversy surrounding the ergogenicity of dietary protein circles around the word "adequate." In the athlete, the ability to maintain body tissue could be impaired if the amino acids of that tissue were being used at high rates for energy production; this possibility has led to the suggestion that the amount of protein required to sustain muscle mass in a physically active individual is greater than that required by a sedentary person. This premise assumes that the absolute amount of amino acids turned over during exercise is greater than at rest and that the amount turned over at rest is the same in active and inactive individuals. Should the exercising individual actually desire to increase body protein mass, it follows that even more protein would be needed.

The question of protein requirement, however, is not related solely to protein intake. If energy sufficient to cover expenditure is not supplied from exogenous sources, body stores of fat, carbohydrate, and protein will be harnessed to provide for essential functions; if energy intake is greater than need, protein will be accumulated along with fat. Thus, the amount of dietary protein required to maintain body protein stores in any circumstance is tied inexorably to the adequacy of the energy supply.

In this chapter, we will explore the metabolism of protein during exercise, evaluate the major methods for determining protein requirement, address the data available regarding protein requirements, and, based on these data, make recommendations for "adequate" dietary protein intake to maintain tissue in the active individual and to augment tissue when desired.

METABOLISM OF PROTEIN

General

Protein consumed as food is mixed in the gut with protein from gastric and intestinal secretions and from sloughed cells (Figure 3–1). Most of this protein is digested into amino acids that are ab-

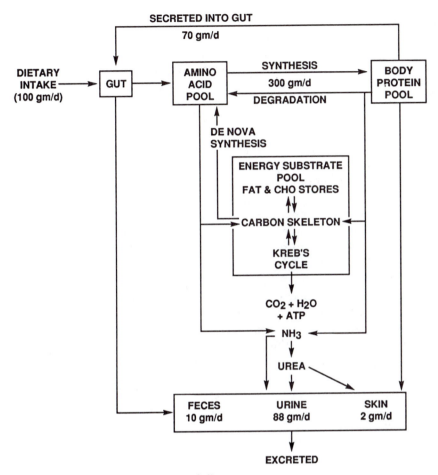

FIGURE 3-1. *Whole body protein metabolism.*

sorbed actively across the lining of the gut. A small portion of the protein in the gut (about 10%) is not absorbed and appears in the feces.

The absorbed amino acids join an elusive body pool from which amino acids are used for synthesis of body proteins. Amino acids are also contributed to the body pool by the degradation of preexisting body proteins and by de novo synthesis from carbon skeletons and transaminated amino groups. In the healthy adult, the rates of synthesis and degradation of body protein, i.e., protein turnover, are fairly well balanced so that the total pool of amino acids and protein is relatively constant.

Perturbation of the constancy of the amino acid pool can occur when the amino acids of the pool are used extensively as substrates for oxidative energy transformations in cellular metabolism. For the adult who is in energy balance, some portion of the pool is irrevocably consumed by oxidation each day. The actual amount oxidized depends on a variety of factors, some of which are related to exercise (see below).

The loss of amino acids from the pool to provide energy is normally replaced by dietary protein or amino acids. If dietary amino acid intake is greater than that needed to replenish the amino acid pool, the excess amino acids can be used for energy. In this process, the nitrogen-containing amino group is removed (deamination), and the carbon skeleton may enter the Krebs cycle. If intake of both energy and protein are greater than need, the excess amino acids may be converted in the liver to fat (lipogenesis) and carbohydrate (gluconeogenesis) and stored. The amino groups released when amino acids are used for energy or for the synthesis of fat and carbohydrate can be transaminated to other carbon skeletons to produce dispensable amino acids, or they can be deaminated and converted to urea in the liver. If dietary protein intake is inadequate to cover the need for mandatory amino acid oxidation, body proteins will be degraded to replenish the amino acid pool. If dietary energy intake is inadequate to cover energy expenditure, the amino acid pool becomes a potential source of additional energy substrate. The major by-product of amino acid oxidation is urea, but a small portion of the amino groups is lost directly as ammonia, which is excreted in the urine.

The situation is complicated by the inability of the body to manipulate the amino groups to manufacture all amino acids necessary for protein synthesis. Of the 22 amino acids making up proteins in the human, nine (called indispensable amino acids) cannot be synthesized in amounts adequate to cover need (Table 3–1). Thus, when these indispensable amino acids are catabolized, they *must* be replaced from the diet. Without adequate dietary intake of each of these building blocks, the amino acid pool is reduced, protein synthesis is slowed, and more body protein is degraded in an attempt to keep the amino acid levels in the pool optimal for protein synthesis. The dispensable amino acids released from the degraded protein will be in excess and will be utilized as substrate, their amino groups ending up as urea.

In summary, maintenance of body protein stores depends on 1) adequacy of dietary protein, 2) adequacy of dietary energy, and 3) adequacy of dietary indispensable amino acids (i.e., high quality protein).

TABLE 3-1. *Summary of estimated requirements and intake of indispensable amino acids* $(mg \cdot kg^{-1} \cdot d^{-1})$

Amino Acid	Estimated Requirement		Estimated Intake	
	WHO/FAO[a]	Young et al.[b]	Dietary[c]	Dietary[d]
Leucine	14	39	100	57
Isoleucine	10	23	63	36
Valine	10	24	70	40
Threonine	9	21	50	29
Phenylalanine & Tyrosine	19	39	55	31
Tryptophan	3.5	6	14	8
Methionine & Cystine	13	16	30	17
Lysine	12	42	84	48
Histidine	8–10	—	31	17

[a] From World Health Organization, 1985
[b] From Young et al., 1989
[c] Estimated from 4 d weighed food records of 6 women who ran 44.8 km (27.8 miles)/week and consumed 77.8 g protein and 8.28 MJ (1980 kcal)/d. From Butterfield et al., 1990.
[d] Estimated from amino acid composition of diets selected by physically active women, assuming a protein intake equivalent to that recommended by National Research Council, Food and Nutrition Board (1989a)

Amino Acid Utilization with Exercise

Although amino acids can be catabolized for energy, the utilization of certain amino acids seems to be localized in certain tissues. Of particular interest to the question of exercise is the use by muscle of the branched chain amino acids (BCAA), i.e., leucine, valine, and isoleucine. These amino acids are first reversibly transaminated, pyruvate and alpha-keto glutarate being the primary recipients of the amino groups. The keto-acids thus produced may be irreversibly oxidatively decarboxylated, and the carbon chain residues can be used as energy substrate. The alanine and glutamate formed by transamination travel to the liver where they are thought to be converted to glucose for release into the blood (Felig & Wahren, 1971).

Localization in specific tissues of the enzymes responsible for amino acid utilization creates the potential for compartmentalization of the processes involved in amino acid utilization. In the rat, muscle tissue has a high concentration of branched chain aminotransferase (Hutson, 1988) but fairly low activity of the branched chain keto-acid dehydrogenase (Khatra et al., 1977; Aftring, 1986); in liver, branched chain aminotransferase levels are very low (Hutson, 1988), and dehydrogenase activity is high (Khatra et al., 1977; Aftring, 1986). This enzyme distribution suggests that in the rat BCAA are primarily deaminated in muscle, but that the resultant keto-acids are

AMINO ACIDS AND HIGH PROTEIN DIETS **91**

released into the blood (Hutson et al., 1978) and travel to the liver, where they are decarboxylated and used for energy. In humans the distribution of enzymes appears to be different, the bulk of the dehydrogenase activity being in muscle (Khatra et al., 1977), suggesting that BCAA decarboxylation occurs there. If the distribution in man of the aminotransferase is similarly opposite to that in the rat, complete degradation of leucine in muscle would be expected. Fielding et al. (1986) have shown that alpha-ketoisocaproic acid, the keto-acid of leucine, can accumulate in muscle during intense exercise, suggesting that the transaminase activity is high in human muscle.

Both acute and chronic exercise in humans and rats have marked effects on BCAA degradation. During exercise, the liver releases BCAA, which are delivered to the muscle (Ahlborg et al., 1974). In addition, significant degradation of muscle protein occurs, giving rise to increased levels of BCAA within muscle (Dohm et al., 1982; Lemon et al., 1985; Pivarnik et al., 1989). The handling of leucine during exercise has been most intensively studied. Its oxidation in muscle increases consequent to increased activity of branched chain keto-acid dehydrogenase (Kasperek et al., 1985). At the same time, muscle release of alanine and glutamine increases, and these amino acids are carried to the liver where they undergo gluconeogenesis (Dohm et al., 1985), contributing to the maintenance of blood glucose levels. Most of the ammonia released is converted to urea in the liver. Serum (Haralambie & Berg, 1976; Lemon & Mullin, 1980; Plante & Houston, 1984) and urinary (Decombaz et al., 1979; Dohm et al., 1982) urea increase significantly during and immediately following an exercise bout, especially under circumstances where carbohydrate stores are compromised (Lemon & Mullin, 1980). The increase in urinary urea after exercise appears to be positively related to exercise intensity (Lemon, 1987). Various authors have estimated that the contribution of amino acids to total energy expenditure during exercise is as high as 5–10% based on tracer studies of leucine oxidation (Young & Torun, 1981; White & Brooks, 1981) or total urea production (Lemon, et al., 1982).

Habitual participation in strenuous exercise, i.e., training, results in adaptive changes that promote some of these degradative activities and minimize others. Leucine oxidation during exercise increases with training in rats (Dohm et al., 1977; White & Brooks, 1981; Henderson, et al., 1985) and in untrained humans (Hagg et al., 1982; Wolfe et al., 1984). Other reports suggest that leucine oxidation may be decreased in the course of further training of well-conditioned humans (Bylund et al., 1977; Young & Torun, 1981). Recently, Stein et al. (1989) observed no rise in leucine flux at initiation of an exercise bout in eight elite triathletes exercising at about 40–50% of V̇O₂max, but an actual decrease in leucine flux was noted after 4 h of exercise, suggesting establishment of a new, lower plateau of leucine turnover. These investigators considered the decline in leucine flux to represent an adaptation of protein turnover toward protein conservation during an extended exercise bout. In the liver, gluconeogenesis is enhanced by training (Turcotte et al., 1990), but the utilization of amino acids as substrates for gluconeogenesis may be superseded by other substances such as lactate.

DETERMINATION OF PROTEIN REQUIREMENT FOR THOSE WHO EXERCISE

The literature previously cited shows that there is an increased utilization of amino acids as an energy source during an acute bout of exercise; this lends support to the hypothesis that athletes need more dietary protein than do sedentary individuals. How the use of individual amino acids during a single exercise bout translates into overall change in protein economy in the untrained or trained individual is not clear. An estimation of protein need from the metabolic data is complicated by the interactions of the amino acid and protein pools and by the interrelationship of protein utilization and energy balance described above.

Methods

Measurements of protein turnover and nitrogen balance have been used to approach the problem of defining protein and amino acid requirements. Each is based on a number of assumptions, and each has its own difficulties in execution and interpretation.

Protein Turnover. This method is based on the assumption that if the rates of synthesis and breakdown are accelerated, the rate of amino acids irrevocably leaving the pool will be increased (Stein et al., 1983b), and thus the need for dietary protein to replace these amino acids will be increased. The procedure involves administering a labelled amino acid, either orally or by intravenous infusion. This amino acid is assumed to equilibrate completely and instantaneously with the existing amino acid pool (Waterlow et al., 1978). In reality, equilibration may take 3–15 h, depending on the amino acid given and the route of administration (Wolfe, 1984). Once equilibrium is established, the rate of exit from the pool can be monitored by evaluating end products (ammonia, urea, or carbon dioxide). Because the rate of entry of radioactive label into the pool is known (the rate of infusion), the rate of flux can be estimated as the input of label divided by the steady-state specific activity (termed "enrichment") of the product (Wolfe, 1984). The rate of protein synthesis is calculated from the flux minus the output, and the rate of protein degradation is the flux minus the input (Waterlow et al., 1978; Wolfe, 1984; Meredith et al., 1989).

The assumption is made that the small amount of labelled amino acid added will be utilized in the same manner as the endogenous amino acid and that its metabolism will be representative of the entire pool. The amino acid considered most representative of whole body protein turnover is ^{15}N-glycine (Stein et al., 1986). Wolfe et al. (1984) demonstrated that ^{13}C-leucine, often used in early turnover studies involving exercise, is not appropriate as a measure of *whole body* turnover given the shifts in metabolism of that amino acid in muscle with exercise. It is, however, an appropriate measure for muscle amino acid oxidation. Wolfe (1984) suggests a multi-amino acid approach to monitor amino acid flux in exercising humans, using ^{15}N-glycine to monitor whole body turnover (primarily splanchnic turnover), and ^{13}C-leucine to evaluate muscle metabolism. Although this method provides a sensitive indicator of the flux of amino acids, and consequently protein, it does not provide a *quantifiable* measure of protein utilization.

Nitrogen Balance. This method is based on the assumption that dietary protein need is the result of the breakdown of some portion of the amino acid pool and that the magnitude of that breakdown can be determined by collecting and measuring all nitrogen-containing degradation products (primarily urea) and comparing that figure with dietary nitrogen intake. The theory states that when dietary nitrogen intake meets the need of the mandatory amino acid turnover, nitrogen equilibrium is established. When nitrogen intake is greater than need, all excess amino acids are deaminated, and nitrogen output continues to equal intake (equilibrium). When dietary nitrogen intake does not meet the need of mandatory breakdown, the balance of synthesis and degradation is perturbed, and nitrogen excretion exceeds intake, resulting in a negative nitrogen balance. Under circumstances of growth, synthesis outstrips degradation, protein is accumulated, and nitrogen is retained, resulting in a positive nitrogen balance. This method is thought to provide a quantifiable measure of the adequacy of a protein intake (World Health Organization, 1985), although in reality the data do not always fit the theory because nitrogen equilibrium is not always attainable (Oddoye & Margen, 1979). Jeejeebhoy (1986) considered nitrogen balance to be more a measure of adaptability of the system than of need.

The major routes of exit of nitrogen from the body are the feces and urine (Figure 3–1), but significant amounts may also be lost by other routes (Table 3–2). Determination of protein requirements from nitrogen balance requires feeding at least two levels of protein, one below need, and one at or above need. A regression line is then drawn between the two points and the point of intersection of the line of nitrogen equilibrium represents the amount of nitrogen theoretically required to achieve balance (Figure 3–2). In reality, the true requirement is thought to be somewhat higher than this intersect, as the efficiency with which protein is utilized falls off as intake approaches need (Munro & Crim, 1980). The accuracy of the determination of protein requirements from nitrogen balance studies depends upon the ability to quantify intake and to make complete collections.

The validity of such determinations depends upon: 1) the quality of protein fed, 2) the period of adaptation to the protein intake (and, to some extent, the quantity of protein fed), and 3) the adequacy of the energy intake.

Protein Quality. Protein sources, such as egg albumin and casein, containing all indispensable amino acids in ratios similar to those found in animal protein, are considered "high quality" proteins which can be fully utilized by the body for protein synthesis. Protein requirements determined using such proteins will be minimized because only "mandatory" amino acid oxidation will occur, resulting in minimal nitrogen excretion. Evaluation with proteins of lesser quality, such as those found in a mixed diet, will predict higher protein requirements because more of the component amino acids will be unused in synthesis and will be degraded for energy, resulting in increased nitrogen excretion. Thus, protein quality is important in the determination of protein requirement.

Adaptation Period. When protein intake is altered, there is a mandatory period of adaptation to the new intake, during which daily nitrogen excretion will be unstable despite constant intake (Figure

TABLE 3-2. *Miscellaneous nitrogen (N) losses in healthy young individuals**

Source	Nitrogen Loss**
Blood (mg N/g)	32.4 ± 1.7
Toothbrushing (mg N/event)	14.0 ± 2.5
Saliva (mg N/g)	1.0 ± 0.1
Semen (mg N/ejaculation)	37.0 ± 10.0
Menstrual blood loss (mg N/d)	43.0 ± 24.0
Exhaled ammonia (mg N/d)	50.0 ± 6.0
Fecal matter on toilet paper (mg N/d)	4.4 ± 2.5

* Modified from Calloway et al., 1971, and from D.H. Calloway and M.S. Kurzer (1982), Menstrual cycle and protein requirements of women, *J. Nutr.* 112:98–108.
** Values are means ± SD

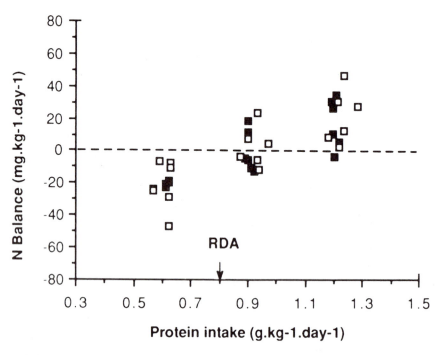

FIGURE 3-2. *Determination of protein requirement using regression analysis. Protein fed at three levels close to estimated need results in nitrogen balance values near equilibrium. Requirement is determined by calculating the best line between points for each subject. Protein requirement estimated for young and middle-aged endurance runners shown in this figure is 0.94 g per kg body weight per day. (From Meredith et al., 1989, with permission.)*

3–3). The length of time necessary to achieve a new steady state will depend to some extent on the magnitude of the change in intake and on the absolute level of nitrogen fed. When nitrogen intake is decreased, a dramatic negative nitrogen balance will be seen the first day, and nitrogen balance will increase toward some equilibrium level over the subsequent days (Figure 3–3). Conversely, when nitrogen intake is increased, there is a large positive balance the first few days, which falls toward the point of balance with time. The Food and Agriculture Organization (FAO) and World Health Organization (WHO) of the United Nations guidelines for determining protein requirements specify a minimum of 10 d adaptation when nitrogen intake is changed (Rand et al., 1984). Oddoye & Margen (1979) found that when nitrogen intake is very high (20 to 25 g nitrogen/d), nitrogen balance fluctuates significantly from day to day, and it is difficult to establish a steady state.

Energy Intake. The protein sparing effect of increased energy in-

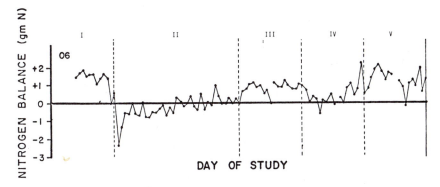

FIGURE 3-3. *Nitrogen balance in one man under various conditions of protein and energy intake. I: Egg white protein intake of 1 g per kg body weight per day; energy intake sufficient to maintain body mass. II: Protein intake decreased to 0.57 g per kg body weight per day; energy intake as in I (note negative nitrogen balance during first few days following diet change). III: Protein intake as in II; energy intake increased by 15% (note that nitrogen balance becomes positive). IV: Protein and energy intake as in III; initiate moderate cycling exercise (40–50% VO₂max) (note initial decline in nitrogen balance, followed by a return to baseline after 12–14 d). V: Protein and exercise as in IV, energy intake increased by an additional 15% (note increase in nitrogen balance). (Modified from Butterfield and Calloway, 1984).*

take has been well established (Calloway & Spector, 1954; Munro, 1964). For any given protein intake, even those below need, increasing energy intake will improve nitrogen balance (Figure 3–4). Conversely, for any protein intake, if energy intake is decreased to less than that expended, some dietary and somatic protein will be used for energy, and nitrogen excretion will increase; this produces a negative balance not necessarily indicative of protein status. Under such circumstances, protein requirement will be over-estimated. Conversely, if energy intake is greater than need, protein synthesis will be promoted over the short term, nitrogen excretion will be diminished, and protein requirement will be under-estimated. Thus, determination of protein requirement from nitrogen balance will depend on the adequacy of energy intake.

Amino Acid Requirements

Because exercise has been shown to acutely elevate the catabolism of some indispensable amino acids (BCAA), an increased requirement for these component amino acids in the physically active individual may be hypothesized. Such speculation has led to inclusion of these amino acids in several commercial products used as food supplements by athletes. The amino acids in question are indispensable, and cannot, therefore, be synthesized in the body or substituted for by other amino acids. Consequently, an increased requirement for these individual protein components could theoretically increase the overall protein requirement.

Indispensable amino acid requirements as presently accepted by the WHO/FAO (Table 3–1) were established using nitrogen balance techniques (World Health Organization, 1985). Bier & Young (1987) have questioned this procedure, suggesting that it represents, at best, an estimation of the amount of these amino acids needed for protein synthesis and does not adequately estimate the amount of these amino acids oxidized on a daily basis. These investigators used stable isotopes of several amino acids and measured oxidation products (primarily carbon dioxide); they have estimated "true" amino acid requirements to be greater than those needed to establish nitrogen balance. Specifically, they estimated that the amount of leucine oxidized during a 2 h exercise bout at 50% of $\dot{V}O_2$max was approximately 90% of the total requirement as determined by nitrogen balance. Other investigators who used different methodologies have suggested similarly high levels of leucine oxidation during exercise (Lemon et al., 1985).

Millward & Rivers (1986) further complicated the controversy by suggesting that amino acid requirements are dependent on meal patterns (timing of synthesis and degradation phases during the day) and total protein intake; they suggested that a higher protein intake results in greater "need" for indispensable amino acids because more will be degraded due to the overall amino acid economy. This hypothesis is supported by the work of Stein et al. (1983b), who found greater protein turnover in oarsmen whose protein intake was high as compared to the turnover in sedentary men with lower protein intakes.

Based on their turnover studies, Young et al. (1989) have made a new set of amino acid recommendations for the general population. The levels of intake suggested by these investigators (Table 3–1) are about twice those previously recommended by WHO/FAO (World Health Organization, 1985) as being necessary for maintenance of protein stores. The new recommendations do not specifically address the possibility of increased need with exercise.

It is important to put these recommendations in perspective in terms of amino acid content of foods. Table 3–1 presents data on the indispensable amino acid content of self-selected diets of a group of physically active women who reportedly consumed smaller quantities of food then would be expected, given their activity level (Mulligan & Butterfield, 1990). These women consumed a mean of 77.8 g protein/d while ingesting 8.28 MJ (1980 kcal)/d and running 44.8 km/d (Butterfield et al., 1990). Clearly, the protein intake of these

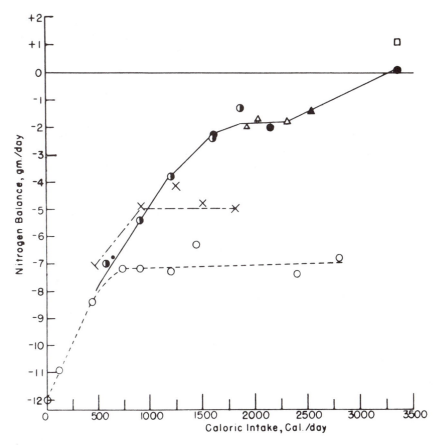

FIGURE 3-4. *Nitrogen balance at various levels of energy intake. Each line represents a different protein intake. Open circles represent data derived on a protein-free diet; crosses represent data derived from an intake of 1–2 g nitrogen/d; top curve represents intakes ranging from 2.4–15 g nitrogen/d. (From Calloway and Spector, 1954, with permission).*

women was adequate to provide the indispensable amino acids in amounts 2.0–2.5 times those suggested by Young et al. (1989). If we assume a similar distribution of indispensable amino acids in protein in general and calculate a theoretical intake of 44 g/d for this group of women based on the currently accepted standard of 0.8 g protein per kg body weight per day (National Research Council, 1989a), estimated intakes as shown in Table 3–1 are above the recommendations of Young et al. (1989).

Thus, even if we assume that indispensable amino acid requirements are double the FAO/WHO estimates in most individuals, and perhaps triple in exercising individuals, the supply of indispensable amino acids in a mixed diet is generally sufficient to meet even these elevated needs, and the major nutritional concern regarding protein becomes meeting the need for total amino acids, i.e., total protein requirement.

Protein Requirements for Endurance Exercise

Determination of protein requirement for exercising individuals by the use of protein turnover and nitrogen balance, when the above considerations are controlled, is still complicated by the kind of exercise performed, the length of training, and the intensity and duration of the exercise performed.

Initiation of Training. Early work focusing on initiation of programs of endurance exercise suggested that protein requirement might be increased under such circumstances. Gontzea et al. (1975) illustrated a decrease in nitrogen balance in previously untrained men in response to initiation of a program of cycling at approximately 50–55% of $\dot{V}O_2$max (Figure 3–5). These men consumed a mixed food diet containing 1 g protein per kg body weight per day and energy estimated to be 10% above need. This decline in nitrogen balance reversed, and after 12 to 14 d of exercise, the men were again in nitrogen balance. The investigators attributed the reversal to an adaption of energy utilization with exercise (possibly an improvement in fitness level) that resulted in protein sparing.

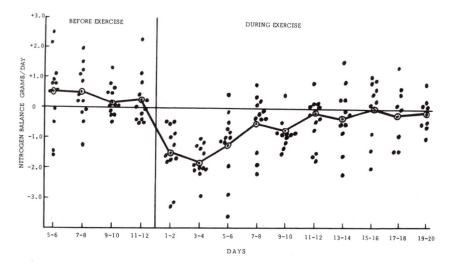

FIGURE 3-5. *Nitrogen balance in men consuming 1 g mixed food protein per kg body weight per day for 12 d before and 20 d after initiation of a cycling program. (From Gontzea et al., 1975, with permission).*

This decline in nitrogen balance following initiation of exercise training could be minimized by increasing protein intake. Thus, Gontzea et al. (1974) found that men initiating an exercise program while consuming a mixed food diet containing 1.5 g protein per kg body weight per day did not go into negative nitrogen balance, whereas those consuming only 1 g/kg did. However, the men consuming the 1.5 g/kg were in positive nitrogen balance before initiation of the exercise, possibly as a result of an inadequate period of adaptation to the increased protein intake, as noted previously. They did experience a drop in nitrogen balance when the exercise program was initiated. The magnitude of decline in nitrogen balance in response to exercise appeared to be the same at both protein intakes.

Other investigators exploring other signs of protein inadequacy found that changes accompanying initiation of an exercise program could be prevented with elevated protein intakes. Yoshimura (1961, 1980) found that the transient anemia accompanying initiation of cycling exercise at 50–60% of VO_2max in men consuming 1–1.4 g animal protein per kg body weight per day could be eliminated by feeding 1.9–3 g/kg. It is interesting to note that the cyclists were in positive nitrogen balance even on the low protein intake.

Early studies of protein turnover in untrained men showed decreased protein synthesis and increased protein degradation during 3.75 h of treadmill running at 50–60% VO_2max (Rennie et al., 1981). During recovery for several hours in the same experiment, protein synthesis increased above pre-exercise values, while degradation remained elevated. The overall result for exercise plus recovery was a net increase in protein synthesis. More recently, Devlin et al. (1990) showed that whole body protein synthesis increased after exercise to exhaustion at 75% of VO_2max, while forearm protein synthesis decreased. These authors suggested that the increase in synthesis during recovery may be confined to the tissues that have increased degradation during exercise.

Garrel et al. (1988), evaluating the efficacy of exercise as a protection against prednisone-induced muscle wasting, found that whole body protein turnover was significantly increased even after adaptation to a moderate jogging program. Turnover, as measured by ^{15}N-glycine, was increased by 19%, and protein synthesis and degradation were elevated by 22% and 16%, respectively, in men after jogging 4 km at 5.6 min/km four times a week for four weeks. These investigators did not attempt to determine nitrogen balance.

Intensity. Studies by Butterfield and colleagues (Butterfield & Calloway, 1984; Todd et al., 1984) of young men initiating a cycling program at 40–50% VO_2max suggest that intensity may be a critical factor in evaluating the effect of exercise on protein requirements. These investigators found the same duration of decline in nitrogen balance with initiation of an exercise program as had been identified by Gontzea et al. (1975) (Figures 3–4 and 3–5), but the men were able to establish nitrogen equilibrium (suggesting adequacy of intake) after two weeks of exercise on 0.57 g egg white protein per kg body weight per day when energy intake was adequate to cover expenditure (Butterfield & Calloway, 1984). Further, even under circumstances of negative energy balance, nitrogen balance could be achieved with 2 h of daily exercise at 40–50% of $\dot{V}O_2$max when only 0.8 g egg white protein per kg body weight per day was consumed (Todd et al., 1984). These investigators concluded that at this low intensity, protein utilization was improved by exercise; they also suggested that protein requirement might be diminished after adaptation to moderate exercise.

Albert et al. (1989) found a similar improvement in protein utilization with low intensity exercise (30% $\dot{V}O_2$max) in normal men fed high quality protein intravenously while participating in a daily program of cycling for 1 h at 75 W. These investigators identified a decrease in the amino acid flux through the forearm and a decrease in protein degradation as measured by ^{15}N-glycine in the exercising men. Energy intake was low (about 1.2 times basal requirement), but protein intake was high (approximately 1.6 g per kg body weight per day).

Trained Athletes. Recent research in trained endurance athletes supports the earlier work that suggested increased protein requirements with initiation of high intensity exercise. Tarnopolsky et al. (1988) estimated protein requirements for endurance athletes in six trained male runners given adequate energy (259 kJ [62 kcal]) and 1.1 or 2.4 g mixed food protein per kg body weight per day during alternate 10 d balance periods. Nitrogen balance was positive under both protein intakes, and regression lines drawn to predict nitrogen intake required for equilibrium suggested a requirement of 1.37 g protein per kg body weight per day. A sedentary control group studied at the same time and given 176 kJ (42 kcal) per kg body weight per day had similarly positive balances on both protein intakes; the predicted protein requirement for nitrogen balance for these controls was 0.73 g per kg body weight per day, a value significantly higher than that generally found to be required for balance in sedentary individuals (World Health Organization, 1985). As pointed out by Tarnopolsky et al. (1985), interpolating requirements from values derived from high protein intakes may have resulted in inflated values. However, the relative relationship of requirements in sedentary and active individuals presented by these investigators is interesting.

Using similar methodology, but feeding moderate levels of egg and milk protein (0.6, 0.9 and 1.2 g per kg body weight per day), Meredith et al. (1989) found a protein requirement of 0.94 g per kg body weight per day in six young and six middle-aged men who had been running for 2–20 y (Figure 3–2). Energy intake was 251 kJ (60 kcal)/kg in the young men and 209 kJ (50 kcal)/kg in the old. However, protein turnover in these men was the same as that found in sedentary men of the same age.

In our own work (Butterfield et al., 1990) on women routinely running 45 km/week and adapted to high quality protein intakes of 0.8 g and 2.0 g per kg body weight per day, we predicted protein requirement to be 1.12 g per kg body weight per day. The inter-individual variation in our experiment was higher (coefficient of variation = 40%) than that usually found in studies of protein requirement (coefficient of variation = 15%); this suggests that our value may be somewhat inflated. Energy intake in these women, although adequate to maintain body weight, was very low (146 kJ [35 kcal] per kg body weight per day).

Brouns et al. (1989) studied 13 highly trained male cyclists under conditions simulating the Tour de France. Based on changes in urinary nitrogen excretion, the authors suggested that nitrogen balance cannot be sustained on 1.4 g protein per kg body weight per day when energy expenditure is 26.6 MJ (6358 kcal)/d. The authors calculated that protein requirements for such activities are about 1.5–1.7 g per kg body weight per day. However, the actual nitrogen balance studies were not presented, nor were any data supporting the authors' conclusions.

Studies of protein turnover in trained athletes do not reflect an increased protein need. Stein et al. (1983b) found no difference in protein synthesis or breakdown in trained oarsmen when compared to sedentary controls. Using ^{15}N-glycine as a tracer and monitoring urinary ammonia, these investigators found that nitrogen flux was higher in the oarsmen, possibly due to their elevated protein intake, but felt the increased flux could not be interpreted as an increase in protein need. The same group (Stein et al., 1983a), using the same method, found no relationship between protein synthesis and energy expenditure in female swimmers and ballet dancers compared to sedentary controls. Rather, synthetic rate was closely correlated to energy intake. A slight tendency toward increased synthesis in the ballet dancers as compared to the sedentary controls was attributed to a 4 h workout performed during the testing period. As noted above, Meredith et al. (1989) found no difference in protein turnover between seasoned endurance athletes and previously studied sedentary men. The different results obtained with the different methods used by Stein et al. and Meredith et al. cast doubt on the assumption that increased protein need is implicated by increased protein turnover.

Protein Requirements for Resistance Exercise

Determination of protein requirements in athletes performing progressive resistance exercise is somewhat more complex than for endurance athletes. In addition to maintaining already existing body protein stores, these athletes want to increase muscle mass for appearance (body builders) or strength (power lifters, field athletes). With regard to increasing protein mass, both absolute accretion of tissue and efficiency of protein retention must be considered.

Maintenance. Early work by Celejowa and Homa (1970) on Polish weight lifters showed 5 of 10 individuals in negative nitrogen balance on self-selected energy intakes of 15.06 MJ (3600 kcal) to 18.00 MJ (4300 kcal)/d and on an average of 1.85 g mixed protein per kg body weight per day. The authors interpreted these results as supporting the need for large protein intakes in weightlifters, and they suggested a requirement of 2.0–2.2 g protein per kg body weight per day. This interpretation has been accepted by other reviewers and is cited as major support for high protein intakes in weight lifters. However, careful perusal of the data suggests an alternative interpretation. Self-selected protein intakes were highly variable from day to day (82 to 197, 97 to 179, and 117 to 221 g/d in each of three weight classes), as were resultant nitrogen balances (coefficient of variation of intra-individual nitrogen balance data ranged from 235% to 2284%). Of the five individuals in negative balance, only two had a mean balance lower than what might be considered the error of the method (±0.5 g nitrogen per day), and even these were not of great magnitude (-2.49 and -1.05 g nitrogen per day). Thus, given the highly variable protein intake and the relatively low mean nitrogen balance values, these individuals might actually have been in nitrogen equilibrium. As indicated above, nitrogen equilibrium will be accomplished at any nitrogen intake greater than need, provided energy intakes are adequate to cover expenditures. Reported energy output (weight lifting values derived by indirect calorimetry using Michaelis-Kofranyi backpacks) and recorded energy intakes were very closely matched. Thus, the paper of Celejowa and Homa (1970) may not tell us the protein requirement for maintenance of nitrogen balance but rather that 1.85 g protein per kg body weight per day is greater than that requirement.

Torun et al. (1977) studied previously untrained men initiating an isometric exercise program while consuming 0.5 or 1.0 g egg and milk protein per kg body weight per day. Energy intakes were adjusted for exercise, and the four men on 0.5 g protein per kg body weight per day appeared to attain nitrogen equilibrium after a 4–5 d period of adaptation to the new exercise program. When protein intake was increased to 1.0 g/kg in two of the men, nitrogen balance became markedly positive. Total body potassium, considered a questionable measure of body cell mass, declined in these individuals while they were consuming the lower protein intake but was restored when protein intake was increased. These latter results have been interpreted to suggest that 1.0 g protein per kg body weight per day is required for maintenance of protein mass with isometric exercise; the nitrogen balance data suggest that maintenance of lean tissue is possible on 0.5 g protein/kg, *provided energy intake is adequate*. Interpretation of this study is hampered by the small number of subjects and the frequent and inconsistent changes in energy and protein intake and in exercise level.

Tarnopolsky et al. (1988) also evaluated protein requirements for maintenance of lean tissue in six seasoned body builders given 1.0 and 2.7 g mixed food protein per kg body weight per day while consuming 20.08 MJ (4800 kcal)/d; protein needs of these body builders were less than those of a group of endurance athletes that was also studied. The predicted protein requirement, 0.82 g per kg per day, may be inflated for reasons previously mentioned.

Thus, the protein requirement for maintenance of body protein mass during resistance exercise training remains uncertain. However, if the protein requirements of endurance athletes are greater than those of resistance athletes, as suggested by Tarnopolsky et al. (1988), the need for protein in resistance-trained athletes would be lower than the 0.94 g per kg body weight per day indicated above for endurance athletes.

Accretion of Tissue. Celejowa and Homa (1970) were unable to show accumulation of lean tissue (positive nitrogen balance) in subjects consuming 1.85 g protein per kg body weight per day, although body weights did increase very slightly over the 11 d of study (mean increase in weight = 230 g or 21 g/d). However, these individuals were very close to energy balance when total energy expended at weight lifting (3.15 MJ [754 kcal]/d), general conditioning (2.95 MJ [704 kcal]/d), and other functions (10.88 MJ [2601 kcal]/d) are totaled (16.98 MJ [4059 kcal]/d) and compared to energy intake (16.32 MJ [3900 kcal]/d). Accretion of lean tissue would require some energy surplus.

In studies where such a surplus has been allowed, lean tissue accretion has been shown. Marable et al. (1979) showed a 3.2 kg increase in weight in college men who initiated a weight lifting program while consuming 0.8 g (n = 2) and 2.4 g (n = 4) protein per kg body weight per day. Energy intakes in the two groups were 285 kJ (68 kcal) and 259 kJ (62 kcal) kg^{-1}·d^{-1}, respectively. No measures were made in this experiment of composition of weight gain, but positive crude nitrogen balances (estimated from reported intakes and urinary losses plus a factor for fecal and sweat losses derived from the literature [Calloway, O'Dell & Margen, 1971]) were 3.06 and 5.90 g/d for groups consuming the normal and high protein diets, respectively. Data thus derived suggest that the accretion of lean tissue was greater on the high protein intake but was possible on the recommended dietary allowance (RDA; National Research Council, 1989a) of 0.8 g protein per kg body weight per day. However, controls in this experiment showed extremely high positive balances (+4.17 g nitrogen/d) on the high protein intake, suggesting that the magnitude of the nitrogen balance was inflated by the high intakes. The efficiency with which protein was accumulated (grams nitrogen retained per gram nitrogen consumed) was higher on the low (32%) than on the high (22%) protein intake, a fact probably attributable to the difference in energy intake between the two groups (low protein group consumed 1.32 MJ [316 kcal] more per day).

Bartels et al. (1989) found an overall increase in nitrogen retention in men initiating a weight lifting exercise program while consuming 1.75 g protein per kg body weight per day when energy intake was increased at a rate designed to promote tissue accretion. The nitrogen balance computed from the data reported was 4.5 g nitrogen/d with 15.06 MJ (3600 kcal)/d, 5.2 g nitrogen/d with 16.32 MJ (3900 kcal), and 5.6 g nitrogen/d with 17.47 MJ (4175 kcal). Clearly, the rate of improvement in nitrogen balance with increasing energy intake decreased as energy intake increased. A similar decline in nitrogen retention per unit energy intake as energy intake increases has been shown in non-exercising men (Calloway, 1975). It is also interesting to note that the mean nitrogen balance (5.1 g nitrogen/ d) found by Bartels et al. (1989), who fed 1.75 g protein per kg body weight per day, was similar to the 5.9 g nitrogen/d observed by Marable et al. (1979), who fed 2.8 g protein per kg body weight per day. This suggests that at some point increasing protein intake has diminishing effects. Consolazio et al. (1975) found essentially no difference in the improvement in nitrogen balance over control values in troops initiating a calisthenic and cycling program when fed 1.4 g milk protein per kg body weight per day (control nitrogen balance = -0.08 g/d; exercise nitrogen balance = 0.53 g/d) or 2.8 g protein/ kg (control balance = 0.96 g/d; exercise nitrogen balance = 1.60 g/

d) (Butterfield, 1987). The high protein group appeared to retain more protein because estimated total body dry protein content was greater in that group. However, this result may be consequent to subject selection as much as diet manipulation. No estimate of interindividual variability is given in the paper, making interpretation difficult. Unfortunately, in no studies were markers for exercise performance measured.

Amino Acids and Growth Hormone

It is the drive for lean tissue that has led many resistance-trained athletes to undertake complicated (and illegal) regimens of steroid injections (Hickson et al., 1990). However, some have looked for an alternative through dietary manipulation of hormone secretion. Specifically, they consume large quantities of the amino acids ornithine and arginine in hopes of stimulating growth hormone (GH) secretion, a manipulation which would not be evidenced during drug testing.

This practice is based on data showing that ornithine and arginine, when given intravenously, are strong stimuli to secretion of various fuel-regulating hormones (Knopf et al., 1965; Merimee et al., 1969; Evian-Brion et al., 1982). In medical practice, these amino acids, injected in at least 30 g amounts, are used as a means of evaluating pituitary and hypothalamic function. Reports in the literature of an effect of oral ingestion of these amino acids on GH secretion are confusing. Most reports suggest that ingestion of the amino acids is not useful in elevating GH levels. One report (Isidori et al., 1981), however, indicates that a combination of arginine and lysine taken orally in doses (1200 mg each) significantly lower than those given intravenously will elevate GH levels 500% above baseline values, although neither amino acid taken alone had any effect.

Bucci et al. (1990) have recently shown that L-ornithine hydrochloride given orally (170 mg/kg) will significantly elevate serum GH by 7 ng/mL above control levels 90 min after the dose. The authors suggest that this elevation may not be physiologically significant, however, as the magnitude of normal diurnal variation is greater than that seen with ornithine ingestion. In addition, the authors recount severe stomach cramping and diarrhea at this intake.

Both resistance and endurance exercise are known to elevate GH secretion. Vanhelder et al. (1984) found a 260% increase in GH secretion after 20 min of strenuous resistance exercise, and Bunt et al. (1986) demonstrated a nearly 600% increase in women and a 900% increase in men after prolonged treadmill running at 60% of $\dot{V}O_2max$. The magnitude of the elevation found with exercise is similar to that claimed by Isidori et al. (1981) for oral ingestion of the combination of arginine and lysine but much greater than that found by Bucci et al. (1990) with ornithine. However, data from Merimee et al. (1969) suggest that exercise and intravenous amino acid stimulation are not additive; rather, once GH levels are elevated by a mechanism, be it exercise or amino acid infusion, it will not be further elevated by additional amino acid infusion. Thus, combining exercise with amino acid ingestion has little chance of magnifying the effect of a good workout on GH secretion.

Elam and colleagues have published two reports regarding the effects of ornithine and arginine supplementation on lean body mass. In one report (Elam, 1988) these investigators suggested that these amino acids, in conjunction with resistance exercise, decrease lean body mass (with weight loss). In 1989, Elam et al. reported that the amino acid supplementation was associated with increases in lean body mass. In both cases body composition was estimated by skinfold measurements, and neither dietary protein nor energy intake were controlled or monitored. In the latter paper only posttraining values were reported, preventing the identification of any causal relationship between amino acid administration and change in lean body mass.

RECOMMENDATIONS

Protein and amino acids are ergogenic aids only as they help in maintaining lean tissue, the tissue necessary for exercise and sport performance. Based on the data presently available, certain recommendations can be made.

Protein

Protein recommendations, as established by the Food and Nutrition Board of the National Research Council, are based on mean values required for nitrogen balance derived in a given population. To this value is added twice the standard deviation of that mean so that 97.5% of all persons will be covered by the recommendation (National Research Council, 1989a). If we take this approach, the following recommendations can be made.

Endurance Athletes. Initiation of an endurance exercise program appears to involve a short period of increased protein catabolism which may be favorably modified by increasing protein intake; however, no specific value has been identified for optimal protein intake during this time. Because initiation of an exercise program usually involves a high rate of energy expenditure relative to the sedentary state, the protein intake recommended below for high intensity exercise is proposed for the first two weeks of any new exercise regimen.

Low-Intensity Exercise. Low-intensity exercise (less than 50% of VO_2max) appears to provide a positive stimulus to protein utilization and does not increase protein requirements. Thus, for those who exercise for fitness at low intensities, e.g., leisurely walking, cycling, dancing, or other such activities, protein requirements are not elevated above the present RDA of 0.8 g protein per kg body weight per day (National Research Council, 1989a).

High-Intensity Exercise. For those who train rigorously for endurance events, such as running, cycling, or strenuous dance routines, protein requirement appears to be slightly increased. Based primarily on the work of Meredith et al. (1989), where energy intake was adequate and constant and protein intake was moderate, a requirement of 0.94 g protein per kg body weight per day could be assumed. Using the method of the National Research Council for setting the protein recommendation, the resultant value for strenuous endurance athletes would be 1.26 g protein per kg body weight per day. Meredith et al. (1989) noted that this intake of protein is not greater than that normally consumed by most North Americans and would not represent an increase in protein intake over normal dietary patterns. They also observed that this recommendation represents an energy intake as protein of only about 6.5% of the total energy intake for the athlete who consumes a high-energy intake.

The above recommendation is based on data derived in men consuming 251 kJ (60 kcal)/kg. Data from our laboratory suggest that the protein requirement for women undertaking endurance training may be slightly higher than the value for men, perhaps because their energy intakes are so much lower (146 kJ [35 kcal]/kg). However, until these data can be confirmed by others, a separate recommendation will not be made for women. In any event, usual protein intakes in women athletes are consistently well above the 1.26 g per kg body weight per day recommended above (Marable et al., 1988).

Resistance Exercise. The data available for resistance exercise are not as abundant nor as clear as those for endurance exercise. Consequently, the following recommendations are conservative and tentative.

Maintenance. There is little evidence to suggest that protein requirement for maintenance of muscle mass is increased in those who perform resistance exercise for body building or strength enhancement. If the relationship between protein utilization in endurance and resistance athletes suggested by Tarnopolsky et al. (1988) is confirmed, the recommendation for resistance exercise would be very close to the RDA. Actually, there are reports in the literature of individuals gaining muscle mass during resistance training on protein intakes equivalent to the RDA (Marable et al., 1979; Todd et al., 1984). However, given the large muscle mass often found in individuals who train with resistance exercise, and because the RDA is expressed per kg body weight, the total protein intake recommended for these individuals will often be higher than that found in many sedentary people.

Augmentation of Tissue. Increasing muscle mass with resistance exercise appears to require a positive energy balance (Marable et al., 1979; Bartels et al., 1989). Adding energy will improve the utilization of even a marginal protein intake so that lean tissue can be accumulated. Adding protein above the RDA to a diet appears to enhance the retention of nitrogen, although data from most studies are confounded by changes in energy intake made concomitant with other experimental manipulations. The efficiency of nitrogen retention is highest at the lower protein intakes, and there may be an upper limit to the rate of accumulation of lean tissue such that increasing protein intake above that level does not enhance nitrogen retention significantly. Thus, the recommendation for accretion of lean tissue with resistance exercise includes both a protein and energy recommendation. Protein intake need not exceed 1.6 g per kg body weight per day (twice the RDA), and energy intake should exceed that needed to maintain body weight by a small daily increment, i.e., as little as 836 kJ (200 kcal)/d or 12.6 kJ (3 kcal)/kg body weight.

A final note of caution regarding hazards of high protein intakes should be made. In its recent report on Diet and Health, The National Research Council (1989b) recommends that protein intake not exceed twice the RDA for anyone because there is convincing evidence for an association between high protein intakes and certain cancers and coronary artery disease. It is as important for the athlete as for the rest of the population to eat in a manner that promotes long-term optimal health.

Amino Acids

There is compelling evidence that current recommendations for amino acid intake do not meet the need generated by oxidation of amino acids, especially during prolonged exercise. However, consumption of twice the RDA for protein as recommended above is more than adequate to meet the increased amino acid requirements proposed by Young et al. (1989)(Table 3–1). There is no reliable evidence that increased intakes of individual amino acids will enhance exercise performance or will significantly stimulate the secretion of GH to enhance protein retention.

Deleterious effects of amino acid imbalances are well-documented. Over-supply of individual indispensable amino acids had led to growth retardation in cats (Hargrove et al., 1988); supplementation of low protein diets with indispensable amino acids can lead to changes in neurotransmitter levels in the brain in rats (Yokogoshi et al., 1987); and excess tryptophan consumption has been linked with liver pathology in rats (Trulson & Sampson, 1986). The recent reports of an association between tryptophan ingestion and the occurrence of eosinophilia-myalgia, a life-threatening condition, are particularly sobering (Anonymous, 1990). Thus, dietary supplementation with individual amino acids may have negative effects and should be done with caution, if at all. Finally, consumption of supplements has been found to substitute for consumption of other foods (Holland, 1987), possibly resulting in inadequate intake of one nutrient while trying to address presumed deficiencies in another.

Energy

If energy intake is inadequate to cover need, protein will be used for energy, and the need for protein will increase. This relationship is important to remember when interpreting the recommendations for protein intake made in the literature, but it is also important for the athlete. If energy intake is not adequate, protein will not be optimally used for maintenance of muscle tissue. Thus, an effort should be made to match energy intake with expenditure. In most cases, *ad libitum* food intake should meet energy need over time (Celejowa & Homa, 1970). In those circumstances where accretion of tissue is desired, a conscious increase in energy intake above energy expenditure may be necessary. In the circumstance where energy intake is curtailed, as in "making weight," some loss of lean tissue is to be expected. Studies on weight loss (Webster et al., 1984) suggest that about 1 g of lean tissue is lost with 3 g of fat, even with only mild caloric restriction. Increasing protein intake to about $1.5 \ g \cdot kg^{-1} \cdot d^{-1}$ will minimize the loss of lean tissue (Stunkard, 1987), but if energy intake is markedly reduced, nitrogen balance cannot be maintained (Yang & van Itallie, 1984). Exercise itself is the best protection against loss of lean tissue under circumstances of negative energy balance (Todd et al., 1984).

Tools for assessing both energy intake and output are available. Energy intake can be quickly estimated by using the Exchange Lists developed by the American Dietetic Association (1986) for use in designing diets for diabetics. These lists categorize foods according to similar macronutrient composition and provide a reasonable estimation of protein, fat, carbohydrate, and energy intake, assuming one is careful about serving sizes. Energy expenditure can be estimated from a calculation of the daily energy requirements of persons plus an estimate of the energy expended during strenuous exercise. Energy needs for inactive individuals are based on basal energy needs plus an estimate for energy expenditure for body maintenance functions. Calculation of basal needs is based on height, weight, and age, using the prediction equations of Harris & Benedict (1919). The value thus derived is multiplied by an age-dependent factor (1.5 for older persons and 1.7 for younger individuals) (Schutz et al., 1981) to obtain a maintenance value. Tables in exercise physiology textbooks provide values for energy expended during various activities; these values can be added to the energy requirements of sedentary persons to estimate total energy expenditure. This estimation of energy expenditure can be compared to energy intake to provide a rough measure of the energy balance. Computer software programs are available to simplify the process.

SUMMARY

It is now an accepted part of the dogma of energy transformations that protein represents a significant energy substrate for muscle at rest and during exercise (Brooks & Fahey, 1984). It is the branched chain amino acids, leucine, isoleucine, and valine, which act as the major protein fuels in muscle. The catabolism of these indispensable amino acids has led to the hypothesis that the utilization of protein in exercising muscle will increase the whole body protein requirement of the physically active individual compared to that of the sedentary person. Estimation of nitrogen balance is the primary technique used to test this hypothesis and to determine protein requirement, but this technique requires careful administration of nitrogen intake and even more rigorous collection of nitrogen output. Aside from the problems of delivery and retrieval of nitrogen, the method is highly sensitive to the direction and magnitude of energy balance, and much of the confusion as to protein requirements with exercise stems from inadequate control of energy balance.

We can make the following recommendations that are based on data from experiments in which nitrogen balance was adequately assessed.

In individuals performing high intensity endurance exercise on a routine basis (exercising three to four times each week at more than 65% of maximum oxygen consumption, $\dot{V}O_2max$), protein intake should be about 1.2–1.3 g per kg body weight per day. In individuals performing moderate or low intensity endurance exercise (three to four times each week at 35–50% of $\dot{V}O_2max$), protein intake should not be increased over that recommended for sedentary individuals, i.e., 0.8 g per kg body weight per day (National Research Council, 1989a). For those individuals initiating even a moderate endurance exercise program, increasing protein intake above the sedentary level (to the level of intense exercise) may help to prevent loss of lean tissue. There is no clear indication in the literature as to the true protein requirement during initiation of an exercise program, but there is evidence that an adaptation will occur, elevated protein intake or not, over a two-week period so that protein intake need not remain elevated in those performing moderate endurance exercise, once the adapted state is attained. It should be noted that the protein intakes recommended here are well within the normal protein intake of most North Americans.

For those individuals performing resistance exercise, two areas of concern arise. One would like to know both the protein intake required to maintain the preexisting lean tissue and the conditions necessary for accretion of lean tissue. Only an inkling of an answer to each of these concerns is available from the present literature. It appears that the protein requirement for maintenance of lean tissue in those performing resistance exercise may be only slightly higher than the present recommendation for protein intake in sedentary individuals. The optimum conditions for accrual of lean tissue with resistance exercise are not known, but surfeit energy intake is necessary (recommended = 12.6 kJ [3 kcal] per kg body weight per day). The National Research Council recommends against consuming protein in amounts greater than twice the RDA because of the association between high protein intakes and certain cancers and heart disease (National Research Council, 1989b).

A final note should be made regarding individual indispensable amino acids, the requirements for which are controversial. Proposals have been made that true requirements are two to three times greater than the levels previously recommended. However, analysis of the amino acid content of food protein shows that even with protein intakes near the RDA, the intake of indispensable amino acids is well above these proposed higher amino acid intakes. Thus, there is no scientific support at this time for increasing intake of individual amino acids when exercising. The proposal that oral consumption of such amino acids may stimulate GH secretion in physiologically significant amounts does not have a scientifically sound base.

ACKNOWLEDGEMENTS

I wish to express my thanks to Lynis Dohm, Peter Lemon, and George Brooks for their initial and final reading of the manuscript. Their thoughtful input is in part responsible for the scope and depth of the finished product. I want also to thank John Grasso for searching out illusive references and thoughtfully reading the finished product. His new perspective kept me on my toes.

AMINO ACIDS AND HIGH PROTEIN DIETS **113**

BIBLIOGRAPHY

Aftring, R.P., K.P. Block and M.C. Buse (1986). Leucine and isoleucine activate skeletal muscle branched chain alpha-keto dehydrogenase in vivo. *Am. J. Physiol.* 250:E599-E604.

Ahlborg, G., P. Felig, L. Hagenfeldt, R. Hendler and J. Wahren (1974). Substrate turnover during prolonged exercise in man: splanchnic and leg metabolism of glucose, free fatty acids and amino acids. *J. Clin. Invest.* 53:1080-1090.

Albert, J.D., D.E. Matthews, A. Legaspi, K.J. Tracey, M. Jeevanandam, M.F. Brennan and S.F. Lowery (1989). Exercise mediated peripheral tissue and whole-body amino acid metabolism during intravenous feeding in normal man. *Clin. Sci.* 77:113-120.

American Dietetic Association (1986). *Exchange Lists for Meal Planning.* Chicago: American Diabetic Association and American Dietetic Association.

Anonymous (1990). L-tryptophan recall broadened to all dosages. *Food Chemical News.* Federal Drug Administration, March 26, p. 45.

Bartels, R.L., D.R. Lamb, V.M. Vivian, J.T. Snook, K. F. Rinehart, J.P. Delaney and K.B. Wheeler (1989). Effect of chronically increased consumption of energy and carbohydrate on anabolic adaptations to strenuous weight training. In: A.C. Grandjean and J. Storlie, (eds), *The Theory and Practice of Athletic Nutrition: Bridging the Gap.* Report of the Ross Symposium. Columbus, Ohio: Ross Laboratories, pp. 70-80.

Bier, D.M. and V.R. Young (1987). A kinetic approach to assessment of amino acid and protein replacement needs of individual sick patients. *J. Parent. Nutr.* 11:95S-97S.

Brooks, G.A. and T.D. Fahey (1984). *Exercise Physiology: Human Bioenergetics and Its Applications.* New York: John Wiley & Sons.

Brouns, F., W.H.M. Saris, J. Stroecken, E. Beckers, R. Thijssen, N.J. Rehrer and F. ten Hoor (1989). Eating, drinking, and cycling. A controlled Tour de France simulation study, Part II. Effect of diet manipulation. *Int. J. Sports Med.* 10(suppl. 1):S41-S48.

Bucci, L., J.F. Hickson, J.M. Pivarnik, I. Wolinsky, J.C. McMahon and S.D. Turner (1990). Ornithine ingestion and growth hormone release in body builders. *Nutr. Res.* 10: 239-245.

Bunt, J.C., R.A. Boileau, J.M. Bahr and R.A. Nelson (1986). Sex and training differences in human growth hormone levels during prolonged exercise. *J. Appl. Physiol.* 61:1796-1801.

Butterfield, G.E. (1987). Whole body protein utilization in humans. *Med. Sci. Sports Exerc.* 19:S157-S165.

Butterfield, G. and D.H. Calloway (1984). Physical activity improves protein utilization in young men. *Brit. J. Nutr.* 51:171-184.

Butterfield, G., J. Gates and L. Holloway (1990). Energy and protein utilization in female runners. *Med. Sci. Sports Exerc.* (In preparation)

Bylund, A.C., T. Bjuro, G. Cederblad, J. Holm, K. Lundholm, M. Sjostrom, K.A. Angquist and T. Scherstein (1977). Physical training in man. *Eur. J. Appl. Physiol.* 36:151-169.

Calloway, D.H. (1975). Nitrogen balance of men with marginal intakes of protein and energy. *J. Nutr.* 105:914-923.

Calloway, D.H., A.C.F. O'Dell and S. Margen (1971). Sweat and miscellaneous losses in human balance studies. *J. Nutr.* 101:775-786.

Calloway, D.H. and H. Spector (1954). Nitrogen balance as related to caloric and protein intake in active young men. *Am. J. Clin. Nutr.* 2:405-411.

Celejowa, I. and M. Homa (1970). Food intake, nitrogen and energy balance in Polish weight lifters during a training camp. *Nutr. Metab.* 12:259-274.

Consolazio, C.F., H.L. Johnson, R.A. Nelson. J.G. Dramise and J.H. Skala (1975). Protein metabolism during intensive physical training in the young adult. *Am. J. Clin. Nutr.* 28:29-35.

Decombaz, J., R. Reinhart, K. Anantharaman, G. von Gultz and J.R. Poortmans (1979). Biochemical changes in a 100 km run: Free amino acids, urea, and creatinine. *Eur. J. Appl. Physiol.* 41:61-72.

Devlin, J.T., I. Brodsky, A. Scrimgeour, S. Fuller and D.M. Bier (1990). Amino acid metabolism after intense exercise. *Am. J. Physiol.* 258:E249-E255.

Dohm, G.L., A.L. Hecker, W.E. Brown, G.J. Klain, F.RE. Puente, E.M. Askew, and G.R. Beecher (1977). Adaptation of protein metabolism to endurance training. *Biochem. J.* 164:705-708.

Dohm, G.L., R.T. Williams, G.J. Kasperek and A.M. vanRij (1982). Increased excretion of urea and N-methylhistidine by rats and humans after a bout of exercise. *J. Appl. Physiol.* 52:27-33.

Dohm, G.L., G.J. Kasperek, E.B. Tapscott and H.A. Barakat (1985). Protein metabolism during endurance exercise. *Federation Proc.* 44:348-352.

Elam, R.P. (1988). Morphological changes in adult males from resistance exercise and amino acid supplementation. *J. Sports Med. and Phys. Fit.* 28:35-39.

Elam, R.P., D.H. Hardin, R.A.L. Sutton and L. Hagen (1989). Effects of arginine and ornithine on strength, lean body mass and urinary hydroxyproline in adult males. *J. Sports Med. Phy. Fit.* 29:52-56.

Evian-Brion, D., M. Donnadieu, M. Roger and J.C. Job (1982). Simultaneous study of soma-totrophic and corticotrophic pituitary secretions during ornithine infusion test. *Clin. Endo.* 17:119–122.

Felig, P. and J. Wahren (1971). Amino acid metabolism in exercising man. *J. Clin. Invest.* 50:2703–2709.

Fielding, R.A., W.J. Evans, V.A. Hughes. L.L. Moldawer and B.R. Bistrian (1986). The effects of high intensity exercise on muscle and plasma levels of alpha-ketoisocaproic acid. *Eur. J. Appl. Physio.* 55:482–485.

Garrel, D.R., P.D. Delmas, C. Welsh. M.J. Arnaud, S.E. Hamilton and M.M. Pugeat (1988). Effects of moderate physical training on prednisone-induced protein wasting: a study of whole-body and bone protein metabolism. *Metabolism* 37:257–262.

Gontzea, I., P. Sutzescu and S. Dumitrache (1974). The influence of muscular activity on ni-trogen balance and on the need of man for protein. *Nutr. Rept. Intern.* 10:35–43.

Gontzea, I., P. Sutzescu and S. Dumitrache (1975). The influence of adaptation to physical effort on nitrogen balance in man. *Nutr. Rept. Intern.* 11:231–236.

Hagg, S.A., E.L. Morse and S.A. Adibi (1982). Effect of exercise on rates of oxidation, turnover and plasma clearance of leucine in human subjects. *Am. J. Physiol.* 242:E407-E410.

Haralambie, G. and A. Berg (1976). Serum urea and amino nitrogen changes with exercise duration. *Eur. J. Appl. Physiol.* 36:39–48.

Hargrove, D.M., Q.R. Rogers, C.C. Calvert and J.G. Morris (1988). Effects of dietary excesses of branched-chain amino acids on growth, food intake and plasma amino acid concentrations in kittens. *J. Nutr.* 11:311–320.

Harris, J.A. and F.G. Benedict (1919). A biometric study of basal metabolism in man. Carnegie Institute of Washington, Publication No. 279.

Henderson, S.A., A.L. Black and G.A. Brooks (1985). Leucine turnover and oxidation in trained rats during exercise. *Am. J. Physiol.* 249:E137-E144.

Hickson, J.F.,T.E. Johnson, W. Lee and R.J. Sidor (1990). Nutrition and the precontest prep-arations of a male bodybuilder. *J. Am. Diet. Assoc.* 90:264–267.

Holland, A. (1987). Dietary intake and nitrogen balance in athletes with and without con-sumption of a protein supplement. *Hum. Nutr.: Appl. Nutr.* 41A:367–372.

Hutson, S.M. (1988). Subcellular distribution of branched-chain aminotransferase activity in rat tissues. *J. Nutr.* 118:1475–1481.

Hutson, S.M., T.L. Coel and A.E. Harper (1978). Regulation of leucine and alpha-ketoisoca-proate metabolism in skeletal muscle. *J. Biol. Chem.* 253:8126–8133.

Isidori, A., A.L. Monaco and M. Cappa (1981). A study of growth hormone release in man after oral administration of amino acids. *Curr. Med. Res. Opin.* 7:475–481.

Jeejeenboy, K.N. (1986). Nutritional balance studies: indicators of human requirements or adap-tive mechanisms. *J. Nutr.* 116:2061–2063.

Kasperek, G.J., G.L. Dohm and Snider (1985). Activation of branched chain keto-acid dehy-drogenase by exercise. *Am. J. Physiol.* 248:R166-R171.

Khatra, B.S., R.K. Chawla, C.W. Sewell and D. Rudman (1977). Distribution of branched-chain alpha-keto acid dehydrogenase in primate tissues. *J. Clin. Invest.* 59:558–564.

Knopf, R.F., J.W. Cann, S.S. Fagans. J.C. Floyd, E.M. Guntsche and J.A. Rull (1965). Plasma growth hormone response to intravenous administration of amino acids. *J. Clin. Endocrinol. Metab.* 25:1140–1144.

Lemon, P.W.R. (1987). Protein and exercise: Update 1987. *Med. Sci. Sports Exerc.* 19:S179-S190.

Lemon, P.W.R., N.J. Benevenga, J.P. Mullin and F.J. Nagle (1985). Effect of daily exercise and food intake on leucine oxidation. *Biochem. Med.* 33:67- 76.

Lemon, P.W.R. and J.P. Mullin (1980). Effect of initial muscle glycogen levels on protein ca-tabolism during exercise. *J. Appl. Physiol.* 48:624–629.

Lemon, P.W.R., F.J. Nagle, J.P. Mullin and N.J. Benevenga (1982). In vivo leucine oxidation at rest and during two intensities of exercise. *J. Appl. Physiol.* 53:947–954.

Marable, N.L., J.K. Hickson, M.K. Korslund, W.G. Herbert, R.F. Desjardins and F.W. Thye (1979). Urinary nitrogen excretion as influenced by muscle-building exercise program and protein intake variation. *Nutr. Rept. Intern.* 19:795–805.

Marable, N.L., N.L. Kehrberg, J.T. Judd, E.S. Prather and C.E. Bodwell (1988). Caloric and selected nutrient intakes and estimated energy expenditures for adult women: Identification of non-sedentary women with lower energy intakes. *J. Am. Diet. Assoc.* 88:687–693.

Meredith, C.N., M.J. Zachin, W.R. Frontera and W.J. Evans (1989). Dietary protein require-ments and body protein metabolism in endurance-trained men. *J. Appl. Physiol.* 66:2850–2856.

Merimee, T.J., D. Rabinowitz and S.E. Fineberg (1969). Arginine-initiated release of human growth hormone: Factors modifying the response in normal man. *New Eng. J. Med.* 280:1434–1438.

Millward, D.J. and J.P. Rivers (1986). Protein and amino acid requirements in the adult human. *J. Nutr.* 116:2559–2561.

AMINO ACIDS AND HIGH PROTEIN DIETS **115**

Mulligan, K. and G. Butterfield (1990). Discrepancies between energy intake and expenditure in physically active women. *Brit. J. Nutr.* (in press).

Munro, H.N. (1964). General aspects of the regulation of protein metabolism by diet and by hormones. In: H.N. Munro and J.B. Allison, (eds), *Mammalian Protein Metabolism.* New York: Academic Press, p. 381.

Munro, H.N. and M. Crim (1980). The proteins and amino acids. In: R.S. Goodhart and M.E. Shils, (eds), *Modern Nutrition in Health and Disease*, 6th ed. Philadelphia: Lea and Febiger.

National Research Council, Food and Nutrition Board (1989a). *Recommended Dietary Allowances.* 10th ed. Washington, D.C.: National Academy Press.

National Research Council, Committee on Diet and Health, Food and Nutrition Board (1989b). *Diet and Health: Implications for Reducing Chronic Disease Risk.* Washington, D.C.: National Academy Press.

Oddoye, A. and S. Margen (1979). Nitrogen balance in humans: long term effect of high nitrogen intake on nitrogen accretion. *J. Nutr.* 109:363–377.

Pivarnik, J.M., J. F. Hickson and I. Wolinsky (1989). Urinary 3-methylhistidine excretion increases with repeated weight training exercise. *Med. Sci. Sports Exerc.* 21:283–287.

Plante, R.I. and M.E. Houston (1984). Exercise and protein catabolism in women. *Ann. Nutr. Metab.* 28:123–129.

Rand, W.M., R. Uauy and N.S. Scrimshaw (1984). *Protein-energy Requirement Studies in Developing Countries. Results of International Research.* Tokyo: United Nations University, p. 1–33.

Rennie, M.J., R.H.T. Edwards. S.Krywawych, C.T.M. Davies, D. Halliday, J.C. Waterlow and D.J. Millward (1981). Effect of exercise on protein turnover in man. *Clin. Sci.* 61:627–639.

Schutz, Y., D.H. Calloway, G. Butterfield and S. Margen (1981). Estimated energy requirements in young and elderly males confined to a metabolic unit. *Internat. J. Vit. Nutr. Res.* 51:194–195.

Stein, T.P., R.W. Hoyr, M. O'Toole, M.J. Leskiw, M.D. Schluter, R.R. Wolfe and W.D.B. Hiller (1989). Protein and energy metabolism during prolonged exercise in trained athletes. *Int. J. Sports Med.* 10:311–316.

Stein, T.P. M.D. Schluter and C.E. Diamond (1983a). Nutrition, protein and turnover and physical activity in young women. *Am. J. Clin. Nutr.* 38:223–228.

Stein, T.P., R.G. Settle, J.A. Albina, D.T. Dempsey and G. Melnick (1986). Metabolism of nonessential ^{15}N-labelled amino acids and the measurement of human whole-body protein synthesis rates. *J. Nutr.* 116:1651–1659.

Stein, T.P., R.G. Settle, K.A. Howard and C.D. Diamond (1983b). Protein turnover and physical fitness in man. *Biochem. Med.* 29:207–213.

Stunkard, A.J. (1987). Conservative treatments for obesity. *Am. J. Clin. Nutr.* 45:1142–1154.

Tarnopolsky, M.A., J.D. MacDougall and S.A. Atkinson (1988). Influence of protein intake and training status on nitrogen balance and lean body mass. *J. Appl. Physiol.* 64:187–193.

Todd, K.S., G. Butterfield and D.H. Calloway (1984). Nitrogen balance in men with adequate and deficient energy intake at three levels of work. *J. Nutr.* 114:2107–2118.

Torun, B., N.S. Scrimshaw and V.R. Young (1977). Effect of isometric exercises on body potassium and dietary protein requirements of young men. *Am. J. Clin. Nutr.* 30:1983–1993.

Trulson, M.E. and H.W. Sampson (1986). Ultrastructural changes in the liver following L-tryptophan ingestion in rats. *J. Nutr.* 116:1109–1115.

Turcotte, L.P., A.S. Rovner, R.R. Roark and G.A. Brooks (1990). Glucose kinetics in gluconeogenesis-inhibited rats during rest and exercise. *Am. J. Physiol.* 258:E203-E211.

Vanhelder, W.P., M.W. Radomski and R.C. Goode (1984). Growth hormone response during intermittent weight lifting exercise in men. *Eur. J. Appl. Physiol.* 53:31–34.

Waterlow, J.C., P.J. Garlick and D.J. Millward (1978). *Protein Turnover in Mammalian Tissue and in the Whole Body.* New York: North-Holland Publishing Company.

Webster, J.D., R. Hesp and J.S. Garrow (1984). The composition of excess weight in obese women estimated by body density, total body water and total body potsssium. *Hum. Nutr. Clin. Nutr.* 38:299–306.

White, T.P. and G.A. Brooks (1981). [U[14]-C]-glucose, -alanine,-leucine oxidation in rats at rest and during two intensities of running. *Am. J. Physiol.* 240:E155-E165.

Wolfe, R.R. (1984). *Tracers in Metabolic Research: Radioisotope and Stable Isotope/mass Spectrometry Methods.* New York: Alan R. Liss, Inc.

Wolfe, R.R., M.H. Wolfe, E.R. Nadel and J.H.F. Shaw (1984). Isotopic determination of amino acid-urea interactions in exercise in humans. *J. Appl. Physiol.* 56:221–229.

World Health Organization (1985). Energy and protein requirements. Report of joint FAO/WHO/UNU meeting. WHO Technical Report Series, No. 724. WHO: Geneva.

Yang, M.U., and T.B. van Itallie (1984). Variability in protein loss during protracted severe caloric restriction: Role of triiodothyronine and other possible determinants. *Am. J. Clin. Nutr.* 40: 611–622.

Yokogoshi, H., T. Iwata, K. Ishida and A. Yoshida (1987). Effect of amino acid supplementation to low protein diet on brain and plasma levels of tryptophan and brain 5-hydroxyindoles in rats. *J. Nutr.* 117:42–47.

Yoshimura, H. (1961). Adult protein requirements. *Federation Proc.* 20:103–110.

Yoshimura, H., T. Inoue, T. Yamada and K. Shiraki (1980), Anemia during hard physical training (sports anemia) and its causal mechanism with special reference to protein nutrition. *World Rev Nutr. Diet.* 35:1–45.

Young, V.R., D.M. Bier and P.L. Pallet (1989). A theoretical basis for increasing current estimates of the amino acid requirements in adult man with experimental support. *Am. J. Clin. Nutr.* 50:80–92.

Young, V.R. and B. Torun (1981). Physical activity: Impact on protein and amino acid metabolism and implications for nutritional requirements. *Nutrition in Health and Disease and International Development: Symposium from XIIth International Congress on Nutrition.* p. 57–85.

DISCUSSION

LEMON: Some endurance training data from the 70s showed an adaptation that resulted in reduced protein intake. Have you calculated the relative exercise intensity over that three-week adaptation period? It is my understanding that the exercise was an absolute workload; therefore, the relative intensity of the exercise would be decreased, and that might have contributed to the adaptation.

BUTTERFIELD: That is correct. You have a valid point, especially based on my data indicating that lower intensity exercise would require less protein. As a consequence, a person who was in negative nitrogen balance would go into positive balance. It is also possible that an adaptation of energy utilization occurs during that initial period of training so that more energy might become available for sparing the protein.

LEMON: I wanted to comment about Fred Broun's work with simulation of the Tour de France where he altered total energy intake by giving a carbohydrate supplement. The group that received normal nutrition was in a negative energy balance and a large negative nitrogen balance. The group that received a carbohydrate supplement beverage in addition to the normal nutrition while they were riding was able to maintain a positive energy balance, but they were still at a negative nitrogen balance. Their requirements were quite a bit higher than anything you presented, and I think they are atypical because of the energy expenditures, but could you comment on those findings?

BUTTERFIELD: I could never find the actual nitrogen balance data presented in a way that was very clear. Can you tell me what actually was happening with nitrogen?

LEMON: They were consuming above 1.7 g protein/kg body weight. Based on their measures of utilization, they came up with values of about 1.5 g/kg measured as fecal nitrogen, urine nitrogen, and sweat nitrogen. The protein requirement in that group was a little bit higher than some of the data you presented.

BUTTERFIELD: Yes, but that would go along with the notion that

AMINO ACIDS AND HIGH PROTEIN DIETS **117**

the higher the intensity, perhaps the higher the protein require- ments. The other thing I worried about in those studies was the degree of muscle protein damage. If this type of intense exercising causes serious muscle protein damage, the protein requirement would be elevated to allow for recovery.

LEMON: Resistance exercise is where most of the abuse of high protein intake occurs. Most of the studies are done in experienced weight lifters as opposed to those beginning a weight lifting pro- gram. Why did you make a recommendation that the protein re- quirement is a little bit higher in beginners?

BUTTERFIELD: The more I think about it, the more I am not con- vinced that even with the initiation of a resistance exercise program that protein requirement is increased as long as energy intake is increased. In most resistance exercise experiments, people have not been concerned about total energy intake. Data from both Tarna- polsky and Bartels showed that energy intakes were very high. If an athlete has a regular job, is working out 2–3 h/d, and is trying to eat a 70% carbohydrate diet, I think it is going to be difficult for him or her to consume adequate energy. We think about resistance exercise as not burning very many calories, but some estimates us- ing indirect calorimetry suggested that a hard workout could require 700–800 kcal/d, and that is a lot of energy to replace.

LEMON: I was amazed at the amount of food that some of these body builders consume. On the other hand, some of them, when trying to get down to a certain weight class, are on relatively low energy diets, and that may be a factor. I was interested, though, in body builders who start a very strenuous program, maybe even an advanced body building program. When they have a lot of muscle damage, do the protein requirements increase?

BUTTERFIELD: I don't know of any published data. Intuitively, I suspect the protein requirement is slightly elevated, but I don't think it is going to be elevated to 3–4 g/kg, which is what a lot of these people consume.

LEMON: We just finished a project using strenuous weight lifting exercise in untrained individuals. We found that they were in neg- ative nitrogen balance and that their protein requirement was ele- vated in the range of about 1.5 g protein/kg/d. But this was in a six days per week program in novices who were trained very, very hard.

BUTTERFIELD: How long did you wait to measure the nitrogen balance relative to when they started the exercise?

LEMON: The nitrogen balance was done 3 1/2 weeks after they started the diet manipulation. But an interesting point is that there was not any change in performance measures with increased protein intake. We had a group that received a carbohydrate supplement and one that received an isocaloric protein supplement. Thus, your point about the importance of energy intake is very important. Despite a negative nitrogen balance in the carbohydrate supplement group, changes in mass and strength over the period of the training were comparable. Above an intake of about 1.3 g protein/kg body weight per day, there seemed to be no advantage of greater protein intake in terms of performance measures.

LOMBARDO: In the first four weeks of a progressive resistance training program in novices, strength gain may be more a function of neuromuscular facilitation than of muscular hypertrophy. Perhaps that's why you didn't find the change in mass and why it did not make much difference in nitrogen balance.

LEMON: That's a good point. We would have preferred to train them longer, but because of some of the dietary controls, it was difficult to do so. Normally, within a month one sees changes in muscle mass, and we did under both diet conditions, but the increases were similar.

DOHM: You make a very nice case for energy balance being a major consideration for increasing muscle mass. If we can get anything across to weight lifters, it is probably that. In a practical sense, weight lifters and wrestlers, especially high school lifters and wrestlers who are trying to make weight, are probably in the biggest deficit of energy at a time when they would like to be maintaining their muscle mass. Someone needs to determine whether low energy, high protein diets can spare muscle mass.

BUTTERFIELD: When you look carefully at the nitrogen balance data in studies of low energy diets, even though the claim of nitrogen equilibrium is made, they don't really take into consideration all the miscellaneous nitrogen losses, so people on low energy diets are probably not in nitrogen equilibrium; they are just not in dire negative nitrogen balance. Increasing the protein intake may improve the situation, but I don't want to give weight lifters or wrestlers who are in negative energy balance the idea that if they eat enough protein, they are not going to lose any lean tissue.

DOHM: We need to answer a question that body builders and weight lifters are asking of us, and that is, can you increase the amount of muscle hypertrophy by any nutritional manipulation? I don't think the ways we are attacking the problem are appropriate at this point. They want to know about whole body protein accretion, and we can't answer that question with nitrogen balance or protein turnover studies. I think we are going to have to use CAT scans across muscles to see whether we are getting hypertrophy and whether we can stimulate hypertrophy with protein supplements.

LEMON: The study that I was discussing did use CAT scans to measure area and muscle biopsies to measure protein content, but between the two supplemented conditions, carbohydrate or protein, there were no differences over the one month.

HICKSON: One of the amino acid supplements that you did not consider that has been receiving a lot of attention, both at the basic experimental level and at the clinical level, is glutamine. Muscle glutamine concentration is considered to be a major regulator of protein synthesis in skeletal muscle. At the clinical level, if you give glutamine by itself, it gets rapidly broken down and probably cannot be used to elevate muscle glutamine concentration. What a number of investigators have done is to infuse something like glutamyl alanyl dipeptide, and this can improve the postoperative state of protein synthesis in humans. I don't know whether it can be used as an ergogenic aid.

LEMON: Gail, do you have any comments about gender differences in protein utilization? There have been a couple of reports, one in animals and one in humans with endurance exercise, suggesting that there may be a difference between men and women in protein use. Do you think that there is a difference?

BUTTERFIELD: We have found a higher protein requirement in the women as compared to men, but the energy intakes for the women were so much lower that I don't want to call that a gender effect. Nitrogen balance will vary in women over the menstrual cycle, so there may be some problem depending on where the nitrogen balance determinations are made. We tried to do ours at the same phase of all menstrual cycles, but that slight variation in the menstrual cycles does not seem to change the protein requirement in sedentary women. Whether or not that pertains to exercise, I am not sure. The really low energy intakes in the women athletes bothered me tremendously, and unless we can feed them equivalent amounts of energy, I wouldn't be able to say there is a gender effect.

LEMON: I was wondering if the requirements might actually be higher in men than women. Perhaps hormonally mediated differences in free-fatty acid use and greater dependence on glycogen utilization in men might have an effect on protein utilization. A recent study suggested that in humans there was a much greater urea excretion in men than women in a prolonged treadmill exercise bout. There were also differences in some of the hormonal data that were consistent with animal studies. But your data suggested that the protein requirement of women was slightly higher than for the men.

BUTTERFIELD: Yes, but the men were taking in 50–60 kcal/kg compared to 35 kcal/kg for the women. I don't think they are comparable at all.

NADEL: Is urea production during endurance exercise intensity dependent? I ask this because in Bob Wolf's study where he showed increases in leucine oxidation, there were no increases in plasma urea nitrogen, but that was with light exercise.

BUTTERFIELD: According to Peter, the urea increase in the blood is intensity dependent. I have never looked at it acutely. I always look at the 24 h urea production.

NADEL: So, is this an important amount of nitrogen?

BUTTERFIELD: From my point of view it isn't. If you look at what happens to the total nitrogen economy over 24 h or over several days, it seems that there must be some adaptation that is counterbalancing the increasing urea production that happens directly after an exercise bout.

NADEL: Is leucine a representative amino acid, so that if leucine oxidation increases during exercise, that tells you what all the amino acids are doing?

BUTTERFIELD: I think that Bob Wolf now feels that leucine can't be used as a means of assessing total body protein utilization. It really represents oxidation going on in the muscle, so you have to use some other marker if you are going to look at total body protein.

HEIGENHAUSER: There are many individuals in the geriatric age range who are now competing in athletics. If you look at the relationship between age and muscle mass, there is a sharp drop off in muscle mass around 65 to 70 years of age. Why is that decrease of muscle mass occurring in relationship to total body nitrogen, total body mass, the intake of protein and inactivity? Are there differences in protein requirements with aging?

BUTTERFIELD: Accompanying the decreased muscle mass, and I don't want to claim any causation, is a decline in growth hormone secretion. We are curious as to whether or not the decline in growth hormone secretion might be responsible for some of that change in body composition. The ability to regain some of that tissue seems to be reduced as one grows older. The protein requirements in elderly, sedentary people are the only ones that have been examined, and the protein requirements to maintain a lower lean body mass are the same in elderly folks as they are in young people. Whether or not an exercising older individual has a change in protein requirements has not been investigated.

TERJUNG: You are building a case to expect a significant oxidation of amino acids and therefore increased protein turnover with exercise. You indicate that as much as 5–10% of the total energy expenditure in exercise can come from amino acids and protein. I think that is an overestimate. The potential for the carbon enrichment from carbohydrate causes an overestimate, and that 5–10% figure should probably be reduced by a factor of 5 to 10.

LEMON: I agree. Leucine is not a good marker of protein utilization. My comments relative to 5–10% protein utilization are based on nitrogen excretion, not leucine oxidation. But others have made estimates based on leucine oxidation even higher than 5–10%, and I think that is misrepresentation of the situation.

WILLIAMS: Can endurance athletes improve their ability to utilize protein as an energy source during exercise?

LEMON: Scott Henderson did some studies with leucine oxidation in trained and untrained animals, both at rest and during exercise. The trained animals showed a greater oxidation of leucine both at rest and during exercise. Lynis Dohm, maybe you could comment on your animal work showing changes with training in leucine oxidation.

DOHM: We just heard that leucine oxidation is not a good marker. Lysine oxidation does not change during exercise, so why should we hang our hats on leucine oxidation?

LEMON: I am not suggesting that we should, but leucine is the amino acid that has been studied in most detail. Oxidation of some of the other branched chain amino acids increases with exercise as well, but I have not seen any training study on the other branched chain amino acids. We did a study with nitrogen excretion in trained and untrained individuals during a prolonged exercise bout, and we got nonsignificantly higher excretion of nitrogen in the trained. That would be more a measure of total amino acid use than oxidation of leucine.

BUTTERFIELD: In any of these studies of nitrogen excretion after exercise, we must know what the energy balance is. If you haven't matched the energy output with the energy intake over the 24 h that you are studying, you are going to get a higher nitrogen excretion than if you do match it. Again, the energy question becomes a critical factor.

SHERMAN: Are there any studies showing that protein intake at the RDA results in a lower ability to gain strength versus protein intakes of 1.3 g/kg per day?

BUTTERFIELD: The reasonably well-designed studies that examined different protein intakes did not report any strength data.

4

Vitamins and Trace Minerals

Priscilla M. Clarkson, Ph.D.

123

INTRODUCTION

Athletes have been targeted as a significant consumer group for vitamin and mineral supplements. Sports magazines are often filled with advertisements for vitamins and minerals purported to enhance performance, delay fatigue, and speed up recovery. These supplements can be costly and contain doses of up to 5,000 times the recommended levels. The effectiveness and safety of vitamin/mineral supplements must be documented to prevent their inappropriate use by athletes, regardless of proven benefits, and to close the door on nutritional quackery (Williams, 1989).

Questionnaires and diet surveys of athletes confirm the widespread use of these supplements. One study showed that of 2,977 high school and college athletes, 44% took vitamin supplements and 13% took mineral supplements (Parr et al., 1984). Thirty-one percent of 80 Australian Olympic athletes (Steel, 1970) and 29% percent of 347 non-elite runners who had participated in a marathon (Nieman et al., 1989) reported that they were taking vitamin and/or mineral supplements. Other studies have documented even higher percentages of athletes taking supplements: 71% and 75% of female runners (Clark et al., 1988 and Barr, 1986, respectively), 92% of a group of world class amateur and professional athletes (Grandjean, 1983), and 100% of female bodybuilders (Lamar-Hildebrand et al., 1989).

Not only are many athletes taking supplements, but the amount consumed by certain athletes is often astounding. Cohen et al. (1985) described a professional ballet dancer who spent $700 per year on vitamin supplements. An adolescent ballet dancer was found to be taking a combination of supplements that resulted in a daily Vitamin A intake of 50,000 IU (Benson et al., 1985). Grandjean (1983) reported that one athlete was using 14 different supplements and consumed 63 tablets each day.

Although some athletes take modest amounts of vitamin and mineral supplements to improve health, others take supplements to enhance performance. In the latter case, when vitamins and minerals are taken in dosages above the recommended levels prescribed for a healthy diet, the supplements would be classified as ergogenic aids.

This paper will examine whether athletes are deficient in certain vitamins or minerals, whether vitamin/mineral status is related to exercise capacity, and whether supplementation affects performance. First, the problems and considerations associated with measurement of vitamin/mineral status and their relationship with physical performance will be addressed.

ASSESSING VITAMIN AND MINERAL STATUS OF ATHLETES

The most common way to assess vitamin and mineral status is to monitor food intake. However, more sensitive means include actual measurement of tissue status or assessment of blood levels of vitamins. Clinical signs of deficiency or excess are also important in evaluation of an individual's vitamin/mineral status. In the following two sections, several of these methods will be discussed along with possible limitations of the techniques.

Food Intake Assessment

The main ways to assess food intake are diet surveys or actually measuring the amount of food that is eaten. Generally diet surveys, or records, have been used to assess the dietary status of athletes. Individuals are asked to describe the type of food ingested and the amounts, and records are often taken for 1 d, 3 d, 7 d, or more (Short, 1989). Despite their widespread use, there are several problems with these surveys. First, they depend on an accurate report by the subject. Either the subject will forget to, or be reluctant to, report certain foods. Also, the amount of food may be over- or under-estimated. Some studies do not account for the vitamin and minerals that are taken in supplements, and only report levels obtained from food.

A record of 1 d may not be as accurate a reflection of an athlete's diet as a record of several days. However, results of a recent study showed that the 7 d diet record method may not rank subjects with the degree of accuracy that was previously assumed (Nelson et al., 1989). For some nutrients, such as iron, zinc, nicotinic acid, and pyridoxine, a number of short separate periods provided a more accurate assessment of food intake than sequential days (Nelson et al., 1989). Thus, the length of time needed to obtain an accurate assessment may differ for different nutrients (Nelson et al., 1989).

The food intakes obtained from the diet records are translated into nutrient intake by use of computerized data bases. Problems exist with the accuracy of this analysis (Short, 1989). A food may vary in its nutrient content due to the source (plant or animal), bioavailability, processing, storage, or preparation of the food, and these are often not taken into account. For some foods there may be no established vitamin and mineral content listed in the data base. Because vitamins and minerals occur in such small amounts, difficulties in interpreting the results are exacerbated.

Despite these problems, the diet record can provide useful information on the approximate mean nutritive intake of a group (Short,

1989). However, the accuracy of the reported vitamin and mineral intakes poses a limitation for assessing ergogenic effects of different levels of these nutrients.

To address whether a diet is adequate for a given vitamin/mineral, the diet record analysis is compared to standards referred to as the Recommended Dietary Allowances (RDA). The RDA represents the level of intake of an essential nutrient "considered to be adequate to meet the known nutritional needs of practically all healthy persons" (National Research Council, 1989). The RDAs were established by determining the average physiological requirement and then adjusting this value by a factor to compensate for incomplete utilization by the body, the variation in requirements among individuals, and the bioavialability of the nutrients from different food sources (National Research Council, 1989). Thus, the RDAs are set fairly high in order to include a safety factor. Furthermore, it should be noted that the RDAs can differ substantially from country to country. For example, the RDA for vitamin C in the US is 60 mg, while in the UK it is 30 mg, in France it is 80 mg, and in the USSR it is 65–70 mg.

The 1989 RDAs for vitamins and trace minerals are listed in Table 4-1. The RDAs are based on an average-size person with an average amount of physical activity. In many instances the studies that were used to set the RDAs for vitamins and minerals did not report the activity level of subjects, or the studies examined subjects who participated in light to no activity (National Research Council, 1989). Therefore there is some question concerning the adequacy of using the RDA to evaluate nutritional needs of athletes.

Because the RDAs are not an absolutely specific recommendation for a given individual, generally deficiencies or excesses are expressed as a percentage of an RDA. Most studies use 66.6% or 75% of the RDA to describe a poor vitamin/mineral intake. Two to three times the RDA is considered to be a high intake, 3–9 times a very high intake, and megadose intakes are generally greater than 10 times the RDA. It should be noted that megadoses of vitamins and minerals can actually function like drugs and have side effects and toxicities (Alhadeff et al., 1984; Aronson, 1986).

For some vitamins and minerals there is no established RDA. These nutrients are known to be essential, but inadequate data exist to establish a specific RDA. However, provisional recommendations titled "Estimated Safe and Adequate Daily Dietary Intakes of Selected Vitamins and Minerals" (ESADDI) have been developed as guidelines. Nutrients that fall under this category are vitamins K, pantothenic acid, and biotin and the trace minerals copper and chromium.

TABLE 4-1. *Recommended Dietary Allowances (RDA) and Estimated Safe and Adequate Daily Dietary Intakes (ESADDI) For Adults (age 19–50)*[+]

	Male	Female
RDA		
Vitamins		
Fat Soluble		
Vitamin A (μg)	1,000	800
Vitamin D (μg)	5[*]	5[*]
Vitamin E (mg)	10	8
Water Soluble		
Thiamin (mg)	1.5	1.1
Riboflavin (mg)	1.7	1.3
Niacin (mg)	19	15
Vitamin B_6 (mg)	2.0	1.6
Folate (μg)	200	180
Vitamin B_{12} (μg)	2.0	2.0
Vitamin C (mg)	60	60
Trace Minerals		
Iron (mg)	10	15
Zinc (mg)	15	12
Selenium (μg)	70	55
ESADDI (intakes the same for males and females)		
Vitamins		
Biotin (μg)	30–100	
Pantothenic (mg)	4–7	
Trace Minerals		
Copper (mg)	1.5–3.0	
Chromium (μg)	50–200	

[*] Vitamin D for male and female 19–24 years old is 10 μg.
[+] (National Research Council, 1989)

In the sections that follow, the information from diet records should be viewed with some caution. Not all studies used the same recall procedures, the RDAs were revised in 1989, and studies completed in other countries do not use the United States version of the RDA. However, the studies do provide an overall picture of diet practices.

Clinical and Biochemical Assessment

For certain vitamins and minerals, the status of the body content can be more accurately assessed by clinical signs or analyzing tissue samples or blood samples. For example, classic symptoms of zinc deficiency include loss of appetite and skin changes (National Research Council, 1989). Although tissue analysis can accurately document a specific deficiency, as in the case of iron deficiency from the analysis of bone marrow (Wishnitzer et al., 1983), these techniques are invasive, time consuming, and costly. Commonly, vitamin levels are measured directly in the blood (serum or plasma) or indirectly by an assessment of erythrocyte enzyme function.

Different means to assess vitamin levels may give different results. For example, one study of college athletes found that a discrepancy existed in the number of subjects who showed vitamin deficiency when thiamin status in the blood was assessed by two different methods (Guilland et al., 1989). Also, the accuracy of some assessment techniques is questionable. For example, the tests for biochemical deficiency are considered to be equivocal for assessment of magnesium, copper, and zinc status from blood samples (Lukaski et al., 1983).

An important consideration in evaluating blood levels of vitamins and minerals is whether what is assessed in the blood is an accurate representation of what is present in the tissues. Since blood levels seem to be affected by several factors, including acute exercise, an accurate interpretation of the results may be difficult. Several of the vitamins and minerals may be mobilized from tissues into the blood during or after exercise. Also, exercise may affect vitamin and mineral levels in the blood by loss in sweat or altered excretion in the urine. While some of these changes after acute exercise are short lived, others may take 24–48 hours before returning to resting levels.

The assessment technique for certain vitamin and mineral concentrations in the blood may not be an entirely accurate measure of the nutrient status of an individual. Therefore, some caution should be used when interpreting these results.

RELATIONSHIP OF VITAMIN/MINERAL STATUS AND PERFORMANCE

One way to assess the relationship of vitamin/mineral status and performance is to examine those subjects who are vitamin or mineral deficient and see whether their performance differs from those who are not deficient. (For a detailed review of studies examining vitamin deficiency and performance see Van der Beek, 1985.) It is difficult to find a group of subjects who will be deficient in only one vitamin or mineral. Generally these types of studies are done in areas where nutrition is poor and subjects may have multiple deficiencies and associated problems (Buzina & Suboticanec, 1985; Powers et al., 1985).

Another version of deficiency-oriented studies is to place subjects on a specific vitamin/mineral deficient diet for a given time, and examine performance criteria before and after the diet regimen. Although these studies provided some useful information, examination of only a few vitamin deficiencies has been done (Keys et al., 1944; Wald et al., 1942). This is probably due to the risks that a subject may incur since most vitamins and minerals are so important to a wide variety of metabolic processes.

Although numerous studies have been done to assess the effectiveness of vitamins and minerals as ergogenic aids, many of these studies are fraught with problems. Often an adequate number of subjects was not tested to be able to discern whether the ergogenic aid was effective. Statistical methods (Cohen, 1969) were not used to establish the sample size needed to detect a significant amount of change in a performance test. In most studies, a complete assessment of the nutritional status of the subjects was not presented. Without assessment of the diet intake, biochemical analysis of blood or tissue samples, and clinical signs or symptoms of deficiency or excess, it is difficult to determine the effectiveness of vitamins and minerals as ergogenic aids. Furthermore, individual variability in the response to vitamin and mineral ingestion has not been adequately examined.

The choice of performance criteria is also of concern. Very few studies of the relationship of exercise capacity, sport performance, and vitamin or mineral status have used the same type of exercise or performance tests. This makes between-study comparisons almost impossible. Exercises range from strength tests to aerobic cycle and treadmill tests. Each test varies not only in the intensity and duration but also in the choice of the criterion measure, i.e. VO_2max, time to exhaustion, work efficiency.

The design of many studies is inadequate. Some are not double blind, lack adequate controls, or have questionable performance criteria. The reliability of performance tests are often not reported. Also, there is some concern that the laboratory tests are not sufficient to determine the effectiveness in field situations. These points are particularly important since the difference between 1st and 5th place in a race can be a matter of tenths or hundredths of a second. A study using unreliable or inappropriate performance criteria or crude performance measurements would not be able to detect a change in performance that may be critical to "winning." Additionally, if the intent of a study is to determine whether supplements affect top class athletic performance, it is important that elite athletes who are highly motivated be used as subjects.

The studies also differ markedly on the length of supplementation, the dosage of supplement, and the form of dosage. The length of time of supplementation in some cases may have been too short to have a beneficial effect. Furthermore, most studies do not assess dietary intake during the course of supplementation period. If the intake changes, then the effectiveness of the supplement may be compromised. The degree of compliance with the supplements is

TABLE 4-2. *Vitamins: Function and Usage with Regard to Exercise*

	Exercise-related Function	Proposed Benefit to Performance
Water Soluble		
Thiamin (mg)	CHO metabolism	enhance endurance performance
Riboflavin	oxidative metabolism, electron transfer reactions	enhance aerobic performance
Niacin	oxidative metabolism, electron transfer reactions	enhance energy metabolism
Vitamin B_6	gluconeogenesis formation of hemoglobin	enhance endurance performance
Pantothenic	oxidation of fatty acids and pyruvate	enhance aerobic performance
Vitamin B_{12}	RBC development	enhance endurance
Folate	nucleic acid synthesis RBC formation	no theoretical benefit
Biotin	fatty acid and glycogen synthesis	no theoretical benefit
Vitamin C	anti-oxidant	prevent tissue damage facilitate repair
Fat Soluble		
Vitamin A	anti-oxidant	prevent tissue damage facilitate repair
Vitamin D	regulates bone mineral metabolism	bone formation during muscle building
Vitamin E	anti-oxidant	prevent tissue damage, facilitate repair

generally not assessed or not reported. Assessment of an individual's activity level over the course of the supplementation period is often not done and a change in activity could confound the results. Also, the effect of supplementation may differ depending on the age, training, and health status of the subjects (Manore & Leklem, 1988).

There are data to suggest, at least for vitamin C (Buzina & Su-

TABLE 4-3. *Trace Minerals: Function and Usage with Regard to Exercise*

	Exercise-related Function	Proposed Benefit to Performance
Zinc	CHO, fat, and protein metabolism, tissue repair	repair of exercise damage
Copper	erythropoiesis, catecholamine regulation, energy metabolism	enhance aerobic performance
Chromium	CHO and fat metabolism, potentiates effects of insulin	delay fatigue muscle anabolism
Selenium	anti-oxidant	protects against exercise damage, delay fatigue
Iron	oxygen transport and delivery	reduce fatigue, enhance endurance

TABLE 4-2 (continued).

Symptoms of a Deficiency	Effects of Supplementation	Possible Toxic Effects
weakness, impaired endurance muscle wasting	does not enhance performance	relatively non-toxic
oral-buccal cavity lesions, skin changes	does not enhance performance	relatively non-toxic
diarrhea, irritability	may impair performance due to reduced fatty acid mobilization	nicotinic acid—vascular dilation, possible liver damage niacinamide—not harmful
dermatitis, convulsions	does not enhance performance	neurological impairment
very rare	data equivocal	relatively non-toxic
megaloblastic anemia, neurological symptoms	does not enhance performance	relatively non-toxic
megaloblastic anemia, fatigue	no studies available	unknown, potentially toxic
very rare	no studies available	relatively non-toxic
loss of appetite, fatigue	data equivocal well controlled studies show no effect	relatively non-toxic
night blindness, loss of appetite, susceptibility to infection	enhanced performance unlikely	anorexia, hair loss, hypercalcemia, and kidney and liver damage
hypocalcemia	does not affect work performance; may affect muscle building (one study)	hypertension, anorexia, nausea, hypercalcemia & hypercalciuria
neuropathy and myopathy	does not enhance performance; may reduce exercise damage due to lipid peroxidation	relatively non-toxic

boticanec, 1985), that a certain threshold level of a vitamin is needed in the body to elicit optimal performance. If subjects' body levels are below this value, performance is improved by supplementation. When this value is reached, further supplementation will not enhance performance. Most studies that have examined the effects of supplementation have not taken into account that a threshold vitamin/mineral status may exist.

TABLE 4-3 (continued).

Symptoms of a Deficiency	Effects of Supplementation	Possible Toxic Effects
loss of appetite, skin changes	may enhance some measures of muscle performance (data from one study)	hypocupremia, impaired immune response
very rare	studies not available	relatively non-toxic
rare, impaired glucose tolerance	studies not available	relatively non-toxic
rare, muscle weakness	studies not available	fingernail changes, hair loss
fatigue, anemia	no effect on performance in non-anemic or non-iron deficient subjects	relatively non-toxic

Most studies that have examined the effectiveness of vitamins and minerals as ergogenic aids have tested adult subjects of approximately college age. However, because diet and nutritional status change with age, there may be a theoretical basis for assessing the effectiveness of vitamin and mineral supplements in older (Masters) athletes.

In the following sections, for each of the vitamins and minerals, there will be a description of the dietary intake and biochemical status of certain athlete groups, exercise-induced changes in vitamin and mineral status, the relationship of performance and vitamin and mineral status, and the effect of supplementation on performance. A summary of the function and usage of vitamins and trace minerals with regard to exercise can be found in Tables 4-2 and 4-3. The scope of this review is limited to research on human subjects and studies published in the English language.

VITAMINS

Vitamins are classified into those that are water soluble and those that are fat soluble. The water soluble are the B complex vitamins and vitamin C (ascorbic acid), and the fat soluble are vitamins A, D, E, and K.

Water Soluble Vitamins

Vitamin B complex consists of 8 vitamins: vitamin B_1 (thiamin), vitamin B_2 (riboflavin), niacin, vitamin B_6 (pyridoxine), vitamin B_{12} (cyanocobalamin), biotin, folic acid, and pantothenic acid. Most of these vitamins are not stored in large quantities in the body and must be ingested on a regular basis. The quantity stored differs among the vitamins. For example, if an individual's diet is deficient in B vitamins, clinical symptoms can sometimes occur in 3–7 days (Guyton, 1986). Vitamin B_{12} is an exception because it can be stored in the liver for a year or longer. A Vitamin C deficient diet can cause deficiency symptoms after a few weeks and can cause death from scurvy in 5–7 months (Guyton, 1986). The B complex vitamins and vitamin C are essential to the body and, in general, cannot be manufactured in the body; therefore, they must be exogenously supplied. Most of these vitamins have theoretical bases for suggesting that they may enhance exercise performance.

Thiamin. Thiamin plays a role in carbohydrate metabolism as a coenzyme in certain biochemical reactions. In the form of thiamin pyrophosphate, it functions specifically as a coenzyme in the conversion of pyruvate to acetyl coenzyme A (CoA) and alpha-ketoglutarate to succinyl CoA, as well as the decarboxylation of branched chain amino acids. Because of thiamin's important role in carbohydrate metabolism, it has been targeted as an ergogenic aid that will increase endurance, delay fatigue, and enhance performance (Aronson, 1986).

The RDA for thiamin is 1.5 mg for adult males and 1.1 mg per day for adult females. Because thiamin is important in energy metabolism, the needed intake varies according to caloric intake (Hunt and Groff, 1990, p 188). Therefore, .5 mg of thiamin/1,000 kcal is recommended for adults (National Research Council, 1989). Thus, athletes who have a high caloric intake would need a concomitantly higher thiamin intake as well. However, for those individuals on a low caloric diet, a minimum of 1.0 mg/day is recommended. There is no evidence for thiamin toxicity through oral ingestion (National Research Council, 1989).

Studies that have assessed diet records of athletes have generally found that most athletes do not have a lower intake of thiamin than the RDA. For example, intake of thiamin for elite nordic skiers (Ellsworth et al., 1985), professional ballet dancers (Cohen et al., 1985), male college athletes (Guilland et al., 1989), national swimmers and college swimmers (Adams et al., 1982; Berning, 1986), elite male triathletes (Burke & Read, 1987), and endurance runners (Peters et al., 1986) were found to be adequate or above the RDA.

However, it appears that athletes who are on calorie restricted diets for weight control are likely to have a less than adequate intake of thiamin. Also, athletes who obtain a high percentage of their calories from low nutrient-density food (candy, sodas, etc.) may be at risk of a thiamin deficiency. The percentage of athletes consuming less than 2/3 of the RDA was 8% of 97 competitive adolescent gymnasts (Loosli et al., 1986), 12% of 92 adolescent ballet dancers (Benson et al., 1985), and 25% of 42 college wrestlers in mid-season (Steen & McKinney, 1986). Short and Short (1983) also found college wrestlers had low thiamin intakes.

Biochemical thiamin deficiency cannot be reliably assessed from blood levels of thiamin (Gubler, 1984). Sauberlich et al. (1979) reported that urinary excretion of thiamin was a reasonably reliable indicator of thiamin nutritional status, although its use has been questioned (Gubler, 1984). However, measurement of coenzyme stimulation of thiamin dependent enzymes from erythrocytes is widely accepted as the most reliable method to determine thiamin status accurately (Hunt and Groff, 1990, p 188). Erythrocyte transketolase (ETK) activity in hemolyzed blood provides an index of the availability of the coenzyme, thiamin diphosphate (Gubler, 1984). In both animal and human studies, good correlations have been found between ETK activity and tissue thiamin levels (Gubler, 1984). The activation of ETK can be assessed by adding thiamin, thiamin diphosphate (TDP), or thiamin pyrophosphate (TPP) to the incubation medium (Hunt and Groff, 1990, p 188). In this case an increase in activity is indicative of a thiamin deficiency.

Studies that have assessed biochemical deficiencies have reported minimal evidence of thiamin deficiency in athletes. Weight et al. (1988a) found that 30 well-trained males were not thiamin deficient, nor were professional ballet dancers (Cohen et al., 1985). However, for male college athletes (N=55), Guilland et al. (1989) have shown that, despite the larger ingested amounts of thiamin for the athletes compared with control subjects, 17% of the athletes had a biochemical deficiency for thiamin (assessed by erythrocyte transketolase activation) while none of the control group did, although the mean values for the two groups were very similar. Part of the discrepancy in these findings may likely be due to the different methodologies used to assess thiamin deficiency. In the Guilland study (1989), although 17% of athletes showed thiamin deficiency when assessed by ETK activation, when TPP was used, 20% of the control subjects but none of the athletes were classified as deficient.

Athletes can achieve the RDA for thiamin and prevent deficiency by ingesting a greater quantity of food and selection of a proper diet (Williams, 1976). Vitamin supplementation, including 7.5 mg of thiamin per day for 30 days, has been shown to improve the thiamin status of athletes and control subjects (Guilland et al., 1989). However, these authors concluded that athletes should be encouraged to consume vitamin-rich foods rather than take supplements. Moreover, vitamin supplements should be used only for athletes with demonstrated biochemical deficiencies (Guilland et al., 1989).

Constant physical exercise may result in an increased need for thiamin (Sauberlich et al., 1979). Nijakowski (1966) found that blood levels of thiamin were lower in sportsmen compared with a control group; however, it is possible that the lower levels were due to higher plasma volume in athletes. After four hours of a skiing excursion, the thiamin levels showed a further decrease. Lower values were also found after three weeks of ski training (Nijakowski, 1966).

Although there is controversy whether thiamin deficiency can alter performance (Williams, 1976, p 123; Williams, 1989), one well-controlled study has shown that performance was not affected by induced thiamin deficiency (Wood et al., 1980). Using a cycle ergometer test, there was no significant difference in exhaustion time between a group who ingested a low thiamin diet (500 μg thiamin) for 4–5 weeks along with a placebo (without thiamin) and a group who had ingested the same low thiamin diet along with a thiamin supplement (5 mg thiamin) (Wood et al., 1980).

However, Steel (1970) noted that of those Olympian athletes who were grouped by high and low (sub-optimal) thiamin ingestion (based on data from questionnaires), the group with the greater thiamin consumption had greater representation among the medal winners and finalists. Steel (1970) recommended that athletes who were ingesting less than adequate amounts of thiamin correct a possible deficiency by ingesting well-balanced meals, rather than taking supplements.

Few studies have assessed the effect of thiamin supplementation as an ergogenic aid (see Keith, 1989). In two controlled studies, the effect of thiamin supplements of 5 mg/day for 1 week on an arm endurance task (Karpovich & Millman, 1942) and .1 mg daily for 10–12 weeks on grip strength and treadmill tests (aerobic and anaerobic work) (Keys et al., 1943) were examined. Both studies found that the supplement had no effect on any measure of work performance.

It seems that most athletes are ingesting proper amounts of thiamin, and few have a biochemical deficiency. Those athletes who are on calorie restricted diets are more likely to have a thiamin deficiency, and a well-balanced diet is recommended to correct it. There seems to be little evidence that thiamin supplementation for athletes consuming a well-balanced diet will have any effect on performance.

Riboflavin. Coenzymes of free riboflavin exist in two forms: flavin mononucleotide (FMN) and flavin adenine dinucleotide (FAD). These are active in cellular oxidation, specifically acting as hydrogen carriers in the mitochondrial electron transport system. This role in mitochondrial function provides the theoretical basis of riboflavin as an ergogenic aid in aerobic metabolism.

The RDA for adults is 1.7 mg/day for males and 1.3 mg/day for females (National Research Council, 1989). Riboflavin is usually linked to caloric intake, and the recommended level is set at .6 mg/1,000 kcal. However, the minimum intake recommended is 1.2 mg/day per adult (National Research Council, 1989). There is no evidence of toxicity from riboflavin ingestion.

Studies that have assessed dietary intake of athletes have found that most adult and adolescent athletes have an adequate or greater than adequate intake of riboflavin (Benson et al., 1985; Berning, 1986; Burke and Read, 1987; Cohen et al., 1985; Ellsworth et al., 1985; Guilland et al., 1989; Loosli et al., 1986; Peters et al., 1986).

Measurement of erythrocyte glutathione reductase (EGR) (an enzyme requiring FAD as a coenzyme) activity in blood samples is considered a sensitive and reliable method for determining riboflavin nutriture (Cooperman & Lopez, 1984; Hunt and Groff, 1990, p 191–192). When the body's riboflavin levels are low, EGR loses its saturation with FAD and its activity drops (Cooperman & Lopez, 1984). The assessment of EGR activity is performed with and without the addition of FAD to the sample. If the addition of FAD produces a marked increase in enzyme activity, riboflavin status is considered inadequate (Hunt and Groff, 1990, p 192).

Biochemical deficiencies of riboflavin are rare. Guilland et al. (1989) have shown that only 4% of male college athletes showed a biochemical deficiency. No biochemical deficiencies were found for professional ballet dancers or competitive swimmers (Cohen et al., 1985; Tremblay et al., 1984). In contrast, Haralambie (1976) found evidence of inadequate riboflavin status in 8 out of 18 athletes.

Exercise and training may increase the need for riboflavin. Belko et al. (1983) found that the need for riboflavin in healthy young women (based on an estimation of riboflavin intake required to achieve normal biochemical status) increased when they participated in jogging exercise for 20–50 minutes a day. However, a mild intensity walking program did not affect riboflavin status in a group of pregnant women (Lewis et al., 1988). Although urinary excretion of riboflavin was shown to decrease after exercise, this appeared to be related to a decrease in blood flow to the kidneys (Tucker et al., 1960).

Keys et al. (1944) placed 6 men students on a riboflavin restricted diet (0.99 mg/day) for a period of 84 days (n = 3) and 152 days (n = 3). Subjects performed an aerobic walking test (60 minutes) and an anaerobic test (60 seconds) on the treadmill and grip strength tests before, every two weeks during, and after the restricted diet period. The performance measures were not adversely affected by the diet regimen. Either riboflavin status has no effect on performance, or the diet was adequate to meet the demands of these exercise tests.

Evidence suggests that supplemental riboflavin has no effect on physical performance or aerobic capacity. Belko et al. (1987) studied two groups of overweight women who participated in an exercise program for 12 weeks. During the training period, one group was ingesting a total of .96 mg/1,000 kcal riboflavin per day while the other group was ingesting 1.16 mg/1,000 kcal per day. No difference in the improvement of aerobic capacity was found between groups. Exercise performance of elite swimmers was examined before and after a 16–20 day period of supplementation of 60 mg of riboflavin per day, and no difference was found in performance (Tremblay et al., 1984).

The results show that exercise may increase the requirement for riboflavin but this need can be adequately satisfied through the athlete's diet. Existing evidence suggests that riboflavin supplementation does not enhance performance.

Niacin. Niacin exists in two forms in foods: nicotinic acid (niacin) and nicotinamide (niacinamide). In the body, niacin is a component of two coenzymes: nicotinamide adenine dinucleotide (NAD) and nicotinamide adenine dinucleotide phosphate (NADP). These coenzymes serve as hydrogen acceptors and donors in glycolysis, fatty acid oxidation, and the electron transport system. From these actions, one might theorize that ingestion of niacin may enhance performance. However, ingestion of nicotinic acid (3–9 g daily) has also been shown to prevent the release of fatty acids (see Keith, 1989, p 237; National Research Council, 1989), and this may adversely affect endurance.

The RDA for niacin is expressed as niacin equivalents (1 mg of niacin is equivalent to 60 mg of dietary tryptophan); it is 19 mg/day for adult males and 15 mg/day for adult females (National Research Council, 1989). As is the case for thiamin and riboflavin, the requirement for niacin is usually linked to energy intake. This means that athletes who have a large caloric intake need a proportionally higher niacin intake. Thus, the recommended intake is 6.6 mg niacin/1,000 kcal. However, for those individuals ingesting less than 2,000 kcal per day, a minimum of 13 mg/day of niacin is recommended (National Research Council, 1989).

Doses of 3 g/day of niacin have been used in the treatment of hypercholesterolemia because they can significantly lower total serum cholesterol, decrease low-density lipoproteins, and increase high density lipoproteins (Hunt and Groff, 1990, pp 194–195). These doses, however, are often associated with undesirable side effects such as flushing, liver damage, increased serum uric acid levels, skin problems, and elevated plasma glucose levels (Hunt and Groff, 1990, pp 194–195). However, niacinamide in large doses is not harmful.

Niacin consumption by adult athletes and dancers has been shown to be adequate (Adams et al., 1982; Berning, 1986; Burke and Read, 1987; Ellsworth et al., 1985; Peters, 1986). However, 7.6% of adolescent ballet dancers (Benson et al., 1985) and 11% of adolescent gymnasts (Loosli et al., 1986) consumed less than 2/3 of the RDA.

No biochemical deficiencies determined from blood samples were found for professional ballet dancers or highly trained male athletes (Cohen et al., 1985; Weight et al., 1988a). However, assessment of niacin status from blood samples is questionable (Hankes, 1984). Measurement of urine levels of niacin metabolites, N'-methylnicotinamide, and N'-methyl-2-pyridone-5-carboxyamide is considered the most promising technique to assess niacin status (Hankes, 1984; National Research Council, 1989). Because of the difficulty in measuring the pyridone compound, the most commonly used method for assessing niacin nutriture is the measurement of N'-methylnicotinamide (mg/g creatinine) for 4–5 h after a 50 mg dose of nicotinamide (Hunt and Groff, 1990, p 196). However, none of these methods is considered a completely accurate reflection of niacin status.

There is some evidence to suggest that exercise may increase the requirement for niacin (see Keith, 1989, p 238). Since most adult athletes have shown no evidence of niacin deficiency, it would seem that an increased requirement is satisfied by the athlete's diet. Poor dietary practices of the adolescent dancers and gymnasts may explain the lower intake of niacin.

In a double-blind placebo experiment, Hilsendager and Karpovich (1964) found that 75 mg of niacin had no effect on arm or leg endurance capacity. Moreover, Bergstrom et al. (1969) found that subjects who were given niacin, 1 g intravenously and .6 g perorally prior to exercise, perceived the workload to be heavier after compared with before the supplement. This finding may be explained by the effect niacin has on fatty acid release from adipose tissue. Nicotinic acid ingestion before exercise has been shown to decrease fatty acid mobilization (Carlson & Oro, 1962; also, for a more detailed review see Williams, 1989). Should this occur during exercise, it would force the muscle to rely more on its muscle glycogen stores. In fact, Bergstrom et al. (1969) found that muscle glycogen content was lower in post-exercise biopsy samples taken from subjects who had received the niacin supplements compared with control subjects.

Most athletes consume an adequate amount of niacin, and any deficiencies may be satisfied by following a sensible diet. There is no evidence that niacin supplementation enhances performance. Moreover, because niacin can reduce fatty acid mobilization during exercise, niacin supplementation may impair performance in prolonged endurance events.

Vitamin B$_6$ (Pyridoxine). Vitamin B$_6$ exists in five forms: pyridoxine, pyridoxal, pyridoxamine, pyridoxal phosphate (coenzyme form), and pyridoxamine phosphate (coenzyme form). They function in protein and amino acid metabolism, gluconeogenesis, and in formation of hemoglobin, myoglobin, and cytochromes. Also, pyridoxine phosphate is a component of glycogen phosphorylase, an enzyme involved in the breakdown of muscle glycogen.

The 1989 RDA for vitamin B$_6$ is 2.0 mg/day for men and 1.6 mg/day for women (National Research Council, 1989). The current 1989 RDA values are lower than those previously established. With only moderate success, pharmacological doses have been used for the treatment of a variety of diseases including atherosclerosis, carpal tunnel syndrome, and muscle fatigue (Hunt and Groff, 1990, p 220). Although the incidence of acute toxicity of vitamin B_6 is low, intakes of 117 mg of this nutrient for more than 6 months can result in neurological impairment (National Research Council, 1989). Chronic ingestion of 2–6 gm of pyridoxine/day has been shown to result in sensory neuropathy (Hunt and Groff, 1990, p 220).

Adequate vitamin B_6 intakes have been reported for 30 well trained men (Weight et al., 1988a). Although 66% of male college athletes were found to consume only 69% of the RDA for vitamin B_6, the value was even lower for the control subjects (59%) (Guilland et al., 1989). Female college athletes (Welch et al., 1987) and female triathletes and endurance athletes (Bazzarre et al., 1986) were reported to have less than acceptable vitamin B_6 intakes. An average of 58% of college wrestlers did not consume 2/3 of the RDA over the training season (Steen & McKinney, 1986). For adolescent gymnasts and ballet dancers, 70% and 42.3%, respectively, consumed less than 2/3 of the RDA (Loosli et al., 1986; Benson et al., 1985). It should be noted that if the 1989 RDA values were used in the above studies, a smaller percentage of athletes may be classified as deficient. Applegate (1989) suggested that women triathletes with low calorie intakes may be at risk for inadequate intake of vitamin B_6 and other micronutrients. Vitamin B_6 intake for the general population of adult women is also low. In 1985, the average intake for adult men and women was 94% and 73% of the present RDA (National Research Council, 1989).

There are several ways to assess vitamin B_6 status (Driskell, 1984). These include 1) direct measurement of the co-enzyme pyridoxal 5'-phosphate (PLP) (the most active form of vitamin B_6) in the blood or direct measurement of 4-pyridoxic acid (a metabolically inactive end product) in the urine; 2) load tests such as the measurement of urinary tryptophan metabolites after giving an oral load of 2–5 g L-tryptophan; and 3) indirect function tests that measure the activity of vitamin B_6-dependent enzymes (National Research Council, 1989). Use of a combination of these methods is considered to provide the best indicator of vitamin B_6 nutriture (National Research Council, 1989).

Biochemical deficiencies for vitamin B_6, assessed by enzyme activation and PLP levels in plasma, were found in 17–35% of male college athletes, which was similar to that found for the control group (Guilland et al., 1989). However, it was also noted in this study that the athletes had a greater intake of vitamin B_6 compared with the control subjects. Blood samples of professional ballet dancers (Cohen et al., 1985) and of 30 well trained men (Weight et al., 1988a) showed them to have adequate vitamin B_6 levels.

There are data to suggest that exercise may alter the blood levels of vitamin B_6. Leklem and Shultz (1983) found that a 4500-meter run dramatically increased the blood levels of pyridoxal 5'-phosphate in trained adolescent males. Also, two studies have reported an increase in blood levels of pyridoxal 5'-phosphate after a 50-minute and after a 20-minute cycling exercise, respectively (Hatcher et al., 1982; Manore & Leklem, 1988). Manore and Leklem (1988) found that pyridoxal-5'-phosphate levels returned to baseline values after only 30 minutes rest.

It has been suggested that pyridoxal phosphate may be released from muscle glycogen during exercise (Manore & Leklem, 1988), and that the increase in pyridoxal 5'-phosphate in the blood after exercise may reflect a need for it as a cofactor for gluconeogenesis (Leklem and Shultz, 1983). Pyridoxal phosphate may be released from glycogen phosphorylase to provide glucose, via the glucose-alanine cycle, for muscle energy needs (Belko, 1987).

The effect of chronic exercise on vitamin B_6 status is unclear. Pregnant women who participated in an eight-week walking program demonstrated an increase in aerobic capacity but no change in blood levels of total vitamin B_6 or pyridoxal phosphate (Yates et al., 1988). Another study found that 4-pyridoxic acid excretion in urine was significantly lower in trained athletes compared with controls (Dreon & Butterfield, 1986). Whether this would indicate an increased requirement for vitamin B_6 or reflect a greater storage capacity in athletes, as suggested by the researchers, is not known.

Despite the exercise-induced changes in vitamin B_6 levels, vitamin B_6 does not appear to be useful as an ergogenic aid. Lawrence et al. (1975b) examined swimming performance of trained swimmers who ingested 51 mg of pyridoxine hydrochloride or a placebo daily for 6 months. No significant difference was found between the groups on 100-yard swimming times.

Because of the role of vitamin B_6 as an integral part of the glycogen phosphorylase enzyme, several studies have examined the relationship between carbohydrate intake and vitamin B_6. Hatcher et al. (1982) found that blood levels of pyridoxal phosphate and vitamin B_6 after exercise were lower in subjects who had consumed a low CHO diet compared with a moderate or high CHO diet 3 days before the exercise. The authors suggested that on the low CHO diet, gluconeogenesis is accelerated which increases the need for pyridoxal phosphate as a cofactor. When the tests were repeated, but with both groups ingesting 8 mg vitamin B_6 supplement each day, the increase in pyridoxal phosphate in blood was 2 times greater and vitamin B_6 was 3 times greater than without the supplement. The authors concluded that, with the supplement, more vitamin B_6 was made available over the course of the exercise.

In a recent study, Manore and Leklem (1988) found that vitamin B_6 supplementation along with an increased CHO consumption resulted in lower free fatty acids during exercise. The authors recommended that athletes who are on a high CHO diet should not supplement their diets with vitamin B_6 above the RDA level. Moreover, deVos et al. (1982) reported that vitamin B_6, because of its role in glycogen phosphorylase activity, may cause a faster depletion of muscle glycogen stores during exercise after ingestion of a low CHO diet.

The evidence suggests that exercise appears to increase the need for vitamin B_6 and that certain athletes have a vitamin B_6 deficiency. Deficiencies should be corrected by a well balanced diet and, if necessary, small amounts of supplements (within the RDA). Because vitamin B_6 supplementation can lower circulating fatty acids during exercise and there is no evidence to suggest that supplementation will enhance performance, the use of vitamin B_6 as an ergogenic aid is contraindicated.

Pantothenic acid. Pantothenic acid acts as a structural component of Coenzyme A (CoA), thus making it important in metabolism involving the Krebs cycle. Since endurance exercise relies predominantly on oxidative energy production via the Krebs cycle, pantothenic acid has been considered by some as a possible ergogenic aid for endurance performance.

Pantothenic acid is among several vitamins and minerals for which there is no established RDA. The ESADDI for pantothenic acid for adults is 4–7 mg/day. Pantothenic acid is excreted as such in the urine, and when excretion is less than 1 mg/day, a deficiency is suspected (Hunt and Groff, 1990, p 197). Although urinary excretion of pantothenic acid correlates with dietary intake, the interindividual variation is large (National Research Council, 1989). Pantothenic acid levels in serum and whole blood have also been used to assess pantothenic acid status (Fox, 1984), although there is some question concerning the accuracy of this technique.

Although only a few studies have examined athletes' intake or biochemical status of pantothenic acid (Calabrese & Kirkendall, 1983; Cohen et al., 1985; Nijakowski, 1966), inadequate intakes of pantothenic acid are rare for anyone consuming a proper diet (Keith, 1989). One notable exception is a study of female professional ballet dancers. Of 25 dancers, 19 were ingesting less than 85% of the ESADDI (Calabrese & Kirkendall, 1983). These dancers also consumed diets very low in calories yet they were taking vitamin supplements. However, the dancers were taking large quantities of isolated vitamins and minerals rather than balanced supplements. Thus, their intake of particular vitamins, like pantothenic acid, remained below the RDA (Calabrese and Kirkendall, 1983).

It is not known whether exercise increases the requirement for pantothenic acid. Nijakowski (1966) found that sportsmen had a higher level of pantothenic acid in the blood than controls and that cycle ergometry exercise of short duration resulted in a decrease. However, blood levels of this vitamin were unchanged after a long duration exercise of 4 hours. Since plasma volume was not corrected, it is difficult to interpret these changes.

The effect of pantothenic acid supplementation on exercise performance is equivocal. Highly trained endurance runners who ingested 2 gm doses of pantothenic acid per day for 2 weeks showed decreased exercise blood lactate levels and decreased oxygen consumption during prolonged exercise (at 75% $\dot{V}O_2max$) compared with the placebo group (Litoff et al., 1985). In contrast, Nice et al. (1984) examined the effect of pantothenic acid supplementation (1 gm per day for 2 weeks) or placebo on run time to exhaustion in 18 highly trained distance runners. In this controlled double blind study, no significant differences were found between groups in run time or any of the standard blood parameters that were assessed (i.e. cortisol, glucose, CPK, electrolytes).

Individuals who consume a well balanced diet are highly unlikely to have a deficiency of pantothenic acid. If exercise does increase the requirement for this vitamin, the increased requirement could easily be corrected by ingestion of a proper diet. There is some evidence that supplementation with pantothenic acid enhances performance but the data are equivocal.

Vitamin B_{12} (Cobalamin). Keith (1989) states that vitamin B_{12} is probably one of the most abused vitamins among athletes. Some athletes may receive injections of 1,000 mg shortly before or 1,000 mg per hour for several hours before competition (Williams, 1989). Other athletes, particularly bodybuilders, are taking sublingual drops of vitamin B_{12} to build muscle and provide extra energy for workouts (Yacenda, 1989). Because of cyanocobalamin's role in the formation and function of red blood cells (RBC), it is thought that vitamin B_{12} supplementation would enhance the oxygen-carrying capacity of RBC and improve endurance.

The RDA for adults is set at 2.0 $\mu g/day$ (National Research Council, 1989). It should be noted that the 1989 RDA for vitamin B_{12} is one-third to one-half lower than that established for the 1980 RDA.

Limited data exist concerning dietary consumption or biochemical status of vitamin B_{12} in athletes. Vitamin B_{12} consumption by ballet dancers was found to exceed the RDA (Cohen et al., 1985). However, Welch et al. (1987) found that female college athletes had a less than acceptable intake of vitamin B_{12}. Also, 16.3% of adolescent dancers (Benson et al., 1985) and 10% of adolescent gymnasts (Loosli et al., 1986) consumed less than 2/3 of the RDA. Thus, there is some evidence that athletes, especially adolescents with low body weights, may not be ingesting proper amounts of this vitamin. However, if these studies were to compare their data to the 1989 RDAs, the percentage of athletes consuming a deficient amount of B_{12} may be less.

Blood levels of vitamin B_{12} are commonly used to assess vitamin B_{12} status, although N-formiminoglutamate excretion is also used (Hunt and Groff, 1990, p 214). A low body content of vitamin B_{12} is associated with low serum levels (Ellenbogen, 1984). Based on analysis of blood samples, Weight et al. (1988a) found well-trained male endurance athletes had adequate vitamin B_{12} status. It should be noted that athletes who are complete vegetarians may acquire a vitamin B_{12} deficiency since vitamin B_{12} only occurs in animal products and some fermented soybean products.

Existing evidence suggests that vitamin B_{12} supplementation has no effect on performance (Williams, 1976, p 129). Montoye et al. (1955), in a well controlled study, placed 51 adolescent boys (age 12–17) into one of three groups: an experimental group that consumed 50 μg of vitamin B_{12} daily, a placebo group, or a control group. No significant difference was found after 7 weeks between the supplemented group or the placebo group in time to run one-half mile or in the Harvard step-test score. Tin-May-Than et al. (1978) studied performance capacity in healthy male subjects before and after injections of cyanocobalamin 3 times a week for 6 weeks. They found no significant improvement in $\dot{V}O_2max$, grip strength, pull ups, leg lifts, or standing broad jump performance. There seems to be no scientific basis for vitamin B_{12} supplementation as an ergogenic aid.

Studies have not fully examined whether the requirement for vitamin B_{12} is increased by exercise or training. The small percentage of athletes who do not ingest adequate amounts of vitamin B_{12} could easily improve their status through a proper diet or ingestion of small amounts of supplement. From the studies that have been done, there are no data to suggest that vitamin B_{12} supplementation will enhance performance.

Folic acid (Folate). This vitamin exists as folic acid (pteroylglutamic acid) and folate (pteroylglutamate), which are involved with DNA synthesis and nucleotide and amino acid metabolism, and are especially important in tissues undergoing rapid turnover such as red blood cells. A folic acid deficiency is suggested to be the most common vitamin deficiency in humans and can result in anemia (Keith, 1989).

The RDA is set at 180 μg for adult females and 200 μg for adult males (National Research Council, 1989). It should be noted, especially when examining the studies cited below, that the 1989 RDAs are about 50% lower than those previously established.

Of 92 adolescent ballet dancers and of 97 adolescent gymnasts, 58.6% and 68%, respectively, consumed less than 2/3 of the RDA of folic acid (Benson et al., 1985; Loosli et al., 1986). In one study of professional ballet dancers, 5 out of 10 men and 2 out of 10 women did not consume 75% of the RDA; however, blood levels were within the normal range (Cohen et al., 1985). In another study of women professional ballet dancers, 20 out of 25 were consuming less than 85% of the RDA (Calabrese et al., 1983). Female college athletes (Welch et al., 1987) and female triathletes and endurance athletes (Bazzarre et al., 1986) had less than acceptable intakes of folic acid. Taking into account an adjustment for the lower 1989 RDA, the folic acid intake for athletes seems to reflect the condition of the U.S. population in general since approximately 10% of the people are reported to have low folate stores (National Research Council, 1989).

Serum folate levels are not considered good indicators of folate status. Tissue levels of folate are assessed by measurement of folate in erythrocytes, although low red blood cell folate may be due to a vitamin B_{12} deficiency as well (Hunt and Groff, 1990, p 214). An increase in N-formiminoglutamate excretion in the urine also indicates either folate or vitamin B_{12} deficiency. To determine whether the deficiency is folate or vitamin B_{12}, the most useful test is the deoxyuridine suppression test. This test measures the activity of thymidylate synthetase in cultured lymphocytes or bone marrow cells upon the addition of one or the other vitamin (Hunt and Groff, 1990, p 214). These latter tests for nutriture status of folic acid have not been performed on athletes.

Despite possible folic acid deficiencies in athletes, no studies have assessed the relationship of folic acid status and exercise performance or the effect of folic acid supplementation on performance.

Biotin. Biotin acts as a coenzyme for several carboxylase enzymes that are important in supplying intermediates for the Krebs cycle and for amino acid metabolism. It is also important in fatty acid and glycogen synthesis. There is no RDA for biotin. However, the ESADDI is set at 30–100 μg/day. Biotin deficiencies are rare in individuals consuming a nutritionally sound diet. In a study of professional ballet dancers, 18 out of 24 were consuming less than

85% of the ESADDI (Calabrese & Kirkendall, 1983). In another group of professional dancers, 6 out of 20 dancers were consuming less than 75% of the ESADDI; however the blood values for biotin were higher than the normal range (Cohen et al., 1985). There was no difference in blood biotin levels in sportsmen compared with controls (Nijakowski, 1966). There have been no studies to examine the effect of biotin supplementation on performance.

"Vitamin" B_{15} (Pangamic acid). "Vitamin" B_{15} was first described as the dimethylaminoacetate of gluconic acid. Bucci (1989) cites studies showing "vitamin" B_{15}, in the form of calcium pangamate, increased oxygen utilization of tissues in animals. Although this substance is not recognized as a vitamin by the scientific community and has no RDA or ESADDI, it has received popular attention by athletes. Bucci (1989) cites a Russian study showing that supplementation with 100–300 mg of calcium pangamate for 3 days produced a decrease in blood lactate at submaximal exercise tests. Furthermore, Russian Olympic athletes used this vitamin as an ergogenic aid in 1964 and 1968.

Black and Sucec (1981) examined the effect of a 2-week supplementation period of calcium pangamate (300 mg/day) or a placebo and found that $\dot{V}O_2$max, $\dot{V}O_2$ at anaerobic threshold, and distance for a 15-minute run were not different between conditions. When supplementation of pangamic acid (or placebo) was given over a longer period, 12 weeks, no difference was found between the placebo or the supplemented group in oxygen kinetics during exercise or recovery, exercise heart rates, and blood lactates (Girandola et al., 1980). Thus, the current evidence shows that "vitamin" B_{15} is not effective as a performance enhancer.

Vitamin B complex. Studies have shown that a deficiency of the B complex vitamins could lead to a decrease in endurance capacity (Van der Beek, 1985; Williams, 1989). Therefore there is some reason to suspect that a combination of B vitamins may enhance performance. Several studies have evaluated the effects of vitamin B complex supplementation (an excellent and detailed review can be found in Williams, 1989).

Van der Beek et al. (1984) placed 6 men on a thiamin, riboflavin, ascorbic acid, and pyridoxine poor diet for 8 weeks. After 8 weeks, this diet caused borderline or moderately deficient blood levels of the 4 vitamins. These deficiencies were associated with a 16% decrease in $\dot{V}O_2$max and a 24% decrease in anaerobic threshold. Van der Beek (1985) concluded that a restricted diet of less than 35–45% of the RDA of the B vitamins may lead to decreased endurance capacity within a few weeks.

Early and Carlson (1969) studied the effect of one dose of a vitamin B supplement, containing vitamin B_1, B_2, niacin, B_6, B_{12}, and pantothenic acid. High school males were given either the supplement or a placebo 30 minutes before running ten 50-yard dashes during hot weather. The running times were recorded for each trial. The group who received the supplement showed less fatigue (drop off in running time) over the trials. These authors suggested that the amount of supplement and the combination of ingredients may be important for a supplement to be effective. However, several confounding variables could have influenced the results since neither the diet intake nor vitamin status of the groups was assessed.

The effect of B complex supplementation on endurance capacity during a treadmill test was examined in physically active male college students (Read & McGuffin, 1983). After 6 weeks of supplementation, there was no significant improvement in endurance.

Although a deficiency of B complex vitamins may decrease performance, research is equivocal with regard to the effectiveness of B complex supplementation. Further investigation is needed to determine the usefulness of B complex vitamins as ergogenic aids.

Vitamin C (Ascorbic Acid). Vitamin C has many known functions including the biosynthesis of collagen, catecholamines, serotonin, and carnitine. It also plays a role as an antioxidant and is needed for non-heme iron absorption, transport, and storage (Keith, 1989). It is probably one of the most studied vitamins and one of the most controversial. The popularly believed benefits of vitamin C supplementation range from curing or preventing the common cold to reducing fatigue and enhancing performance capacity (Keith, 1989; Pike & Brown, 1984, p 134; National Research Council, 1989).

The RDA for vitamin C is 60 mg/day for adults (National Research Council, 1989). Although many potentially harmful effects have been attributed to megadoses of vitamin C, studies have shown that high intakes of ascorbic acid are relatively harmless (Hunt and Groff, 1990, p 182).

Most athlete groups studied were exceeding the RDA for vitamin C, and these included endurance runners (Peters et al., 1986), nordic skiers (Ellsworth et al., 1985), professional ballet dancers (Cohen et al., 1985), college male athletes (Guilland et al., 1989), elite male triathletes (Burke and Read, 1987), and elite national swimmers (Berning, 1986). College swimmers were found to have 530% the RDA for vitamin C (Adams et al., 1982). A small percentage of athletes have been shown to have a less than adequate intake of vitamin C. For example, 10% of adolescent gymnasts (Loosli et al., 1986), 7.6% of adolescent ballet dancers (Benson et al., 1985), and 23% of college wrestlers during mid-season (Steen & Mc-

Kinney, 1986) consumed less than 2/3 of the RDA for vitamin C. These athletes are known for their poor dietary practices.

Ascorbic acid can be measured in the serum or plasma, and urine; however, these methods are not completely satisfactory to determine a vitamin C deficiency (Jaffe, 1984). The content of vitamin C in white blood cells is considered to reflect the body's actual stores (Hunt and Groff, 1990, p 182). Professional ballet dancers (Cohen et al., 1985), female endurance athletes (Bazzarre et al., 1986), highly trained male athletes (Weight et al., 1988a), and male college athletes (Guilland et al., 1989) had adequate blood levels of vitamin C. These data provide no evidence to suggest that athletes have a vitamin C deficiency.

Acute exercise appears to increase blood levels of ascorbic acid. Plasma and lymphocyte ascorbic acid levels increased in 9 men who completed a 21 km race (Gleeson et al., 1987). This study also found that the increase in plasma ascorbic acid levels correlated significantly with an increase in plasma cortisol. The authors suggested that exercise may cause ascorbic acid to be released from the adrenal glands into the circulation along with the release of cortisol.

Few studies have examined the effect of acute exercise on ascorbic acid levels, and little information exists on the relationship of vitamin C deficiency and exercise performance (Williams, 1976). Thus, the overwhelming number of investigations of the effects of vitamin C supplementation on performance is surprising. An excellent and comprehensive review of studies concerning the effect of ascorbic acid supplementation on performance can be found elsewhere (Keith, 1989; Williams, 1989). Keith (1989) cited 19 studies, many from outside the US, that have shown a positive effect and 18 that have shown no effect of vitamin C supplementation on performance. A sampling of the studies will be presented here.

Howald et al. (1975) found a significant, but small (8%), increase in submaximal working capacity on a cycle ergometer when vitamin C supplements were given during a training program. Thirteen athletes ingested a placebo for 14 days and then ingested 1 g vitamin C daily for 14 days. Since the vitamin treatment was always given last, the observed effect after the vitamin treatment may have been due to an accumulated training time.

In contrast, Gey et al. (1970) and Keren and Epstein (1980) found that vitamin C supplementation did not affect endurance performance. Gey et al. (1970) placed 286 Air Force officers into two groups: one received 1000 mg vitamin C and the other received a placebo daily for 12 weeks during moderate training. After 12 weeks, the groups did not differ on their improvement in performance of the Cooper 12 minute walk-run test. Also, the group taking the vitamin

C supplements did not have any reduced injury rate compared with the group without the supplementation. Keren and Epstein (1980) examined aerobic capacity, as assessed by the Astrand ergometer test, in 17 subjects who had taken vitamin C supplements of 1000 mg daily compared with 16 subjects who ingested a placebo during a 21-day training program. There was no difference in the increase in aerobic capacity between the two groups. In a well controlled, double blind study, vitamin C supplementation (300 mg daily) for 21 days did not affect workload or other physiological performance measures during a treadmill test (Keith and Driskell, 1982).

The effects of one dose of vitamin C have also been examined. Keith and Merrill (1983) gave subjects a single dose of 600 mg of ascorbic acid or placebo 4 hours before a muscular endurance and a grip strength test. No significant difference was found in the test scores between the groups. Van Huss (1966) had 10 subjects ingest either vitamin C supplemented drinks (2.98 or 15 mg ascorbic acid/kg body weight) or a placebo drink. One to three hours after each drink was consumed, subjects ran to exhaustion on a treadmill. The supplement did not enhance performance but did produce a faster recovery of heart rate and oxygen consumption.

Buzina and Suboticanec (1985) studied adolescent boys from a rural community in Yugoslavia who had vitamin C deficiencies. Other vitamin and iron deficiencies were corrected prior to examining the effect of vitamin C supplementation on performance. The supplement resulted in an increase in oxygen intake during cycle ergometry exercise. However, when a threshold blood level of vitamin C was reached during the supplementation period, there was no further increase in oxygen consumption. The authors suggested that vitamin C enhances performance in only those subjects who were vitamin C deficient.

Vitamin C also acts as an antioxidant to protect cells from free radical damage (see vitamin E section) (Machlin & Bendich, 1987). Since muscle soreness after exercise seems to result from damage to the muscle tissue (Ebbeling & Clarkson, 1989), it could be hypothesized that vitamin C supplementation may affect the development of soreness. Staton (1952) placed 103 male college students into three groups: vitamin C supplemented (33), control (37), and placebo (33). The supplement consisted of 100 mg of vitamin C/day for 30 days. At the 30-day point, the subjects performed a sit-up exercise that required subjects to perform as many repetitions as possible within 3 minutes. The following day they repeated the sit-up test. The number of fewer repetitions that the subjects were able to perform on the second day was taken to indicate the amount of soreness experienced. No significant difference was found between groups in the ratio of sit-ups performed on test days 1 and 2. Therefore Staton (1952) concluded that vitamin C had no effect on soreness. Whether the criterion score did reflect an individual's soreness is uncertain. Also, because the exercise used in this study may not have produced significant muscle damage, especially with regard to the generation of free radicals, further study of the relationship of vitamin C and muscle damage is warranted.

Whether exercise or training will change an athlete's requirement for vitamin C is unclear. However, athletes ingesting a well balanced diet apparently will ingest adequate amounts of vitamin C to prevent a deficiency. Although several studies have shown that vitamin C supplementation will enhance performance, these studies are flawed by poor designs or they have studied subjects deficient in vitamin C. There are equally as many studies, and often better controlled, to demonstrate that vitamin C supplementation has no effect.

Fat Soluble Vitamins

Vitamins A, D, E, and K are fat soluble vitamins, and these can be stored in appreciable amounts in the body. Because their function is predominantly independent of energy metabolism, it may make them less suitable as performance enhancers (Keith, 1989). Since no studies have been uncovered that examined the effect of vitamin K (a vitamin necessary for blood clotting) on performance, this vitamin will not be discussed in the following sections. However, because vitamin D is involved in calcium metabolism (Williams, 1976), vitamin A can function as an antioxidant, and recent evidence suggests that vitamin E (also an antioxidant) may be useful in reducing muscle damage from strenuous exercise (Keith, 1989), there may be reason to suspect that these vitamin supplements would be of value to athletes.

Vitamin A. Vitamin A designates a group of compounds including retinol, retinaldehyde, and retinoic acid. The body's need for vitamin A can be met by intake of preformed retinoids with vitamin A activity and these are generally found in animal products (National Research Council, 1989). Also, the body's need can be met by ingestion of carotenoid precursors of vitamin A (beta-carotene, alpha-carotene, and cryptoxanthin) commonly found in plants (National Research Council, 1989). The primary function of vitamin A is for maintenance of vision and epithelial tissues. Vitamin A is also involved in the growth process and functions in the body's immune response. Beta-carotene, the major carotenoid precursor of vitamin A, plays a role as an antioxidant.

The RDA for vitamin A is expressed in retinol equivalents (RE);

one RE equals 1 μg retinol or 6 μg beta-carotene. The RDA for vitamin A is 1,000 RE (1,000 μg retinol or 6,000 μg beta-carotene) for adult males and 800 RE (800 μg retinol or 4,800 μg beta-carotene) for adult females (National Research Council, 1989). Megadoses of vitamin A are particularly toxic and can result in several pathological conditions including anorexia, hair loss, hypercalcemia, and kidney and liver damage (Aronson, 1986). Sustained daily intakes exceeding 15,000 μg of retinol can produce signs of toxicity (National Research Council, 1989). However, carotenoids are not know to be toxic (National Research Council, 1989).

Group means of endurance runners (Peters et al., 1986), professional ballet dancers (Cohen et al., 1985), female college athletes (Welch et al., 1987), elite national swimmers (Berning, 1986), college swimmers (Adams et al., 1982), and male college athletes (Guilland et al., 1989) showed vitamin A intakes that exceeded the RDA. However, most of these athletes were below the amount considered to be toxic. When examining individual athletes, 9.5% of male college athletes from the group cited above were ingesting less than adequate amounts of vitamin A (Guilland et al., 1989). In a study of several athlete groups, 20% of certain teams, especially wrestlers, had low vitamin A intakes (Short & Short, 1983). Forty-eight percent of college wrestlers (Steen & Mckinney, 1986), 9.7% of adolescent ballet dancers (Benson et al., 1985), and 15% of adolescent gymnasts (Loosli et al., 1986) consumed less than 2/3 of the RDA for vitamin A. Thus, those athletes who were generally following calorie restricted diets showed evidence of lower vitamin A intakes.

Vitamin A (retinol) can be measured from the blood and provides a relatively good index of total body stores. When the liver stores of vitamin A are low, the plasma levels fall (Olson, 1984). Interestingly, Guilland et al. (1989) found that despite the lower intakes of vitamin A in college athletes, biochemical deficiencies based on serum retinol levels were not found. Also, analysis of blood retinol levels showed no deficiencies in highly trained males (Weight et al., 1988a). The lack of deficiency can most probably be due to the body's relatively large storage capacity for vitamin A.

Only one study was found that examined vitamin A supplementation on exercise performance. Five males were placed on a vitamin A deficient diet for about 6 months followed by vitamin A supplementation for 6 weeks (Wald et al., 1942). Exercise performance was examined during a treadmill run to exhaustion. No significant differences in performance criteria were found between the deficient and supplemented condition. However, it should be noted that the 6-month period of vitamin deficiency may not be long enough to deplete the body's stores of vitamin A. Moreover, the study did not assess whether deficiencies were produced since neither blood levels of vitamin A nor clinical symptoms were assessed.

An antioxidant supplement containing 10 mg beta-carotene, 1,000 vitamin C, and 800 I.U. of vitamin E was given to subjects before downhill running exercise on a treadmill (Viguie et al., 1989). Although the details of the study are not available since this was a published abstract, it seems that the subjects performed the same exercise twice, the first time without the supplement and the second time with the supplement. The results showed that the supplement enhanced glutathione status (antioxidant status) and diminished indicators of exercise-induced damage. However, studies have shown that when a damage-inducing exercise is repeated, the indices of damage are always diminished on the second bout regardless of any treatment (Clarkson and Tremblay, 1988).

Although a small percentage of athletes are ingesting diets that are not adequate in vitamin A, there seems to be no evidence that athletes have serious biochemical deficiencies or that exercise increases the need for vitamin A. Whether beta-carotene, because of its antioxidant properties, has any effect on reducing exercise damage due to free radical activity (see discussion of vitamin E), remains to be determined. Also, although only one study is available, it is unlikely that vitamin A supplementation will enhance performance, and megadoses of vitamin A are potentially toxic.

Vitamin D. The major function of vitamin D is its action as a hormone in the process of mineralization of bones and teeth (Keith, 1989). When the skin is exposed to UV radiation of the sun, a sterol (7-dehydrocholesterol) is converted into vitamin D (cholecalciferol). Eventually vitamin D is converted to its hormone forms 25-hydroxycholecalciferol $(25(OH)D_3)$ and 1,25-hydroxycholecalciferol $(1,25(OH)_2D_3)$ by the liver and kidney, respectively. Also, vitamin D is obtainable from a few food sources including fortified milk and milk products. Because of its role in calcium and phosphate metabolism, it could be speculated that vitamin D may be useful as an ergogenic aid.

The RDA for vitamin D set for adults is 5 μg/day (National Research Council, 1989). Megadoses of vitamin D can be potentially toxic and result in hypercalcemia and hypercalciuria (National Research Council, 1989). Although toxic levels have not been adequately established for adults, levels of 5 times the RDA are considered dangerous (National Research Council, 1989). Intakes of 2,000 IU/day (50 μg) for a prolonged time may pose considerable risk (Hunt and Groff, 1990, p 245). Circulating levels of the vitamin $25(OH)D_3$ provide a reasonable estimate of vitamin D status but do not fully reflect the extent of tissue storage (Hunt and Groff, 1990, p 245).

Few studies have examined the dietary intakes or the biochemical status of vitamin D in athletes. Nineteen out of 20 professional ballet dancers were found to have intakes that exceeded the RDA (Cohen et al., 1985). However, college swimmers were consuming only 19% of the RDA (Adams et al., 1982). It is generally believed that vitamin D deficiencies are rare for those individuals with adequate consumption of milk and exposure to sunlight. For the professional ballet dancers, 9 of the 20 dancers were ingesting less than 75% of the RDA from their normal diets but when vitamin supplements were taken into account, only one dancer still fell below this level. The low vitamin D intakes for dancers (without the vitamin supplements) and swimmers were largely due to their inadequate milk consumption (Adams et al., 1982; Cohen et al., 1985). Also, athletes who do not exercise or spend time outside in the sun may be at some risk for inadequate vitamin D nutriture.

Existing evidence suggests that vitamin D supplementation does not affect work performance (Keith, 1989, p 248). However, Bell et al. (1988) found that blood levels of Gla-protein, an indicator of bone formation, and vitamin D were higher in subjects who were involved in muscle building training compared to controls. The authors suggested that the muscle building exercises stimulated: 1) osteoblastic bone formation, and 2) the production of vitamin D, possibly to provide calcium for newly forming muscle tissue. Whether these data indicate a greater vitamin D requirement for athletes involved in muscle building exercise is not known but warrants further investigation.

There seems to be little theoretical basis for use of vitamin D as an ergogenic aid (Keith, 1989; Williams, 1976). Athletes maintaining nutritionally sound diets and adequate exposure to sunlight should have no vitamin D deficiencies. There are insufficient data to show that vitamin D status is affected by exercise or training, other than muscle building. Moreover, megadoses of vitamin D would seem to cause more harm than good.

Vitamin E. Vitamin E comprises at least four compounds known as tocopherols. The most active and well known of these is alpha-tocopherol. Although the exact biological action has not been fully documented, vitamin E has been shown to function as an antioxidant of polyunsaturated fatty acids in cellular and subcellular membranes (Machlin & Bendich, 1987). In this role it serves as a free radical scavenger to protect cell membranes from lipid peroxidation. Free radicals are chemical species with one or more unpaired electrons in their outer orbit making them highly reactive. Vitamin E may be theorized to enhance exercise performance by maintaining the integrity of cell membranes (for an excellent and detailed description of vitamin E action see Kagen et al., 1989).

The RDA for vitamin E is 10 mg of alpha-tocopherol per day for males and 8 mg/day for females (National Research Council, 1989). Vitamin E is relatively non-toxic up to 800 mg/day (National Research Council, 1989).

From assessment of dietary records, 53% of college male athletes (Guilland et al., 1989), 50% of adolescent gymnasts (Loosli et al.,1986), and 38% of adolescent ballet dancers (Benson et al., 1985) consumed less than 2/3 of the RDA. In the Guilland et al. (1989) study, the mean value for vitamin E intake for the athletes was 77% of the RDA, while the value was only 60% for the controls.

Two functional tests of vitamin E status have been developed recently and both relate to the peroxidation of polyunsaturated fatty acids (PUFA) (Hunt and Groff, 1990, p 252). One test measures peroxidation of PUFA *in vitro* from erythrocytes exposed to hydrogen peroxide. The other test is an *in vivo* one in which peroxidation of PUFA in the body is determined by measuring the hydrocarbon gas, pentane, that is produced (Hunt and Groff, 1990, p 252). Analysis of vitamin E levels from adipose tissue biopsy samples is considered a reliable technique because of the slow turnover of alpha-tocopherol in this tissue (Machlin, 1984). Most common tests measure plasma or serum tocopherol levels which can provide a general index of vitamin E status (Machlin, 1984). However, because alpha-tocopherols are carried by lipoproteins, the plasma lipid content can influence the tocopherol concentration. This factor is often not taken into account.

When vitamin E status was assessed from tocopherol levels in blood samples, only 7% of college male athletes (Guilland et al., 1989) and none of the professional dancers or well trained males (Cohen et al., 1985, Weight et al., 1988a, respectively) showed vitamin E deficiency. Vitamin E deficiencies are considered to be rare (Kagen et al., 1989).

Acute exercise has been shown to affect blood levels of tocopherol. Pincemail et al. (1988) found that plasma tocopherol levels were significantly increased in 9 men during intense cycle ergometer exercise. The authors suggested that tocopherol was mobilized from adipose tissue into the blood to be distributed to exercising muscles. At the muscle level, tocopherol would act to prevent lipid peroxidation induced by the exercise. However, since this study did not correct for hemoconcentration and the small increase in plasma tocopherol was back to baseline after 10 minutes rest, the results may simply be due to changes in hemoconcentration.

To study the effects of vitamin E deficiency, Bunnell et al. (1975) fed subjects who were employed in jobs of hard physical labor a low vitamin E diet for 13 months. Although vitamin E levels dropped significantly over the course of the study, subjects did not perceive any muscle weakness, pain, or cramps. Work capacity was not assessed.

Several studies have examined the effect of vitamin E supplementation on exercise performance (for a more detailed review see Williams, 1989). Using well controlled experiments, several researchers have found that vitamin E supplementation did not affect: 1) the performance of standard exercise tests, including bench step tests, a 1-mile run, 400-meter swim, and motor fitness tests in adolescent male swimmers given 400 mg of alpha-tocopherol daily for six weeks (Sharman et al., 1971); 2) VO_2max or muscle strength in college swimmers given 1200 IU daily for 85 days (Shephard et al., 1974); 3) VO_2max in ice hockey players given 1200 IU daily for 50 days (Watt et al., 1974); 4) a swimming endurance test and blood lactate in competitive swimmers given 900 IU daily for 6 months (Lawrence et al., 1975a, 1975b); 5) motor fitness tests, cardiorespiratory efficiency during cycle ergometry exercise, and bench stepping, and 400 meter swim times in male and female trained swimmers given 400 mg daily for 6 weeks (Sharman et al., 1976); or 6) swimming performance time of the 100- or 400-meter freestyle (Talbot and Jamieson, 1977).

Two studies examined the effect of Vitamin E supplementation on performance at high altitudes. Nagawa et al. (1968) reported that supplementation of 300 mg per day for at least 4–5 weeks had no effect on several exercise tests, including cycle ergometry exercise, running sprints, and a series of races from 3–20 kilometers, performed at altitudes of 2700 and 2900 meters. However, in a few observations they noted increases in VO_2max. Kobayashi (1974), using a better controlled design, examined the effect of vitamin E supplementation of 1200 IU daily for 6 weeks on submaximal cycle ergometry exercise. Testing was done at altitudes of 1525 m and 4570 m. Submaximal oxygen intake, oxygen debt, and blood lactate levels were significantly lower in the vitamin E supplemented group compared with the placebo group or the control trials. This positive effect may be due to the antioxidant properties of vitamin E (Williams, 1989). At the higher altitudes, the decreased availability of oxygen may increase lipid peroxidation of the red blood cell membranes and thereby enhance their destruction. Vitamin E could counteract this effect (Williams, 1989).

Vitamin E may play a role in reducing muscle damage from strenuous exercise. Studies have shown that exhaustive exercise that produces muscle damage is associated with an increase in free radical activity (Kanter et al., 1988; Maughan et al., 1989). Maughan et al. (1989) found that subjects who showed an increase in muscle enzymes in the blood following 45 minutes of downhill running also showed the greatest increase in products of lipid peroxidation. The increase in muscle enzymes in the blood is considered to indicate a disruption in membrane integrity. After the downhill run, the time course of changes in lipid peroxidation products was similar to that of serum enzyme activities.

The data suggest a relationship between free radical activity and loss of membrane integrity following exercise. However, results are equivocal on whether muscle damage is reduced by vitamin E supplementation. Helgheim et al. (1979) found that vitamin E (447 IU/day) supplementation for 6 weeks did not reduce the increase in serum enzymes following strenuous exercise. Also, muscle soreness, a general indicator of muscle damage, was not reduced in subjects taking vitamin E supplements (600 IU/day) for 2 days before performing a strenuous exercise (Francis & Hoobler, 1986). Although Sumida et al. (1989) did find that 4 weeks of vitamin E supplementation (447 IU/day) resulted in a reduced serum enzyme response to exercise, a balanced design was not used. Rather, subjects performed the same exercise before supplementation and then again after supplementation. It is well known that serum enzyme response is substantially reduced the second time an exercise regimen is performed regardless of any treatment (Clarkson & Tremblay, 1988; Ebbeling & Clarkson, 1989).

Goldfarb et al. (1989) examined the effect of 800 IU of vitamin E per day for 4 weeks on measures of lipid peroxidation (lipid hyperperoxide and malondialdehyde) in blood samples taken after a run at 80% $\dot{V}O_2$max. Compared to the placebo group, the vitamin E supplemented group showed reduced levels of lipid peroxidation at rest and after running.

Vitamin E deficiency may be rare in athletes ingesting a well-balanced diet. Although there are data to suggest that exercise may increase the requirement for vitamin E, the results are not definitive. The weight of the evidence for vitamin E supplementation as a performance enhancer falls heavily on the side of vitamin E having no effect on several types of performance tests (see also, Shephard, 1983). Although vitamin E appears to act in the prevention of lipid peroxidation, results are still equivocal with regard to the use of vitamin E supplementation in the reduction of exercise-induced muscle damage in humans. Moreover, although megadoses of vitamin E intake are relatively harmless compared with vitamins A and D, some individuals experience gastric disturbances and weakness when taking vitamin E supplements ranging from 200 IU to 1,000 IU (Kagen et al., 1989).

TRACE MINERALS

Nine trace minerals have been found to be essential to the body, and RDAs or ESADDIs have been established for them (National Research Council, 1989). Five of these have been suggested to enhance exercise performance: zinc, copper, chromium, selenium, and iron.

Advertisements appear in popular magazines touting the benefits of trace mineral supplements as performance enhancers. In the following sections, the interpretation of dietary records for trace mineral intake should be viewed with caution. This assessment of trace mineral intake is problematic because of the bioavailability of the trace minerals in different foods, the effect of food processing, and the weak data bases used to assess trace mineral levels.

Zinc

The many functions of zinc include serving as a component of more than 100 enzymes involved in carbohydrate, lipid, and protein metabolism and playing a role in tissue repair (Anderson & Guttman, 1988; Campbell & Anderson, 1987; Lane, 1989). In addition to its valuable role in many biological processes, the interest in zinc as a supplement stems from the findings of inadequate consumption by the general population (Campbell & Anderson, 1987) and the loss of zinc in sweat (Anderson & Guttman, 1988).

The RDA for zinc is 15 mg/day for adult men and 12 mg/day for adult women (National Research Council, 1989). Prior to 1989, the RDA for zinc was 15 for women. The nutritional status of zinc in the US population seems to be well maintained (Lane, 1989). Zinc intakes of greater than 15 mg/day can result in hypocupremia (impairment in the copper status) and impairment in the body's immune response (National Research Council, 1989).

From assessment of diet records, 52% of college wrestlers consumed less than 2/3 of the RDA during mid-season (Steen & McKinney, 1986), all of 25 professional ballet dancers consumed less than 85% of the RDA (Calabrese & Kirkendall, 1983), and over 75% of 40 highly trained women runners had an inadequate intake (Deuster et al., 1986). Of adolescent ballet dancers and gymnasts, 75% and 78%, respectively, consumed less than 2/3 of the RDA (Benson et al., 1985; Loosli et al., 1986). Male endurance runners averaged slightly below the RDA during a 20-day road race, but met the RDA during a control period (Peters et al., 1986). If the above studies compared the ingestion of zinc to the 1989 RDA standards, fewer women athletes may be considered deficient. Measurement of neutrophil zinc provides an accurate assessment of zinc status (Hunt and Groff, 1990, p 305). However, the most common means to assess zinc status is from serum or plasma samples, although these levels can be affected by several factors such as stress, infection, and oral contraceptives (Hunt and Groff, 1990, p 305). Studies have found that endurance athletes had relatively low resting blood levels of zinc (Deuster et al., 1986; Dressendorfer & Sockolov, 1980; Dressendorfer et al., 1982; Hackman & Keen, 1983; Haralambie, 1981). On the other hand, female triathletes and endurance athletes were found to have lower than adequate intakes of zinc but blood levels of zinc were adequate (Bazzarre et al., 1986), and highly trained males were shown to have adequate blood zinc levels (Weight et al., 1988a).

Strenuous exercise alters zinc concentration in the blood. Anderson et al. (1984) found that serum zinc levels were unchanged immediately following a strenuous 6-mile run but were significantly decreased 2 hours later. The decrease may be due to a redistribution of zinc from the blood into the tissues (Anderson et al., 1984). In contrast, Ohno et al. (1985) reported that zinc levels in the blood were increased immediately after 30 minutes of cycle ergometry exercise at 75% $\dot{V}O_2$max, and Hetland et al. (1975) reported that serum zinc concentrations were significantly increased after a 5-hour cross-country ski race. Blood levels of zinc had returned to baseline within 30 minutes after exercise (Ohno et al., 1985).

Dressendorfer et al. (1982) examined plasma zinc levels over a 20-day road race and found that levels increased for the first two days and then returned to near baseline levels for the remainder of the race. The authors attributed this to an intravascular breakdown of red blood cells (RBC), since zinc is found in greater quantities in RBCs than plasma. Ohno et al. (1985) suggested that brief physical exercise may induce a movement of zinc from tissues into the blood.

There is no clear explanation for the above contrasting findings. However, it has been noted that post-exercise changes in plasma zinc levels are sensitive to zinc status of the individual (Lukaski et al., 1984) and show considerable individual variability (Aruoma et al., 1988). Lukaski et al. (1984) found that the postexercise change in plasma serum zinc concentrations were reduced when subjects followed a zinc deficient diet for 120 days compared to when they followed a zinc supplemented diet for 30 days. The authors suggested that in the zinc depleted state there was an impairment in the mobilization of zinc from tissues. Zinc may also leak out of exercise damaged muscle (Anderson & Guttman, 1988) in much the same way as muscle proteins (i.e. creatine kinase, myoglobin).

Zinc is mainly excreted from the body in urine and sweat (Anderson & Guttman, 1988). Exercise that produces sweating will enhance the loss of zinc from the body. Also, exercise results in an increased excretion of zinc in urine. Anderson and Guttman (1988) noted that there was a 1.5-fold increase in urinary zinc excretion after a 6-mile run compared with resting levels. Thus, exercise can result in a sizable loss of zinc which would thereby increase the requirement.

Since zinc may act in many biological processes and it is apparently altered by physical activity, it seems likely that a relationship between zinc status and performance may exist. However, Lukaski et al. (1983) reported no correlation between blood zinc levels and $\dot{V}O_2max$.

Krotkiewski et al. (1982) found that zinc supplementation of 135 mg daily for 14 days resulted in a significant increase in isokinetic strength at 180°/s of angular velocity and increase in isometric endurance. No change was found for dynamic endurance or isokinetic strength at 60 or 120°/sec. Because zinc supplementation seemed to affect only the fast velocity exercise and isometric endurance, Krotkiewski et al. (1982) suggested that zinc may have an effect on anaerobic work with high lactate production. The role zinc plays as a cofactor for the enzyme lactate dehydrogenase (LDH) (that functions in the interconversion of pyruvate and lactate) supports this suggestion. It should be noted that the levels of zinc used in this study are very high and taken for an extended period could lead to renal damage.

With the amount of information available concerning the effects of exercise on zinc status, it is curious that so few studies have investigated the effect of zinc supplementation on performance. However, it should be noted that excessive zinc consumption can produce several negative effects including an inhibition of copper absorption from the diet possibly leading to anemia, and a reduction in circulation high density lipoproteins (McDonald & Keen, 1988).

Copper

Copper serves as a co-factor in many enzymatic reactions and plays a key role in erythropoiesis, catecholamine regulation, energy metabolism, and the formation of connective tissue. Although there is no RDA for copper, the ESADDI is 1.5–3 mg/day for adults (National Research Council, 1989). Intake of copper of up to 10 mg/day is safe, and overt toxicity from dietary copper ingestion is rare (National Research Council, 1989).

Studies have not adequately examined dietary intake of copper in athletes. Moreover, studies that have examined resting serum copper levels in trained subjects are equivocal. Interpretation of the results from these studies is difficult because there is no completely accurate index of copper status (Lukaski et al., 1983). A recently developed technique that involves the determination of erythrocyte superoxide dismutase activity may provide a more accurate assessment of copper status (National Research Council, 1989).

Compared with sedentary controls, runners (Hackman & Keen, 1983; Olha et al., 1982) and a variety of college athletes (Lukaski et al., 1983) were found to have higher resting blood levels of copper. Conn et al. (1986) and Dressendorfer and Sockolov (1980) reported no difference in plasma copper levels between runners and controls. Dowdy and Burt (1980) found that serum copper levels decreased over 6 months of training in men swimmers and suggest that copper nutriture may have been altered by the intensive training. Endurance athletes have been shown to have adequate levels of copper in blood samples (Bazzarre et al., 1986; Weight et al., 1988a). Most of the studies cited above did not control for, assess, or report the dietary intake of copper, thus it is difficult to interpret their results. Although the findings are somewhat disparate, the weight of the data suggests that copper deficiency is rare in trained athletes.

The effect of acute exercise on blood copper concentration has been examined and the findings are also equivocal. Graded cycle ergometry exercise to exhaustion (Olha et al., 1982) and 30 minutes of cycle ergometry exercise at 70–80% VO_2max (Ohno et al., 1984) resulted in a significant increase in blood levels of copper immediately after the exercise. Dressendorfer et al. (1982) examined plasma copper concentration during a 20-day road race and found a substantial increase over the first 8 days and levels remained elevated throughout the duration of the race. In contrast, Anderson et al. (1984) found no change in serum copper immediately or 2 hours after a 6-mile run.

Most of plasma copper is bound to the protein ceruloplasmin. Ceruloplasmin is a glycoprotein of the $alpha_2$-globulin fraction of human plasma. Ceruloplasmin is considered to exert a protective effect against cellular damage due to accumulation of free radicals (Anderson & Guttman, 1988). Dressendorfer et al. (1982) suggested that the increase in copper that was found during the 20-day road race may be due to an increase in the liver's production of ceruloplasmin in response to exercise stress. In this way ceruloplasmin would act as an acute phase protein to neutralize free radicals.

Conn et al. (1986) reported that for trained athletes, there was no correlation between VO_2max and plasma copper levels. No studies have examined the effect of copper supplementation on performance. Definitive data do not exist to show that athletes ingest less than adequate amounts of copper. Although copper can be lost in sweat (Gutteridge et al., 1985), it is not certain that exercise and training will lead to a deficiency. Therefore, there is no basis to recommend copper supplementation for athletes. Because excessive copper ingestion is potentially toxic, such supplementation should be discouraged.

Chromium

Chromium functions in carbohydrate, protein, and lipid metabolism and in blood glucose homeostasis by potentiating the effects of insulin. Although there is no RDA for chromium, the ESADDI is 50–200 μg daily for adults. Oral supplementation of chromium appears to have no toxic effects (Hunt and Groff, 1990, p 317). Accurate methods to assess chromium status in the body are lacking (National Research Council, 1989).

Dietary intakes of chromium in athletes have not been assessed. However, results have shown that dietary intake of chromium is suboptimal for the general population (Anderson & Guttman, 1988). There is some reason to believe that exercise would increase the requirement for chromium in athletes. Anderson et al. (1984) found that serum chromium was increased immediately after and at 2 hours after a 6-mile run, and that urinary concentration and excretion of chromium were increased at 2 hours after the run.

Further research from the same laboratory found that the basal urinary chromium excretion was significantly less for trained subjects compared to untrained subjects either on a self-selected diet (Anderson & Kozlovsky, 1985) or a controlled diet (Anderson et al., 1988). The lower levels of chromium excretion for the trained subjects may be due either to a deficiency of chromium or to an adaptive response to conserve chromium (Anderson et al., 1988). However, after exercise, the trained subjects showed an increase in chromium excretion but the untrained subjects did not.

Recently, chromium in the form of chromium picolinate has been shown to affect the gain in muscle mass for subjects participating in strength training (Evans, 1989). In a double blind study, football players ingested either supplements containing 1.6 mg chromium picolinate or a placebo for six weeks. During this period they also followed a weight-lifting program. Body composition was estimated from anthropometric measurements. At the end of 6 weeks, the placebo group had increased their lean body weight by 1.8 kg while the chromium supplemented group increased lean body weight by 2.6 kg. Also, the chromium supplemented group lost 3.4 kg of body fat while the placebo group lost 1 kg of fat. Similar results were obtained when the same study design was used for subjects who had just begun weight training. Evans (1989) attributed these changes to chromium's role in potentiating the effects of insulin. In this way insulin would increase the uptake of amino acids, increase the assembly of amino acids into protein, decrease the breakdown of muscle protein, and regulate the efficiency of deposition of lipid in adipose cells (Evans, 1989).

Although the results of the Evans' studies (Evans, 1989) are attractive, they should be viewed with some caution. One important problem is that the percent body fat and lean body mass were estimated by skinfold measurements. The equations used to predict percent body fat and lean mass from skinfold measures were based on data derived from an average population. These equations provide only an indirect estimate, and for football players the accuracy of this method is questionable. It is possible that the small differences reported in lean body mass between the chromium supplemented group and the placebo group may be due to errors in the estimation techniques.

Although dietary intake of chromium for the general population is about one half of the minimum suggested (Anderson & Guttman, 1988), this deficiency could be made up by wise selection of foods high in chromium. The effect of chromium supplementation in athletes has not been adequately examined, and there are no data to suggest a relationship exists between performance and chromium status. Studies on exercise/training and chromium are needed before any rationale can be made for recommending chromium supplements to enhance performance. However, the recent evidence linking chromium picolinate supplementation with increases in muscle mass is intriguing and warrants further investigation.

Selenium

Selenium is a component of the enzyme glutathione peroxidase which functions to reduce lipid peroxidation (Lane, 1989). Selenium seems to play a synergistic role with vitamin E to protect cell membranes from free radical damage. Certain muscle diseases are associated with a deficiency of vitamin E and selenium (Anderson & Guttman, 1988).

The RDA for selenium is 70 μg/day for males and 55 μg/day for females (National Research Council, 1989). There are some data to suggest that intake of selenium over 1 mg/day for an extended period of time may have negative effects such as thickened but fragile fingernails and hair loss (National Research Council, 1989). Selenium status can be reliably measured from biological fluids using graphite-furnace atomic absorption spectrophotometry (Hunt and Groff, 1990, p 313). The activity of glutathione peroxidase in platelets has been used to assess selenium status, but this method may be accurate only for populations with low selenium intakes (National Research Council, 1989).

Since exercise has been shown to increase lipid peroxidation, it is possible that a relationship exists between performance and selenium intake or status (Lane, 1989). However, no studies are available that have assessed the dietary intake of selenium in athletes nor have any studies examined relationships among exercise performance, training, and selenium in human subjects. Since the diet of the general population is adequate in selenium and excessive intake of selenium may be toxic (Lane, 1989), at this time there is no sound justification for recommending selenium supplements as an ergogenic aid.

Iron

Iron is an essential trace mineral for the formation of hemoglobin, myoglobin, cytochromes, and many metabolically important enzymes. Iron deficiency is considered to be the most common nutritional deficiency in the world, and there is evidence that some athletes may be deficient. Because iron plays a major role in oxygen delivery to the tissues as well as in energy metabolism, it could be suggested that a deficiency may seriously affect performance, and that supplements may enhance performance. The RDA for iron is 10 mg per day for males and 15 mg per day for females (National Research Council, 1989). It should be noted that prior to 1989, the RDA for women was 18 mg. Therefore, studies of women athletes' nutrient status that were done before this change use a higher RDA standard for iron than the current one. Adults can tolerate 25–75 mg of iron per day without deleterious effects (National Research Council, 1989). Iron toxicity is rare in healthy adults who do not have genetic deficiency that causes increased iron absorption (National Research Council, 1989).

Numerous studies have assessed iron nutrition of athletes and excellent reviews on this subject are available (Clement & Sawchuk, 1984; Eichner, 1986; Haymes, 1987; Pate, 1983; Sherman & Kramer, 1989). The following discussion provides an overview of the relationship of iron status and exercise performance.

Several studies have found that iron intake of athletes is considerably below the RDA. Adult athletes who have been shown to ingest lower than recommended amounts of iron (generally less than 2/3 RDA) are female college athletes (Welch et al., 1987), male college wrestlers in mid-season (Steen & McKinney, 1986), female college swimmers (Adams et al., 1982), and female endurance athletes (Bazzarre et al., 1986; Clement & Asmundson, 1982). Seventy-five percent of female adolescent ballet dancers (Benson et al., 1985) and 53% of adolescent female gymnasts (Loosli et al., 1986) consumed less than 2/3 of the RDA for iron. Although the number of athletes deficient in iron intake would be less if the current RDA were used for comparison, there would still remain a sizable number of athletes showing a less than adequate iron ingestion.

On the other hand, adequate iron intakes have been found for male endurance runners over a 20-day race (Peters et al., 1986), elite male and female nordic skiers (near adequate intake)(Ellsworth et al., 1985), professional male and female ballet dancers (Cohen et al., 1985), male runners (Clement & Asmundson, 1982), elite male triathletes (Burke and Read, 1987), and female runners (Deuster et al., 1986). Low iron intake in some of the athlete groups is due to poor dietary practices while adequate intake is often related to the use of vitamin supplements (Cohen et al., 1985; O'Toole et al., 1989).

The most accurate means to assess iron status is to determine iron content of bone marrow samples obtained via aspiration. Because this procedure is so invasive, other techniques are generally used to assess iron biochemical deficiencies from blood samples (Haymes, 1987). Poor iron status is indicated by low levels of serum ferritin, increased levels of free erythrocyte protoporphyrin (FEP), reduced hemoglobin levels, and increased levels of transferrin. Serum ferritin levels are a good indication of iron stored in bone marrow. A reduction in serum ferritin levels would indicate **iron depletion**, the first stage of iron deficiency. Continued iron deficiency results in an impairment in erythrocyte formation. This is the second stage in iron deficiency and is termed **iron-deficient erythropoiesis**. When iron is not available to bind with the protoporphyrin FEP (free erythrocyte protoporphyrin), which is used in the formation of the heme molecule, FEP will increase in the blood. Thus, increased FEP is a good indication of depressed erythrocyte formation. As the inability to form erythrocytes progresses, hemoglobin levels begin to fall. This final stage is termed **iron deficiency anemia**. Transferrin is a protein that carries iron in the blood and when iron is not available, levels of transferrin will increase. Transferrin levels, however, are also affected by other factors such as infection and inflammation.

There is a controversy over whether athletes are iron depleted. Low serum ferritin levels have been shown for male middle and long distance runners (Dufaux et al., 1981); female distance runners (Clement & Asmundson, 1982); female endurance athletes (Bazzarre et al., 1986); female track, softball, and hockey players (Parr et al.,

1984); and male and female endurance runners (Casoni et al., 1985). Moreover, Ehn et al. (1980) who studied 8 male runners and Wishnitzer et al. (1983) who studied 11 male runners and 1 female runner found that the runners had only small quantities of iron stored in bone marrow.

Recent studies, however, have shown that athletes are not iron depleted any more so than the general population (Balaban et al., 1989; Risser et al., 1988; Selby and Eichner, 1989). Balaban et al. (1989) reported that serum ferritin levels in 35 male and 37 female elite runners were similar to levels found for the general population. In a sample of 100 female varsity athletes, Risser et al. (1988) found that the incidence of iron deficiency was less (31%) for the athlete group compared with the controls (45.5%), but this was not statistically significant. Selby and Eichner (1989) assessed plasma ferritin levels in 114 athletes and concluded that athletes demonstrate the same age-related increase in storage iron as the general population and that the risk of iron depletion in athletes as a group seems to be no greater than that for non-athletes. Plowman and McSwegin (1981) found that iron deficiency, as assessed by serum iron levels and total iron binding capacity of the blood, was evident in 33.3 % of high school and cross country runners and 28.6 % of the controls. Ballet dancers and ultraendurance athletes were found to have adequate serum iron or ferritin levels (Cohen et al., 1985; O'Toole et al., 1989).

The cause of iron depletion in some athletes is not entirely known. Ehn et al. (1980) suggested that a low absorption and an increased elimination of iron could explain the depleted iron stores. Snyder et al. (1989) found that the low bioavialability of iron in vegetarian diets contributed to the lower serum ferritin levels for athletes following a modified vegetarian diet. Whether significant amounts of iron are lost in sweat is questionable. Brune et al., (1986) found that iron lost in sweat induced by a sauna was marginal. However, Lamanca et al. (1988) showed that during exercise iron is lost in sweat, and although males produce more sweat than females, females had higher sweat iron concentrations. Thus, the type of diet, a low iron absorption, and an increased elimination could produce a negative iron balance, especially for women. It is also possible that low serum ferritin levels reported for endurance athletes may be due to adaptive expansions in myoglobin, hemoglobin, and plasma that can dilute serum ferritin.

Iron deficiency erythropoiesis and iron deficiency anemia (indicated by low serum ferritin and low hemoglobin levels) do not seem to be prevalent in the athlete population (Sherman & Kramer, 1989). In fact, the marginal or low hemoglobin and the low serum ferritin levels found in athletes could be due to other factors than clinically defined iron deficiency anemia. One adaptation to endurance exercise is an expansion of plasma volume which then results in a dilution of hemoglobin. This condition has sometimes been termed pseudoanemia (Eichner, 1986). There is no decrease in red cell mass so oxygen-carrying capacity is not impaired. Furthermore, the increase in plasma volume could reduce viscosity and increase cardiac output, thereby enhancing performance. Therefore, without an empirical trial of iron ingestion, it is difficult to discern the meaning of borderline hemoglobin (or serum ferritin levels) in endurance athletes because a low value may simply reflect dilution.

Eichner (1986) points out another factor that could affect iron status. The hemolysis that occurs from foot strike, or pounding on the feet during running, could result in low hemoglobin levels. However, with normal training the degree of hemolysis is mild and transitory (McDonald & Keen, 1988).

Strenuous exercise has been shown to alter blood iron levels. Dressendorfer et al. (1982) found that plasma levels of iron increased significantly over the first 2 days of a 20-day road race and then decreased. Since the increase was coincident with a fall in hemoglobin, increased iron was considered to be due to intravascular hemolysis. After the marathon, serum ferritin was shown to be elevated for three days (Lampe et al., 1986).

Ricci et al. (1988) and Lampe et al. (1986) reported no change in serum ferritin levels during endurance training in male long distance runners and during 11 weeks of training in female marathon runners, respectively. Studies have also examined changes in serum ferritin levels in untrained subjects who were participating in new training programs. Blum et al. (1986) reported that serum ferritin levels decreased by a small amount after a 13-week aerobic exercise program in previously untrained women. Using a more intense training regimen, Magazanik et al. (1988) found that serum ferritin levels decreased by 50% after 4 weeks of training. These data suggest that training can result in iron depletion or "sport anemia." Magazanik et al. (1988) concluded that iron status of athletes involved in intense training should be examined regularly for iron deficiency. However, it should be noted that several of the athletes in this study had only modest falls in serum ferritin which could be due to plasma volume expansion.

Substantial evidence exists that iron deficiency anemia can compromise performance (Haymes, 1987). However, Matter et al. (1987) found that there was no difference in maximal treadmill performance between female marathon runners with low serum ferritin levels and those with high levels. These data suggest that early stages of iron deficiency may not affect performance but as the deficiency progresses to anemia, performance will be impaired (Haymes, 1983). Although Clement & Sawchuk (1984) present some evidence, albeit inconclusive, that iron deficiency without anemia can adversely affect performance, a more recent study by the same laboratory did not support these data (Newhouse et al., 1989).

Furthermore, Celsing et al. (1986) found that non-anemic iron deficiency did not affect treadmill run time to exhaustion. They induced iron deficiency in 9 healthy male subjects by repeated venesection over a 9-week period followed by a transfusion to reestablish normal hemoglobin levels. Treadmill run times to exhaustion assessed prior to the venesection were not significantly different from the run times assessed after the transfusion. Thus, when the anemia was corrected, but not the iron deficiency, performance time was unaltered.

When iron supplements are given to subjects with iron deficiency anemia, the iron status is improved and so is exercise and work performance (Haymes, 1987; Sherman & Kramer, 1989). However, results are equivocal concerning the effects of supplementation on performance for those subjects with evidence of iron depletion without anemia. Matter et al. (1987) found that 1 week of iron therapy corrected biochemical evidence of iron deficiency but did not influence maximal exercise performance or blood lactic acid levels in female marathon runners. Other studies have also reported no change in exercise performance due to iron therapy in athletes who had mild iron deficiencies (Newhouse et al., 1989; Schoene et al., 1983).

On the other hand, Rowland et al. (1988) found that adolescent non-anemic iron deficient runners did show improvements in endurance time when given iron supplements compared to those given a placebo. However, there may be problems with the interpretation of the data. For example, hemoglobin values did rise during the supplementation period (although not significantly) which may indicate an early stage of anemia. Also, the placebo group (but not the iron-treated group) showed a significant increase in VO_2max but a decrease in endurance time. Haymes (1987) suggested that the equivocal results among studies may be due to the amount of iron supplements used. However, properly controlled studies seem to agree that "non-anemic iron deficiency" does not impair performance.

Some athletes, especially females, show evidence of iron depletion, but the incidence of iron deficiency anemia is uncommon. A poor diet plus iron lost in sweat could produce a negative iron balance. Minimal iron depletion does not seem to affect exercise performance although iron deficiency anemia does. Although the data are equivocal, performance is not enhanced by iron supplements in adult athletes with minimal iron deficiencies, but may affect performance of adolescents. Moreover, an excessive iron intake can inhibit the absorption of zinc (McDonald & Keen, 1988). There is little basis to suggest that iron supplementation for subjects without serious iron deficiency will have any ergogenic effect.

MULTIVITAMIN AND MINERAL SUPPLEMENTATION

From the above studies it can be suggested that most vitamins and minerals taken singularly do not enhance performance. However, since several vitamins and minerals can act synergistically (Bates et al., 1989), it is possible that multivitamin-mineral combinations may affect exercise capacity. Powers et al. (1985) examined the effect of a multivitamin and iron supplement or a placebo given to Gambian children (West Africa) twice a week for 10 weeks. Treadmill exercise performance deteriorated in the group receiving the placebo but was improved in the group receiving the supplement, such that energy cost was lower. Bates et al. (1989) cite other studies where multivitamins were more effective than singular vitamins in children with poor diets.

In a double-blind cross over study, 30 well-trained males received either a placebo or a vitamin/mineral supplement for three months (Weight et al., 1988a). Blood levels of vitamins and minerals and hematological variables were within the normal range throughout the study. The authors concluded that vitamin and mineral supplements were unnecessary in athletes consuming well-balanced diets. Furthermore, Weight et al. (1988b) examined the effect of the vitamin/mineral supplement on running performance in these same subjects. The performance test was a treadmill run to exhaustion. Maximal oxygen consumption, peak running speed, blood lactate turnpoint, peak post-exercise lactate, and a 15-km time trial were assessed. These variables were not altered by the 3 months of supplementation.

Barnett and Conlee (1984) examined the effect of 4 weeks of a vitamin and mineral dietary supplement or a placebo given to well trained males. They found that the supplement did not alter metabolic profiles during a submaximal endurance test and did not enhance VO_2max. The authors concluded that the multivitamin/ mineral supplement was ineffective as an ergogenic aid for endurance performance in athletes on nutritionally sound diets.

The effect of 12 weeks of ingestion of a commercial vitamin/ mineral supplement or a placebo on performance was examined in football players and physical education majors (Nelson, 1960). Performance tests were a 10-yard sprint, the vertical jump, and maximum number of revolutions (in 60 seconds) on a cycle ergometer. There was no significant difference between the placebo group and the supplemented group on any performance measure.

The effect of four months of vitamin and iron supplementation on $\dot{V}O_2$max, heart rate, and the Cooper test was examined in physically active college students (Schrijver et al., 1987). The study design was placebo controlled and double-blind. The supplement contained 10 times the Dutch recommended daily intakes. The supplements did not result in an increase in physical performance capacity. However, the authors point out that beneficial effects of longer term supplementation cannot be ruled out.

Although there are studies that have shown an improvement in performance after ingesting some form of vitamin/mineral supplement for a period of time, these studies are poorly designed or lack statistical analysis of the data (see Williams, 1989). Long term supplementation seems to have no effect on exercise performance in persons who do not have serious vitamin/mineral deficiencies. The weight of the data fall on the side of vitamin/mineral supplements being ineffective as ergogenic aids.

Most experts agree that vitamin and mineral supplements are ineffective as ergogenic aids. However, Wilmore and Freund (1984) noted that better controlled studies with proper experimental designs and more relevant criteria of performance are necessary before a final conclusion could be made regarding the effects of vitamin supplementation on performance.

WHY ATHLETES TAKE SUPPLEMENTS

One reason why athletes take supplements may be that they have limited knowledge of proper nutrition. Studies of college wrestlers (Steen & McKinney, 1986) and adolescent gymnasts (Loosli et al., 1986) found that many of the athletes had serious misconceptions about diet. Parr et al. (1984) studied questionnaires completed by 2,977 college and high school athletes concerning nutrition knowledge and practices and found that a high percentage were unfamiliar with dietary guidelines, other than the basic food groups. Most studies confirm that athletes do not have an adequate knowledge of proper dietary practices (Short, 1989). An early study indicated that Australian Olympic athletes had not received qualified dietary advice (Steel, 1970). Furthermore, Steel (1970) suggested that many of the athletes may be psychologically dependent on high doses of vitamin supplements.

The athlete's source of information on nutrition has also been examined. Parr et al. (1984) found that 77% of college and high school athletes ranked parents as the first or second source of nutritional information. Sixty-seven percent ranked television commercials, magazines, and advertisements as the first or second source. Coaches and athletic trainers were ranked 1st or 2nd by 28–36% of the athletes. Because such a large percentage of athletes acquire their nutrition knowledge from advertisements, it is no wonder that so many athletes are taking supplements!

Wolf et al. (1979) reported that 35% of coaches in the Big Ten prescribed vitamin supplements to their players and 14% prescribed mineral supplements. Since a sizable portion, about a third, of the college and high school athletes did receive their information on nutrition from coaches and trainers (Parr et al., 1984), sound information on nutrition should be directed at coaches and trainers.

However, most athletes ranked parents as a major source of information. Thus, an important way to improve the dietary practices of college and high school athletes may be to provide information on nutrition, especially with regard to vitamin and mineral supplements, to the parents of athletes.

SUMMARY

Although studies have shown that exercise can increase the need for some vitamins and minerals, and some athlete groups have specific vitamin/mineral deficiencies, these studies for the most part agree that the deficiency can easily be corrected by a well-balanced diet. Of the numerous studies that have assessed the effect of vitamin/mineral supplementation on performance, few studies have documented any beneficial effects. Moreover, megadoses of certain vitamins and minerals can be toxic.

Because many studies dealing with the effects of vitamin and mineral supplements on performance are not well controlled, have weak experimental designs, test inappropriate performance criteria, and have not used elite athletes as subjects, more research is needed before final conclusions can be made. This is particularly important since only a very small increase in performance may make the difference between winning and losing.

Despite the lack of evidence that vitamins or minerals have any positive effect on performance, many athletes take supplements, and some take very large doses. Why athletes take these supplements is not exactly clear, but it may be due to their lack of sound information on nutrition. Coaches and trainers can play a significant role in instructing athletes on proper nutritional habits. Moreover, since

many high school and college athletes acquire nutritional information from their parents, it may be worthwhile to prepare material
for parents concerning proper nutrition for young athletes.
Providing athletes with sound information on vitamins and
minerals can be a challenge since the message may not be one that
all athletes want to hear. Perhaps it is more tempting to believe that
a pill will provide the "winning edge" than to believe that success
is largely based on hard work and a good diet.

ACKNOWLEDGEMENTS

I wish to acknowledge the kind assistance of E. Randy Eichner, Linda Houtkooper, and
Melvin H. Williams who provided expert, comprehensive, and valuable reviews of this manuscript. Thank you to Glenn Drabik who assisted in collecting articles. Also a special thank you
to Mary Massei, my mother, who generously volunteered her time to assist me with the collection and xeroxing of most of the articles cited, and who, about 35 years ago, provided me
with the last 11 words of this manuscript.

BIBLIOGRAPHY

Adams, M.M., L.P. Porcello, and V.M. Vivian (1982). Effect of a supplement on dietary intakes
of female collegiate swimmers. *Physician Sportsmed.* 10:122–134.
Alhadeff, L., C.T. Gualtieri, and M. Lipton (1984). Toxic effects of water-soluble vitamins. *Nutrition Reviews* 42: 33–40.
Anderson, R.A., N.A. Bryden, M.M. Polansky, and P.A. Deuster (1988). Exercise effects on
chromium excretion of trained and untrained men consuming a constant diet. *J. Appl. Physiol.*
64: 249–252.
Anderson, R.A., M.M. Polansky, and N.A. Bryden (1984). Strenuous running: Acute effects
on chromium, copper, zinc, and selected clinical variables in urine and serum of male runners. *Biol. Trace Element Res.* 6: 327–336.
Anderson, R.A., and A.S. Kozlovsky (1985). Chromium intake, absorption and excretion of
subjects consuming self selected diets. *Am. J. Clin. Nutr.* 41: 1177–1183.
Anderson, R.A., and H.N. Guttman (1988). Trace minerals and exercise. In: E.S. Horton and
R.L. Terjung (eds.) *Exercise, Nutrition, and Energy Metabolism.* New York: Macmillan Pub. Co.,
pp. 180–195.
Applegate, E. (1989). Nutritional concerns of the ultraendurance athlete. *Med. Sci. Sports Exerc.*
21: S205-S208.
Aronson, V. (1986). Vitamins and minerals as ergogenic aids. *Physician and Sportsmed.* 14: 209–
212.
Aruoma, O.I., T. Reilly, D. MacLaren, and B. Halliwell (1988). Iron, copper and zinc concen-
trations in human sweat and plasma; the effect of exercise. *Clin. Chim. Acta* 177:81–88.
Balaban, E.P., J.V. Cox, P. Snell, R.H. Vaughan, and E.P. Frenkel (1989). The frequency of
anemia and iron deficiency in the runner. *Med. Sci. Sports Exerc.* 21:643–648.
Barnett, D.W., and R.K. Conlee (1984). The effects of a commercial dietary supplement on
human performance. *Am. J. Clin. Nutr.* 40:586–590.
Barr, S.I. (1986). Nutritional knowledge and selected nutritional practices of female recreational
athletes. *J. Nutrition Education* 18:167–174.
Bates, C.J., H.J. Powers, and D.I. Thurnham (1989). Vitamins, iron, and physical work. *Lancet*
Aug 5;2(8658):313–314.
Bazzarre, T.L., L.F. Marquart, M. Izurieta, and A. Jones (1986). Incidence of poor nutritional
status among triathletes, endurance athletes and control subjects. *Med. Sci. Sports Exerc.* 18:S90
(abstract).
Belko, A.Z., E. Obarzanek, H.J. Kalwarf, M.A. Rotter, S. Bogusz, D. Miller, J.D. Haas, and
D.A. Roe (1983). Effects of exercise on riboflavin requirements of young women. *Am. J. Clin.
Nutr.* 37:509–517.
Belko, A.Z. (1987). Vitamins and exercise—an update. *Med. Sci. Sports Exerc.* 19: S191–196.
Bell, N.H., R.N. Godsen, D.P. Henry, J. Shary, and S. Epstein (1988). The effects of muscle-
building exercise on vitamin D and mineral metabolism. *J. Bone Miner. Res.* 3: 369–373.

Benson, J., D.M. Gillien, K. Bourdet, and A.R. Loosli (1985). Inadequate nutrition and chronic calorie restriction in adolescent ballerinas. *Physician and Sportsmed.* 13: 79–90.

Bergstrom, J., E. Hultman, L. Jorfeldt, B. Pernow, and J. Wahren (1969). Effect of nicotinic acid on physical working capacity and on metabolism of muscle glycogen in man. *J. Appl. Physiol.* 26:170–176.

Berning, J. (1986). Swimmers' nutrition, knowledge and practice. *Sports Nutr. News* 4:1–4.

Black, D.G., and A.A. Sucec (1981). Effects of calcium pangamate on aerobic endurance parameters, a double blind study. *Med. Sci. Sports Exerc.* 13:93 (abstract).

Blum, S.M., A.R. Sherman, and R.A. Boileau (1986). The effects of fitness-type exercise on iron status in adult women. *Am. J. Clin. Nutr.* 43: 456–463.

Brune, M., B. Magnusson, H. Persson, and L. Hallberg (1986). Iron losses in sweat. *Am. J. Clin. Nutr.* 43:438–443.

Bucci, L.R. (1989). Nutritional ergogenic aids. In: J.E. Hickson and I. Wolinsky (eds.) *Nutrition in Exercise and Sport.* Boca Raton, Florida:CRC Press, Inc., pp. 107–184.

Bunnell, R.H., E. DeRitter, and S.H. Rubin (1975). Effect of feeding polyunsaturated fatty acids with a low vitamin E diet on blood levels of tocopherol in men performing hard physical labor. *Am. J. Clin. Nutr.* 28: 706–711.

Burke, L.M., and R.S.D. Read (1987). Diet patterns of elite Australian male triathletes. *Physician Sportsmed.* 15:140–155.

Buzina, R., and K. Suboticanec (1985). Vitamin C and physical working capacity. *Int. J. Vit. Nutr. Res.* (Suppl.) 27:157–166.

Calabrese, L.H., and D.T. Kirkendall (1983). Nutritional and medical considerations in dancers. In: G.J. Sammarco (ed.) *Clinics in Sports Medicine* 2(3). Philadelphia: W.B. Saunders Company, pp. 539–548.

Calabrese, L.H., D.T. Kirkendall, M. Floyd, S. Rapoport, G.W. Williams, G.G. Weiker, and J.A. Bergfeld (1983). Menstrual abnormalities, nutritional patterns, and body composition in female classical ballet dancers. *Physician Sportsmed.* 11:86–98.

Campbell, W. W., and R.A. Anderson (1987). Effect of aerobic exercise and training on the trace minerals chromium, zinc, and copper. *Sports Med.* 4:9–18.

Carlson, L.A., and L. Oro (1962). The effect of nicotinic acid on the plasma free fatty acids. *Acta Med. Scand.* 172:641–645.

Casoni, I., C. Borsetto, A. Cavicchi, S. Martinelli, and F. Conconi (1985). Reduced hemoglobin concentration and red cell hemoglobinization in Italian marathon and ultramarathon runners. *Int. J. Sports Med.* 6:176–179.

Celsing, F., E. Blomstrand, B. Werner, P. Pihlstedt, and B. Ekblom (1986). Effects of iron deficiency on endurance on muscle enzyme activity in man. *Med. Sci. Sports Exerc.* 18: 156–161.

Clark, N., M. Nelson, W. Evans (1988). Nutrition Education for elite female runners. *Physician Sportsmed.* 16:124–136.

Clarkson, P.M., and I. Tremblay (1988). Rapid adaptation to exercise induced muscle damage. *Journal of Applied Physiology* 65:1–6, 1988.

Clement, D.B., and R.C. Asmundson (1982). Nutritional intake and hematological parameters in endurance runners. *Physician Sportsmed.* 10:37–43.

Clement, D.B., and L.L. Sawchuk (1984). Iron status and sports performance. *Sports Med.* 1:65–74.

Cohen, J. (1969). Statistical Power Analysis for the Behavioral Sciences. New York:Academic Press.

Cohen, J.L., L. Potosnak, O. Frank, and H. Baker (1985). A nutritional and hematological assessment of elite ballet dancers. *Physician Sportsmed.* 13: 43–54.

Conn, C.A., E. Ryder, R.A. Schemmel, P. Ku, V. Seefeldt, and W.W. Heusner (1986). Relationship of maximal oxygen consumption to plasma and erythrocyte magnesium and to plasma copper levels in elite young runners and controls. *Fed. Proc.* 45:972 (abstract).

Cooperman, J.M., and R. Lopez (1984). Riboflavin. In: L.J. Machlin (ed.). *Handbook of Vitamins. Nutritional, Biochemical and Clinical Aspects.* New York: Marcel Dekker, pp 299–327.

Deuster, P.A., S.B. Kyle, P.B. Moser, R.A. Vigersky, A. Singh, and E.B. Schoomaker (1986). Nutritional survey of highly trained women runners. *Am. J. Clin. Nutr.* 44: 954–962.

deVos, A.M., J.E. Leklem, and D.E. Campbell (1982). Carbohydrate loading, vitamin B_6 supplementation, and fuel metabolism during exercise in man. *Med. Sci. Sports Exerc.* 14:137 (abstract).

Dowdy, R.P., and J. Burt (1980). Effect of intensive, long-term training on copper and iron nutriture in man. *Fed. Proc.* 39:786 (abstract).

Dreon, D.M., and G.E. Butterfield (1986). Vitamin B_6 utilization in active and inactive young men. *Am. J. Clin. Nutr.* 43:816–824.

Dressendorfer, R.H., C.E. Wade, C.L. Keen, and J.H. Scaff (1982). Plasma mineral levels in marathon runners during a 20-day road race. *Physician Sportsmed.* 10: 113–118.

Dressendorfer, R.H., and R. Sockolov (1980). Hypozincemia in runners. *Physician Sportsmed.* 8:97–100.

Driskell, J.A. (1984). Vitamin B$_6$. In: L.J. Machlin (ed.) *Handbook of Vitamins. Nutritional, Biochemical and Clinical Aspects.* New York: Marcel Dekker, pp. 379–401.

Dufaux, B., A. Hoederath, I. Streitberger, W. Hollmann, and G. Assmann (1981). Serum ferritin, transferrin, haptoglobin, and iron in middle- and long-distance runners, elite rowers, and professional racing cyclists. *Int. J. Sports Med.* 2:43–46.

Early, R.G., and B.R. Carlson (1969). Water-soluble vitamin therapy in the delay of fatigue from physical activity in hot climatic conditions. *Int. Z. Angew. Physiol.* 27:43–50.

Ebbeling, C.B., and P.M. Clarkson (1989). Exercise-induced muscle damage and adaptation. *Sports Med.* 7: 207–234.

Ehn, L., B. Carlmark, and S. Hoglund (1980). Iron status in athletes involved in intense physical activity. *Med. Sci. Sports Exerc.* 12:61–64.

Eichner, E.R. (1986). The anemias of athletes. *Physician Sportsmed.* 14:122–130.

Ellenbogen, L. (1984). Vitamin B$_{12}$. In: L.J. Machlin (ed.) *Handbook of Vitamins. Nutritional, Biochemical and Clinical Aspects.* New York: Marcel Dekker, pp. 497–547.

Ellsworth, N.M., B.F. Hewitt, and W.L. Haskell (1985). Nutrient intake of elite male and female nordic skiers. *Physician Sportsmed.* 13: 78–92.

Evans, G.W. (1989). The effect of chromium picolinate on insulin controlled parameters in humans. *Int. J. Biosci. Res.* 1:163–180.

Fox, H.M. (1984). Pantothenic Acid. In: L.J. Machlin (ed.) *Handbook of Vitamins. Nutritional, Biochemical and Clinical Aspects.* New York: Marcel Dekker, pp. 437–457.

Francis, K.T., and T. Hoobler (1986). Failure of vitamin E and delayed muscle soreness. *J. Med. Assoc. Alabama* 55:15–18.

Gey, G. O., K. H. Cooper, and R.A. Bottenberg (1970). Effect of ascorbic acid on endurance performance and athletic injury. *JAMA* 211: 105.

Girandola, R.N., R.A. Wiswell, and R. Bulbulian (1980). Effects of pangamic acid (B-15) ingestion on metabolic response to exercise. *Biochemical Medicine* 24: 218–222.

Gleeson, M., J.D. Robertson, and R.J. Maughan (1987). Influence of exercise on ascorbic acid status in man. *Clin. Sci.* 73: 501–505.

Goldfarb, A.H., M.K. Todd, B.T. Boyer, H.M. Alessio, and R.G. Cutler (1989). Effect of vitamin E on lipid peroxidation at 80% V̇O$_2$max. *Med. Sci. Sports Exerc.* 21: S16 (abstract).

Grandjean, A.C. (1983). Vitamins, diet, and the athlete. *Clin. Sports Med.* 2:105–114.

Guilland, J., T. Penaranda, C. Gallet, V. Boggio, F. Fuchs, and J. Klepping (1989). Vitamin status of young athletes including the effects of supplementation. *Med. Sci. Sports Exerc.* 21: 441–449.

Gubler, C.J. (1984). Thiamin. In: L.J. Machlin (ed.) *Handbook of Vitamins. Nutritional, Biochemical and Clinical Aspects.* New York: Marcel Dekker, pp. 245–297.

Gutteridge, J.M.C., D.A. Rowley, B. Halliwell, D.F. Cooper, and D.M. Heeley (1985). Copper and iron complexes catalytic for oxygen radical reactions in sweat from human athletes. *Clin. Chim. Acta* 145: 267–273.

Guyton, A.C. (1986). *Textbook of Medical Physiology,* 7th Ed. Philadelphia: W.B. Saunders Company, pp. 867–872.

Hackman, R.M., and C.L. Keen (1983). Trace element assessment of runners. *Fed. Proc.* 42:830 (abstract).

Hankes, L.V. (1984). Nicotinic acid and Nicotinamide. In: L.J. Machlin (ed.) *Handbook of Vitamins. Nutritional, Biochemical and Clinical Aspects.* New York: Marcel Dekker, pp. 329–377.

Haralambie, G. (1981). Serum zinc in athletes in training. *Int. J. Sports Med.* 2: 135–138.

Haralambie, G. (1976). Vitamin B$_2$ status in athletes and the influence of riboflavin administration on neuromuscular irritability. *Nutr. Metabol.* 20: 1–8.

Hatcher, L.F., J.E. Leklem, and D.E. Campbell (1982). Altered vitamin B$_6$ metabolism during exercise in man: effect of carbohydrate modified diets and vitamin B$_6$ supplements. *Med. Sci. Sports Exerc.* 14:112 (abstract).

Haymes, E.M. (1983). Proteins, vitamins, and iron. In: M. Williams (ed.) *Ergogenic Aids in Sport.* Champaign:Human Kinetics Pub., pp.27–55.

Haymes, E.M. (1987). Nutritional concerns: need for iron. *Med. Sci. Sports Exerc.* 19:S197–200.

Helgheim, I., O. Hetland, S. Nilsson, F. Ingjer, and S.B. Stromme (1979). The effects of vitamin E on serum enzyme levels following heavy exercise. *Eur. J. Appl. Physiol.* 40:283–289.

Hetland, O., E.A. Brubak, H.E. Refsum, and S.B. Stromme (1975). Serum and erythrocyte zinc concentrations after prolonged heavy exercise. In: H. Howard and J. Poortmans (eds.) *Metabolic Adaptation to Prolonged Physical Exercise.* Basel:Birkhausen Verlag, pp. 367–370.

Hilsendager, D. and P. Karpovich (1964). Ergogenic effect of glycine and niacin separately and in combination. *Research Quarterly* 35:389–392.

Howald, H., B. Segesser, and W.F. Korner (1975). Ascorbic acid and athletic performance. *Ann. N.Y. Acad. Sci.* 258:458–463.

Hunt, S.M. and J.L. Groff (1990). *Advanced Nutrition and Human Metabolism.* St. Paul:West Publishing Company.

172 *PERSPECTIVES IN EXERCISE SCIENCE*

Jaffe, G.M. (1984). Vitamin C. In: L.J. Machlin (ed.) *Handbook of Vitamins. Nutritional, Biochemical and Clinical Aspects.* New York: Marcel Dekker, pp. 199–244.

Kagen, V.E., V.B. Spirichev, and A.N. Erin (1989). Vitamin E, physical exercise, and sport. In: J.E. Hickson and I. Wolinsky (eds.) *Nutrition in Exercise and Sport.* Boca Raton, Florida:CRC Press, Inc., pp. 255–278.

Kanter, M.M., G.R. Lesmes, L.A. Kaminsky, J. La Ham-Saeger, and N.D. Nequin (1988). Serum creatine kinase and lactate dehydrogenase changes following an eighty kilometer race. *Eur. J. Appl. Physiol.* 57: 60–63.

Karpovich, P.V. and N. Millman (1942). Vitamin B_1 and endurance. *N. Engl. J. Med.* 226:881–882.

Keith, R.E., and E. Merrill (1983). The effects of vitamin C on maximum grip strength and muscular endurance. *J. Sports Med.* 23: 253–256.

Keith, R.E., and J.A. Driskell (1982). Lung function and treadmill performance of smoking and nonsmoking males receiving ascorbic acid supplements. *Am J. Clin. Nutr.* 36: 840–845.

Keith, R.E. (1989). Vitamins in sport and exercise. In: J.E. Hickson and I. Wolinsky (eds.) *Nutrition in Exercise and Sport.* Boca Raton, Florida:CRC Press, Inc., pp. 233–253.

Keren, G., and Y. Epstein (1980). The effect of high dosage vitamin C intake on aerobic and anaerobic capacity. *J. Sports Med.* 20: 145–148.

Keys, A., A.F. Henschel, O. Mickelsen, and J.M. Brozek (1943). The performance of normal young men on controlled thiamine intakes. *J. Nutr.* 26:399–415.

Keys, A., A.F. Henschel, O. Mickelsen, J.M. Brozek, and J.H. Crawford (1944). Physiological and biochemical functions in normal young men on a diet restricted in riboflavin. *J. Nutr.* 27: 165–178.

Kobayashi, Y. (1974). Effect of Vitamin E on aerobic work performance in man during acute exposure to hypoxic hypoxia. Ph.D. Dissertation, University of New Mexico, Albuquerque.

Krotkiewski, M., M. Gudmundsson, P. Backstrom, and K. Mandroukas (1982). Zinc and muscle strength and endurance. *Acta Physiol. Scand.* 116:309–311.

Lamanca, J.J., E.M. Haymes, J.A. Daly, R.J. Moffatt, and M.F. Waller (1988). Sweat iron loss of male and female runners during exercise. *Int. J. Sports Med.* 9:52–55.

Lamar-Hildebrand N., L. Saldanha, and J. Endres (1989). Dietary and exercise practices of college-aged female bodybuilders. *J. Am. Dietetic Assoc.* 89: 1308–1310.

Lampe J.W., J.L. Slavin, and F.S. Apple (1986). Poor iron status of women runners training for a marathon. *Int. J. Sports Med.* 7: 111–114.

Lane, H.W. (1989). Some trace elements related to physical activity: zinc, copper, selenium, chromium, and iodine. In: J.E. Hickson and I. Wolinsky (eds.) *Nutrition in Exercise and Sport.* Boca Raton, Florida:CRC Press, Inc., pp. 301–307.

Lawrence, J.D., R.C. Bower, W.P. Riehl, and J.L. Smith (1975a). Effects of alpha-tocopherol acetate on the swimming endurance of trained swimmers. *Am. J. Clin. Nutr.* 28: 205–208.

Lawrence, J.D., J.L. Smith, R.C. Bower, and W.P. Riehl (1975b). The effect of alpha-tocopherol (vitamin E) and pyridoxine HCL (vitamin B_6) on the swimming endurance of trained swimmers. *J. Am. Coll. Health Assoc.* 23: 219–222.

Leklem, J.E., and T.D. Shultz (1983). Increased plasma pyridoxal 5' -phosphate and vitamin B_6 in male adolescents after a 4500-meter run. *Am. J. Clin. Nutr.* 38:541–548.

Lewis, R.D., C.Y. Yates, and J.A. Driskell (1988). Riboflavin and thiamin status and birth outcome as a function of maternal aerobic exercise. *Am. J. Clin. Nutr.* 48:110–116.

Litoff, D., H. Scherzer, and J. Harrison (1985). Effects of pantothenic acid supplementation on human exercise. *Med. Sci. Sports Exerc.* 17:287 (abstract).

Loosli, A.R., J. Benson, D.M. Gillien, and K. Bourdet (1986). Nutrition habits and knowledge in competitive adolescent female gymnasts. *Physician Sportsmed.* 14: 118–130.

Lukaski, H.C., W.W. Bolonchuk, L.M. Klevay, D.B. Milne, and H.H. Sandstead (1983). Maximum oxygen consumption as related to magnesium, copper, and zinc nutriture. *Am. J. Clin. Nutr.* 37:407–415.

Lukaski, H.C., W.W. Bolonchuk, L.M. Klevay, D.B. Milne, and H.H. Sandstead (1984). Changes in plasma zinc content after exercise in men fed a low-zinc diet. *Am. J. Physiol.* 247:E88-E93.

Machlin, L.J. (1984). Vitamin E. In: L.J. Machlin (ed.) *Handbook of Vitamins. Nutritional, Biochemical and Clinical Aspects.* New York: Marcel Dekker, pp. 99–145.

Machlin, L.J., and A. Bendich (1987). Free radical tissue damage: protective role of antioxidant nutrients. *FASEB J.* 1:441–445.

Magazanik, A., Y. Weinstein, R.A. Dlin, M. Derin, and S. Schwartzman (1988). Iron deficiency caused by 7 weeks of intensive physical exercise. *Eur. J. Appl. Physiol.* 57:198–202.

Manore, M.M., and J.E. Leklem (1988). Effect of carbohydrate and vitamin B_6 on fuel substrates during exercise in women. *Med. Sci. Sports Exerc.* 20: 233–241.

Matter, M., T. Stittfall, J. Graves, K. Myburgh, B. Adams, P. Jacobs, and T.D. Noakes (1987). The effect of iron and folate therapy on maximal exercise performance in female marathon runners with iron and folate deficiency. *Clin Sci.* 72:415–422.

Maughan, R.J., A.E. Donnelly, M. Gleeson, P.H. Whiting, and K.A. Walker (1989). Delayed-onset muscle damage and lipid peroxidation in man after a downhill run. *Muscle and Nerve* 12:332–336.

McDonald, R., and C.L. Keen (1988). Iron, zinc and magnesium nutrition and athletic performance. *Sports Med.* 5: 171–184.

Montoye, H.J., P.J. Spata, V. Pinckney, and L. Barron (1955). Effect of vitamin B_{12} supplementation on physical fitness and growth of young boys. *J. Appl. Physiol.* 7:589–592.

Nagawa, T., H. Kita, J. Aoki, T. Maeshima, and K. Shiozawa (1968). The effect of vitamin E on endurance. *Asian Medical Journal* 11: 619–633.

National Research Council (1989). *Recommended Dietary Allowances*, 10th Edition. Washington: National Academy Press.

Nelson, D. (1960). Effects of food supplement on the performance of selected gross motor tasks. *Research Quarterly* 31:627–630.

Nelson, M., A.E. Black, J.A. Morris, and T.J. Cole (1989). Between- and within-subject variation in nutrient intake from infancy to old age: estimating the number of days required to rank dietary intakes with desired precision. *Am. J. Clin. Nutr.* 50: 155–167.

Newhouse, I.J., D.B. Clement, J.E. Taunton, and D.C. McKenzie (1989). The effects of prelatent/latent iron deficiency on physical work capacity. *Med. Sci. Sports Exerc.* 21:263–268.

Nice, C., A.G. Reeves, T. Brinck-Johnsen, and W. Noll (1984). The effects of pantothenic acid on human exercise capacity. *J. Sportsmed.* 24: 26–29.

Nieman, D.C., J.R. Gates, J.V. Butler, L.M. Pollett, S.J. Dietrich, and R.D. Lutz (1989). Supplementation patterns in marathon runners. *J. Am. Dietetic Assoc.* 89:1615–1619.

Nijakowski, F. (1966). Assays of some vitamins of the B complex group in human blood in relation to muscular effort. *Acta Physiol. Pol.* 17:397–404.

Ohno, H., T. Yahata, F. Hirata, K. Yamamura, R. Doi, M. Harada, and N. Taniguchi (1984). Changes in dopamine-Beta-hydroxylase, and copper, and catecholamine concentrations in human plasma with physical exercise. *J. Sports Med.* 24:315–320.

Ohno, H., K. Yamashita, R. Doi, K. Yamamura, T. Kondo, and N. Taniguchi (1985). Exercise-induced changes in blood zinc and related proteins in humans. *J. Appl. Physiol.* 58:1453–1458.

Olha, A.E., V. Klissouras, J.D. Sullivan, and S.C. Skoryna (1982). Effect of exercise on concentration of elements in the serum. *J. Sports Med.* 22:414–425.

Olson, J.A. (1984). Vitamin A. In: L.J. Machlin (ed.) *Handbook of Vitamins. Nutritional, Biochemical and Clinical Aspects.* New York: Marcel Dekker,Inc., pp. 1–43.

O'Toole, M.L., H. Iwane, P.S. Douglas, E.A. Applegate, and W.D.B. Hiller (1989). Iron status in ultraendurance triathletes. *Physician Sportsmed.* 17:90–102.

Parr, R.B., M.A. Porter, and S.C. Hodgson (1984). Nutrition knowledge and practices of coaches, trainers, and athletes. *Physician Sportsmed.* 12:126–138.

Pate, R.R. (1983). Sports anemia: a review of the current research literature. *Physician Sportsmed.* 11:115–131.

Peters, A.J., R.H. Dressendorfer, J. Rimar, and C.L. Keen (1986). Diet of endurance runners competing in a 20-day road race. *Physician Sportsmed.* 14: 63–70.

Pike, R.L., and M.L. Brown (1984). *Nutrition, An Integrated Approach*, 3rd Ed. New York: Macmillan Publishing Company.

Pincemail, J., C. Deby, G. Camus, F. Pirnay, R. Bouchez, L. Massaux, and R. Goutier (1988). Tocopherol mobilization during intensive exercise. *Eur. J. Appl. Physiol.* 57:189–191.

Plowman, S.A., and P.C. McSwegin (1981). The effects of iron supplementation on female cross country runners. *J. Sports Med.* 21: 407–416.

Powers, H.J., C.J. Bates, W.H. Lamb, J. Singh, W. Gelman, and E. Webb (1985). Effects of a multivitamin and iron supplement on running performance in Gambian children. *Hum. Nutr. Clin. Nutr.* 39C:427–437.

Read, M.H., and S.L. McGuffin (1983). The effect of B-complex supplementation on endurance performance. *J. Sports Med.* 23:178–184.

Ricci, G., M. Masotti, E. DePaoli Vitali, M. Vedovato, and G. Zanotti (1988). Effects of exercise on haematologic parameters, serum iron, serum ferritin, red cell 2,3-diphosphoglycerate and creatine content, and serum erythropoietin in long-distance runners during basal training. *Acta Haemat.* 80:95–98.

Risser, W.L., E.J. Lee, H.B.W. Poindexter, M.S. West, J.M. Pivarnik, J.M.H. Risser, and J.F. Hickson (1988). Iron deficiency in female athletes: its prevalence and impact on performance. *Med. Sci. Sports Exerc.* 20: 116–121.

Rowland, T.W., M.B. Deisroth, G.M. Green, and J. F. Kelleher (1988). The effect of iron therapy on the exercise capacity of nonanemic iron-deficient adolescent runners. *Am. J. Dis. Child.* 142:165–169.

Sauberlich, H.E., Y.F. Herman, C.O. Stevens, and R.H. Herman (1979). Thiamin requirement of the adult human. *Am. J. Clin. Nutr.* 32: 2237–2248.

Schoene, R.B., P. Escourrou, H.T. Robertson, K.L. Nilson, J.R. Parsons, and N.J. Smith (1983). Iron repletion decreases maximal exercise lactate concentrations in female athletes with minimal iron-deficiency anemia. *J. Lab. Clin. Med.* 102:306–312.

Schrijver, E.J., E.J. van der Beek, and H. van den Berg (1987). Effect of vitamin and iron supplementation on physical performance. Presented at: International Symposium on Elevated Dosage of Vitamins: Benefits and Hazards. Interlaken, Switzerland. September, 1987.

Selby, G.B., and E.R. Eichner (1989). Age-related increases of iron stores in athletes. *Med. Sci. Sports Exerc.* 21:S78 (abstract).

Sharman, I.M., M.G. Down, and R.N. Sen (1971). The effects of vitamin E and training on physiological function and athletic performance in adolescent swimmers. *Br. J. Nutr.* 26: 265–276.

Sharman, I.M., M.G. Down, and N.G. Norgan (1976). The effects of vitamin E on physiological function and athletic performance of trained swimmers. *J. Sports Med.* 16: 215–225.

Shephard, R.J., R. Campbell, P. Pimm, D. Stuart, and G.R. Wright (1974). Vitamin E, exercise, and the recovery from physical activity. *Eur. J. Appl. Physiol.* 33:119–126.

Shephard, R.J. (1983). Vitamin E and athletic performance. *J. Sports Med.* 23: 461–470.

Sherman, A.R., and B. Kramer (1989). Iron nutrition and exercise. In: J.E. Hickson and I. Wolinsky (eds.) *Nutrition in Exercise and Sport*. Boca Raton, Florida:CRC Press, Inc., pp. 291–300.

Short, S.H., and W.R. Short (1983). Four-year study of university athletes' dietary intake. *J. Am. Diet. Assoc.* 82:632–645.

Short, S.H. (1989). Dietary surveys and nutrition knowledge. In: J.E. Hickson and I. Wolinsky (eds.) *Nutrition in Exercise and Sport*. Boca Raton, Florida:CRC Press, Inc., pp. 309–343.

Snyder, A.C., L.L. Dvorak, and J.B. Roepke (1989). Influence of dietary iron source on measures of iron status among female runners. *Med. Sci. Sports Exerc.* 21:7–10.

Staton, W.M. (1952). The influence of ascorbic acid in minimizing post-exercise muscle soreness in young men. *Research Quarterly* 23: 356–360.

Steel, J.E. (1970). A nutritional study of Australian Olympic athletes. *Med. J. Aust.* 2: 119–123.

Steen, S.N., and S. McKinney (1986). Nutritional assessment of college wrestlers. *Physician Sportsmed.* 14: 101–116.

Sumida, S., K. Tanaka, H. Kitao, and F. Nakadomo (1989). Exercise-induced lipid peroxidation and leakage of enzymes before and after vitamin E supplementation. *Int. J. Bioch.* 21: 835–838.

Talbot, D., and J. Jamieson (1977). An examination of the effect of vitamin E on the performance of highly trained swimmers. *Can. J. Applied Sport Sciences.* 2: 67–69.

Tin-May-Than, Ma-Win-May, Khin-Sann-Aung, and M. Mya-Tu (1978). The effect of vitamin B_{12} on physical performance capacity. *Br. J. Nutr.* 40:269–273.

Tremblay, A., B. Boilard, M.F. Breton, H. Bessette, and A.G. Roberge (1984). The effects of riboflavin supplementation on the nutritional status and performance of elite swimmers. *Nutr. Res.* 4: 201–208.

Tucker, R.G., O. Mickelsen, and A. Keys (1960). The influence of sleep, work, diuresis, heat, acute starvation, thiamine intake and bed rest on human riboflavin excretion. *J. Nutr.* 72:251–261.

Van der Beek, E.J., W. Van Dokkum, J. Schrijver, J.A. Wesstra, H. Van der Weerd, and R.J.J. Hermus (1984). Effect of marginal vitamin intake on physical performance of man. *Int. J. Sports Med.* 5: 28–31.

Van der Beek, E.J. (1985). Vitamins and endurance training:food for running or faddish claims? *Sports Med.* 2: 175–197.

Van Huss, W.D. (1966). What made the Russians run? *Nutr. Today* 1: 20–23.

Viguie, C.A., L. Packer, and G.A. Brooks (1989). Antioxidant supplementation affects indices of muscle trauma and oxidant stress in human blood during exercise. *Med. Sci. Sports Exerc.* 21:S16 (abstract).

Wald, G., L. Brouha, and R.E. Johnson (1942). Experimental human vitamin A deficiency and the ability to perform muscular exercise. *Am. J. Physiol.* 137:551–556.

Watt, T., T.T. Romet, I. McFarlane, D. McGuey, C. Allen, and R.C. Goode (1974). Vitamin E and oxygen consumption. *Lancet* 2:354–355 (abstract).

Weight, L.M., T.D. Noakes, D. Labadarios, J. Graves, P. Jacobs, and P.A. Berman (1988a). Vitamin and mineral status of trained athletes including the effects of supplementation. *Am. J. Clin. Nutr.* 47: 186–191.

Weight, L.M., K.H. Myburgh, and T.D. Noakes (1988b). Vitamin and mineral supplementation: effect on the running performance of trained athletes. *Am. J. Clin. Nutr.* 47: 192–195.

Welch, P.K., K.A. Zager, J. Endres, and S.W. Poon (1987). Nutrition education, body composition, and dietary intake of female college athletes. *Physician Sportsmed.* 15: 63–74.

Williams, M.H. (1976). *Nutritional Aspects of Human Physical and Athletic Performance*. Springfield:Charles C. Thomas, p. 113–152.

Williams, M.H. (1989). Vitamin supplementation and athletic performance, an overview. *International Journal of Vitamin Nutrition Research* 30: 161–191.

Wilmore, J.H., and B.J. Freund (1984). Nutritional enhancement of athletic performance. *Nutrition Abstracts and Reviews, Reviews in Clinical Nutrition* 54: 1–16.

Wishnitzer, R., E. Vorst, and A. Berrebi (1983). Bone marrow iron depression in competitive distance runners. *Int. J. Sports Med.* 4: 27–30.

Wolf, E.M.B., J.C. Wirth, T.G. Lohman (1979). Nutritional practices of coaches in the Big Ten. *Physician and Sportsmed.* 7:113–124.

Wood, B., A. Gijsbers, A. Goode, S. Davis, J. Mulholland, and K. Breen (1980). A study of partial thiamin restriction in human volunteers. *Am. J. Clin. Nutr.* 33: 848–861.

Yacenda, J. (1989). What are members taking to boost performance? *Fitness Management.* February, 5:11–12.

Yates, C.Y., L.M. Boylan, R.D. Lewis, and J.A. Driskell (1988). Maternal aerobic exercise and vitamin B-6 status. *Am. J. Clin. Nutr.* 48:117–121.

DISCUSSION

WILLIAMS: Last year a professor in Minnesota reported rather significant improvements in muscle mass with chromium supplementation. Would you comment on this?

CLARKSON: This is the Evans (1989) study. The companies who promote chromium for athletes must have gotten their information from this study. It is amazing that from one study there would be such a mass production of chromium.

WILLIAMS: I believe that he gave chromium to a football team and showed improvement in muscle mass and strength in comparison to a placebo. He hypothesized that chromium increased insulin and was thus anabolic in nature.

LOMBARDO: I think this all started with a study on disodium chromolactate in diabetics. When a control group of diabetics was given only chromium, they increased their lean body mass and had better control of their insulin. Somebody then took this the next step.

GISOLFI: Can you tell us what the mechanism is for decreasing performance with supplementation of niacin?

CLARKSON: There is not actually a decrease in performance— only a perception that performance was more difficult. It is thought that the nicotinic acid may lower free fatty acids in the blood by decreasing their mobilization from fat stores.

WILLIAMS: There was one study done in Scandinavia in which the researchers gave niacin supplements to endurance athletes when they were about 2 h into an endurance run; niacin significantly impaired performance compared to a placebo trial, presumably by blocking free fatty acid release.

NADEL: Niacin is a profound vasodilator. If it steals blood flow from muscle, then it is going to inhibit performance.

ROBERTSON: In some pilot work that we performed using fairly large doses of niacin, which did produce a profound vasodilation, subjects perceived exertion to be harder, probably because there is a fairly strong input to perceived exertion from skin temperature. The skin of these people was literally red from cutaneous vasodilatation.

NADEL: The heart rate should also be higher at a constant exercise intensity if you have a lot of blood flow to the skin and reduced filling pressure to the heart.

SAWKA: Investigators at our institute used niacin as a vasodilator for work in the heat. If my memory is correct, they showed that when they gave niacin prior to exercise to people exposed to the heat, they had a number of episodes of syncope, and many of these subjects were not able to exercise. Those who could exercise had a drop in blood pressure and increased heart rate. If given niacin during the exercise test, subjects had a higher heart rate and a higher skin blood flow, a slight reduction in sweating, and no major thermal effects.

WILMORE: I think we need to be very sensitive to what we accept as performance variables. I am not sure that changes in $\dot{V}O_2$max or other laboratory tests are really all that important. We need to try more field tests and also use more elite athletes. I am not suggesting that we should have athletes use supplements, but we really should not close the door on anything until we have done systematic testing in the field in highly controlled conditions with elite athletes.

CLARKSON: On the other hand, even the studies that have used highly trained athletes have not shown performance benefits for several of these supplements.

COGGAN: I agree that in order to make adequate performance measures we need to deal with people who are highly motivated, but if you have those conditions in a laboratory setting, performance tests are highly reproducible, both for very short-term, 30–60 s performance measures, and for those that are over in 3 h. Laboratory tests may not adequately simulate what goes on in the field, but they are reproducible.

BUTTERFIELD: I want to reemphasize what Priscilla said about how the RDA's are set. The recommended dietary allowances are exactly that, recommendations for a population; they are determined by taking the requirements for some small group of people and adding a factor to help ensure that they cover 98% of the population. So when you are comparing individual intakes with the RDA, you should be aware that the RDA is already set very high. Also, niacin, thiamine, and riboflavin are usually recommended based on energy intake. For individuals who have a very low energy intake, there is a minimum requirement that should be met. For people who take in five or six times the normal caloric intake, niacin, thiamine, and riboflavin requirements should be five or six times higher. Most of the studies of vitamin intake versus RDA don't take that into consideration. They look at the stated RDA but not at the total energy intake. Therefore, for those three nutrients, more people may actually be borderline in meeting their requirements than it first appears.

CLARKSON: In 1989, the recommendations for folate were almost 50% lower than they were two years before. All the studies on folate have reported that the athletes were not ingesting adequate amounts, but if you recalculate based on the revised RDA, they probably were.

HEIGENHAUSER: Would you adequately meet the mineral and vitamin requirements if you took in the amounts of carbohydrate and protein that are recommended in earlier chapters in this book?

CLARKSON: The only information I have on that is for vitamin B-6. On a high protein diet, there seems to be an increased need for B-6, but not on a high carbohydrate diet.

HEIGENHAUSER: How would you get adequate vitamin B intake if you were on a high carbohydrate diet?

BUTTERFIELD: If you were to take in the suggested amounts of protein, energy intake adequate to cover the activity level, and 70–75% of energy as complex carbohydrate, you would get the thiamine, riboflavin, and niacin, and probably the folic acid and B-6 you need. As long as the energy intake is high enough to cover the energy expenditure and the food eaten is normal food, the vitamin and mineral needs will probably be met. The people I worry about are 1) those who take carbohydrate primarily in the form of glucose drinks or other liquid supplements that do not supply adequate vitamins and trace minerals and 2) anorexic female athletes who have such incredibly low energy intakes that if they meet their protein requirement, it is going to be 20–25% of their caloric intake. They are not going to be able to meet the vitamin and trace mineral requirements.

EICHNER: I think the same concern might be voiced for women who follow vegetarian diets and have normal or heavy menses. They may not, despite eating a fair number of calories, get enough iron to match menstrual blood loss. This is particularly true if they drink coffee or tea with their meals. Caffeine chelates the grain iron and holds it in the stomach. There are a lot of techniques that can be used to maximize iron absorption, but these women do not necessarily know them.

ROBERTSON: You said that in previous studies there were few true vitamin supplementation paradigms where an added amount of a vitamin was given to individuals known to be consuming the RDA for that vitamin. Were these supplementation paradigms then in individuals who were vitamin deficient?

CLARKSON: The nutritional status of subjects was usually simply assumed to meet the RDA. If I were to do a study right now and give half of you a certain dose of a vitamin, I would have no idea what your current nutritional status is. I assume you are healthy, but half of you may have a deficiency that we do not know about. Investigators rarely assess the nutritional status of the subjects before they begin the "supplementation."

ROBERTSON: But if the RDA's are an overestimate, even people who are considered to be deficient by the RDA may actually be at some adequately nourished level.

BUTTERFIELD: To do a good study, the status of the vitamins and minerals should be assessed biochemically, and the dietary vitamin intake should be measured at the beginning, during, and after the study. The investigator needs to know whether giving the supplement changes the dietary patterns.

POWERS: There have been several papers from Lardy's group, particularly from Li Li Ji, that demonstrated mitochondrial enzymatic down-regulation following an acute bout of exercise. The postulated mechanism for this is damage to sulfhydryl groups close to the active site of the enzyme. Do you know of studies that have investigated supplementation of anti-oxidants, such as vitamin C, glutathione, or vitamin E, prior to exercise to determine if this prevents the mitochondrial enzymatic down-regulation observed in animals on their normal diets?

CLARKSON: I do not believe there are any studies in humans.

HEIGENHAUSER: There is some work from the University of Michigan on damage in mouse muscle caused by eccentric contractions. They gave some anti-oxidants and found that the muscle damage was reduced.

SHERMAN: We just completed a study at Ohio State in which we measured anti-oxidant parameters in blood and muscle of rowers whom we trained for four weeks. They exercised 5 d/week for 90 min at 70–75% of $\dot{V}O_2$max and then for 30 min or more at 90–120% $\dot{V}O_2$max. Measuring indices of lipid peroxidation, we were unable, using this intense training, to detect any evidence of significant oxidant stress.

Related to the supplementation of diets of individuals who are on high carbohydrate diets, we usually set daily protein intake for our subjects at 1.0–1.5 g/kg. Then we start our daily carbohydrate content at 5–10 g/kg. For those diets, about 50–60% of the carbohydrate energy comes from foods that we normally eat. To increase the carbohydrate contribution, we supplement with maltodextrin solutions. With the basic diet of normal foods, we have more than adequate vitamins, minerals, and trace elements, so it is possible to design high carbohydrate diets and meet all the RDAs and not have to use vitamin and mineral supplements.

GISOLFI: If you wanted to do a biochemical assessment for multiple vitamins, how would you go about this?

CLARKSON: You'd have to test one at a time. Blood analyses would be adequate for many vitamins, but you might need bone, muscle, or hair samples for some of the minerals or vitamins, especially if you wanted to know the precise levels in those tissues. To assess the status of all the vitamins and minerals would be a very complex matter.

WILMORE: Should a coach give a multi-vitamin supplement to athletes who are known to be getting inadequate nutrition at home? This is particularly pertinent to high school and junior high school athletes who live in economically depressed areas. Do you have any recommendations for these people?

CLARKSON: There is little or no scientific evidence that I know of that can guide us, but a good example of this scenario is provided by young male ballet dancers. They leave home, usually in ninth grade, to go to New York City. They live in New York on their own in an apartment throughout high school and have to take care of themselves, with no parental guidance.

WILLIAMS: One of the vitamins taken by older master athletes is vitamin E. Should aging athletes take vitamin E supplements?

CLARKSON: I don't think there are any data on older adults.

LOMBARDO: In taking care of athletes who are on weight reduction diets, e.g., wrestlers, gymnasts and ballet dancers, we routinely suggest that they take a daily multiple vitamin supplement with minerals. This way, we assume there will be some limit on their vitamin supplementation as opposed to having them take mega doses of every individual vitamin.

I'd like your opinion on iron therapy. Does an individual with a low or relatively low serum ferritin need iron supplementation, and if so, what will the supplementation do to performance?

CLARKSON: Nothing. Without iron deficiency anemia, there is little basis for iron supplementation. Rowland did a study where he gave iron to adolescents who were determined to be iron depleted without iron deficiency anemia, and he found a positive effect on performance. However, their hemoglobin also increased when they were given the supplement, indicating that they may have been borderline anemic. That is the only study that shows a performance effect on subjects who were not frankly iron-deficient anemic. They may have been borderline anemic, or the positive effect could somehow be a function of age of the subjects.

EICHNER: Two kinds of patients ask about vitamins—cancer patients and athletes. Operationally, I give exactly the same answer to both groups: Most people don't need vitamin supplements, but we don't know for sure; if you take a daily general vitamin pill, it is fine with me.

The ferritin issue was born from misinterpreted animal research, and it was always a myth. It was never correct that low ferritin adversely affected performance in humans. It didn't in animals either. The subjects in early animal research were rodents who were anemic from birth and then were transfused to obviate the anemia. But, of course, their muscles were severely iron deficient because they had not had any iron since the time they were born. The question we are asking is totally opposite. If we are asking whether low ferritin impairs performance in the athlete who is just now beginning to run out of iron but is not yet anemic, the answer there clearly is "no." But for women iron deficiency anemia is common—at least one woman in 20; for men it's 1 in 500. The chance of getting hemochromatosis in men is twice that of getting iron deficiency anemia; men should be eating less iron, not more. But women with a hemoglobin of 13 might be anemic. We define anemia on a population basis, but it would be better if we could define it on an individual basis. If your hemoglobin normally is 15, you're anemic if it drops to 13. With a hemoglobin of 13 g/dL, you have a ferritin of 12 or 10, and if you take iron, it is going to improve your athleticism. Hemoglobin will go right back up to 15 in two months. The answer I give is that when in doubt, use iron, but only use it for two months. If the hemoglobin does not go up at least a gram per deciliter, the athlete wasn't iron deficient anemic.

HEIGENHAUSER: In a highly trained male endurance athlete, a hemoglobin of 15 looks like a normal hemoglobin level. But if he had an iron supplement, would his hemoglobin be higher than that?

EICHNER: It's very doubtful because with a hemoglobin at 15, he is probably iron sufficient. If he were 13.5—14.0, I would say it might be possible.

HICKSON: I would like to comment on the vitamin D effect on muscle mass. If my memory is right, vitamin D is a member of the family of steroid hormone receptors. The genes of the steroid hormone receptors have a large degree of homology. With these two bits of information, it seems likely that the vitamin D effect on muscle mass is operating directly on the muscle. Vitamin D could act through an androgen-receptor-mediated mechanism, or it could inhibit a glucocorticoid-mediated mechanism directly at the muscle level.

WILLIAMS: There was one study from West Germany, in which pistol shooters were given a vitamin B complex supplementation—B-1, B-6, and B-12, and this improved pistol shooting performance. The author speculated that the B vitamins were enhancing neurotransmitter production and reducing anxiety. So there may be a particular class of athlete who may benefit from vitamin B beyond the typical endurance or strength type of athlete. I think there is only the one study, and it needs replication, but it was a well-designed experiment.

COYLE: Some of the elite coaches at our institution were using vitamins effectively as an ergogenic aid by using them as a placebo. They were giving athletes vitamins right before their hard workouts and suggesting that the vitamins would give them quick energy. The athletes seemed to be doing better workouts. When we finally convinced one of the coaches that he was not correct in assuming that vitamins provided quick energy, I think that person was a less effective coach. In the real world, many coaches rely on these types of placebos to help in their coaching.

NADEL: I think the scientific community is obligated to come out with the best information it can and not to perpetuate myths. I think in telling the coach the fallacy of his thinking, you did the right thing.

COYLE: There are plenty of myths to come up with, so athletes will just move on to something else. At least with vitamins, they probably won't hurt themselves.

LOMBARDO: It is well known that a placebo positively affects about 30% of the pain-control patients, who are not highly motivated individuals. What percentage do you think would be positively affected in a highly motivated athletic situation? I expect it would be extremely high, and that is where a lot of the myths for the vitamins come from. I would rather see athletes given vitamins for a placebo than something else, but I don't think we should advocate that.

SHERMAN: Why not recommend that coaches give their athletes a placebo pill as opposed to vitamins? Just call it a placebo pill.

SPRIET: I think it's a mistake to advocate taking any kind of pills because such advice suggests that taking supplements is necessary and acceptable.

5

Bicarbonate Loading

GEORGE J.F. HEIGENHAUSER, PH.D., AND NORMAN L. JONES, M.D.

INTRODUCTION

The formation of lactic acid in exercising muscle was first described in the muscles of hunted stags by Berzelius in 1848. He noted that the amount of lactic acid that accumulated in the muscle was proportional to the extent to which the animal had previously exercised. In 1859, DuBois-Reymond observed that resting muscle was neutral or slightly alkaline and became acidic on activity. During the next decade, Ranke (1865) injected lactic acid into frogs, promoting muscle fatigue. Paralleling this work, Bernard (1859) described the presence of glycogen in muscles and postulated that glycogen was possibly the source of lactic acid production; subsequently, Nasse (1877) showed that glycogen decreased with muscle activity.

In the early part of the 20th century, Parnas and Wagner (1914) and Meyerhof (1920a) demonstrated that glycogen loss was proportional to lactic acid formation, concluding that glycogen was probably the precursor of lactic acid. Hill and Lupton (1923) noted that fatigue in stimulated frog muscle was related to the accumulation of lactic acid in muscle; due to its low pKa, lactic acid was shown to exist primarily as hydrogen ion (H^+) and lactate ion (Lac^-). Meyerhof (1920b) showed that by placing frog muscle into an alkaline solution, more lactic acid would accumulate prior to fatigue. Thus, by the 1920s, evidence was being amassed to show that lactic acid formation from glycogen was the energy source of muscle contraction, that accumulation of H^+ in muscle was associated with fatigue, and that alkalosis could influence lactate production. This led Hill and Lupton (1923) to suggest that buffering of H^+ in exercising muscle could counteract the fatiguing effects of lactic acid and thus prolong the duration of short-term exercise.

Even though it was recognized that proteins and the breakdown of phosphocreatine could buffer the H^+ being produced in heavy exercise, most of the early research during exercise in humans focused on carbon dioxide-combining reactions in the blood that occurred with increasing blood $[Lac^-]$. Barr and colleagues (1923) observed that with mild exercise, little or no change occurred in either $[H^+]$ or $[HCO_3^-]$ in plasma; however, with severe exercise, there was always a decrease in $[HCO_3^-]$ associated with increased $[H^+]$ and $[Lac^-]$. Even though the CO_2 produced when H^+ combined with HCO_3^- was eliminated by the lungs, this buffer system could not prevent significant acidification of the plasma during intense exercise.

With this background, several investigators (Dennig et al., 1931; Jervell, 1928; Margaria et al., 1933) hypothesized that if the buffer-combining capacity of blood could be increased by ingestion of $NaHCO_3$, exercising man could accumulate a greater oxygen debt and increase the duration of exercise prior to fatigue. However, their results were inconsistent, and the hypothesis lay dormant until studies at McMaster University (Jones et al., 1977; Sutton et al., 1976) tested it; in the past 12 y, there has been a renewed interest in this area of research.

The purpose of this chapter is to discuss the ergogenic effects on exercise performance in humans of increasing plasma $[HCO_3^-]$ by $NaHCO_3$ loading. Whenever possible, the discussion will focus on the physiological effects on human performance. However, since most human studies have been primarily descriptive and have focused on the effects of exercise intensity and duration, extrapolation from animal studies will be necessary to explain the mechanisms by which NaHCO₃ loading may affect performance. Before describing studies of NaHCO₃ ingestion, we will review the relationship between increases in [H⁺] and reductions in exercise performance.

EFFECTS OF [H⁺] ON MUSCLE PERFORMANCE

Early studies by Dennig and colleagues (1931) suggested that acidosis induced in men by NH_4Cl ingestion may lower the capacity to perform heavy exercise, but these results were not confirmed in subsequent studies by Asmussen and coworkers (1948). In the late 1970s, two studies (Jones et al., 1977; Sutton et al., 1981) confirmed the work of Dennig and associates in 1931, showing that acidosis induced by ingestion of NH_4Cl reduced both exercise endurance time at 95% of VO_2max and the appearance of lactate in the plasma. Similar results were observed by Kowalchuk and colleagues (1984), who found that induced metabolic acidosis reduced the maximum power output attainable during progressive exercise. However, induced metabolic acidosis had little effect on either the initial peak power output or the total work achieved during 30 s of maximal effort (McCartney et al., 1983). Thus, it appears that induced acidosis has little effect on humans' ability to perform very short-term exercise (<30 s), but is detrimental to the ability to attain maximal performance during progressive exercise and to sustain exercise at intensities approaching VO_2max.

During heavy exercise, when resynthesis of ATP occurs primarily by glycolysis, the pH of human muscle drops from 7.0 at rest to 6.5–6.4 following exercise (Hermansen & Osnes, 1972; McCartney et al., 1985; Spriet et al., 1989). This increase in intramuscular [H⁺] during heavy exercise has been implicated in the fatigue process through allosteric regulation of rate-limiting glycolytic enzymes, impairment of excitation-contraction coupling, and impaired cross-bridge cycling.

Several studies have suggested that H⁺ ions may allosterically inhibit glycolytic flux at the level of the flux-generating enzyme, phosphorylase (Chasiotis et al., 1983; Danforth, 1965), or the rate-limiting enzyme, phosphofructokinase (PFK) (Trivedi & Danforth, 1966). In vitro studies of rabbit skeletal muscle by Krebs (1964) showed that the transformation of the inactive "b" to active "a" form of phosphorylase was decreased as [H⁺] increased. Danforth (1965) found that in electrically-stimulated frog muscle, there was a decrease in transformation of phosphorylase to the active "a" form in muscle made acidic by prior stimulation. Chasiotis (1983) found similar results in human muscle; transformation of phosphorylase inactive "b" by epinephrine to the active "a" form was decreased in muscle made acidic by previous stimulation. Similar effects of [H^+] have been found in frog muscle for PFK, i.e., increases in [H^+] decrease its activity.

Although elevated [H^+] has an inhibitory effect on glycogenolysis and on glycolytic flux, it appears that ATP levels in heavy exercise are not limiting (Spriet et al., 1989). In addition, positive glycolytic modulators such as decreases in ATP and elevation of fructose-2,6–bis-phosphate, glucose-1,6–phosphate, NH_4^+, and cyclic AMP may reverse the H^+ inhibition of PFK and permit ATP production via glycolysis to continue (Dobson et al., 1986; Spriet et al., 1987; Trivedi & Danforth, 1966). Thus, the reduction of force output associated with increased intramuscular [H^+] may not be due to reduced glycolytic flux but rather to a general reduction in excitation-contraction coupling at the level of Ca^{++} activation of the contractile proteins (Donaldson et al., 1978).

Hydrogen ions may act at several loci in which Ca^{++} is involved in excitation-contraction coupling. In 1970, Fuchs and colleagues suggested that H^+ might cause fatigue by competing with Ca^{++} for the Ca^{++}-binding site on troponin C. Later, Fabiato and Fabiato (1978) showed that it took higher concentrations of Ca^{++} to produce a given tension output in skinned muscle fibers when [H^+] was high. The negative effects of the elevated [H^+] could not be counteracted by increasing the bath [Ca^{++}], leading to the suggestion that [H^+] acts by modifying the conformation of the tropomyosin molecule. Nakamaru and Schwartz (1972) observed that an increase in [H^+] increased the binding of calcium to isolated sarcoplasmic reticulum vesicles. These studies suggested that H^+ may lead to a reduction in the number of actin-myosin interactions by affecting the excitation-contraction process, thus decreasing the overall force output of contracting muscle.

The decreased ability of muscle to sustain force as fatigue develops is related to increases in both intramuscular [H^+] and inorganic phosphate ([Pi]). Using nuclear magnetic resonance, Dawson and colleagues (1978) showed a decreased ATP turnover rate in isometrically contracting frog muscle that was associated with increases in [H^+] and [Pi]. At present, it is unclear whether changes in intramuscular [Pi] or [H^+] act independently or in concert with one another to induce fatigue at the level of cross-bridge interaction. In 1988, Cooke and coworkers found that increases in [H^+] decreased isometric maximum contraction velocity and ATPase activity in rabbit skeletal muscle, whereas elevations in [Pi] only led to decreased maximal isometric tension. They suggested that [P_i] elevations would increase the number of cross-bridges in the weakly bound state, resulting in reduction of tension development. It was suggested that the effect of increased H^+ was induced via changes in conformation of the contractile proteins. However, Cooke et al. did not propose that a link between the increases in intramuscular $[H^+]$ and $[P_i]$ was a causal factor for fatigue.

Nosek and colleagues (1987) suggested that the diprotonated form of intramuscular P_i caused the fatigue and that $[H^+]$ contributed to the fatigue process by converting more of the intramuscular P_i from HPO_4^- to the diprotonated form, $H_2PO_4^-$. These workers also argued that $[H^+]$ could independently inhibit force production at the cross-bridge level, but Wilson and associates (1988) presented evidence that reduced force results primarily from increased diprotonated intramuscular P_i rather than from increased $[H^+]$. By preceding a maximal bout of exercise with 2 min of submaximal exercise, they found that the relationship of diprotonated intramuscular $[P_i]$ and force output remained unchanged compared with 4 minutes of maximal exercise (control), whereas the developed force was similar to control levels, despite significantly higher $[H^+]$. From this evidence, it appears that diprotonated $[P_i]$ directly affects the force output; however, it is not clear whether $[H^+]$ affects force production directly or by increasing the amount of P_i in diprotonated form.

Investigators have argued that alkalosis induced by $NaHCO_3$ loading should enhance performance in short-duration, high-intensity exercise either by decreasing intramuscular $[H^+]$ directly or by increasing the buffering of H^+ produced by glycolysis. The evidence for this argument has been based on the following observations:

(1) induced acidosis will decrease exercise performance in intense exercise that is dependent on glycolysis for energy production;

(2) the intramuscular $[H^+]$ observed during intense exercise will result in inhibition of rate-limited enzymes of glycolysis

(3) increased $[H^+]$ will impair Ca^{++}-activated steps in excitation-contraction coupling; and

(4) increased $[H^+]$ and elevated diprotonated $[P_i]$ will impair cross-bridge cycling.

EFFECTS OF NaHCO$_3$ LOADING ON EXERCISE PERFORMANCE

The hypothesis that increasing the buffering capacity of the body by ingestion of $NaHCO_3$ will counteract the detrimental effects of increasing $[H^+]$ during intense exercise is not new. However, studies of human exercise performance have produced contradictory results, due partly to the intensity and duration of exercise used in different studies and partly to the dosage of $NaHCO_3$ (Table 5-1).

In the first two studies (Dennig et al., 1931; Margaria et al., 1933),

TABLE 5-1. *Summary of NaHCO₃ Studies*

Study	n	Activity	Intensity
Dennig et al. (1931)	1	Treadmill running	9.3 mph
Margaria et al. (1933)	1	Treadmill running	87.7 kph (5% grade)
Johnson & Black (1953)	11	Cross-country running	"All-out"
Sutton et al. (1976)	7	Cycling	90% $\dot{V}O_2$max
Jones et al. (1977)	5	Cycling	95% $\dot{V}O_2$max
Kindermann et al. (1977)	10	Running	"All-out"
Sutton et al. (1981)	5	Cycling	95% $\dot{V}O_2$max
Wilkes et al. (1983)	65	Running	"All-out"
McCartney et al. (1983)	6	Cycling	"All-out"
Costill et al. (1984)	10	Intermittent cycling	100% $\dot{V}O_2$max
Katz et al. (1984)	8	Cycling	125% $\dot{V}O_2$max
Kowalchuk et al. (1984)	6	Cycling	Progressive to exhaustion
Wijnen et al. (1984)	4	Intermittent cycling	125% $\dot{V}O_2$max
McKenzie et al. (1986)	65	Running	"All-out"
Parry-Billings & MacLaren (1986)	6	Intermittent cycling	Maximal
Bouissou et al. (1988)	6	Cycling	125% $\dot{V}O_2$max
Goldfinch et al. (1988)	6	Running	"All-out"
Horswill et al. (1988)	9	Cycling	"All-out"
Iwaoko et al. (1988)	6	Cycling	95% $\dot{V}O_2$max

only one subject in each study was used to ascertain the influence of NaHCO₃ ingestion on duration of exercise of sufficient intensity to produce blood lactate levels of 9–10 mmol/L, leading to fatigue in approximately 4–5 min. Both subjects increased their running duration over control values. In 1953, Johnson and Black found no effects of ingesting NaHCO₃ on performance of a 1.5 mile cross-country run. Thus, by the early 1950s, there had been only three studies with a limited number of subjects, and no conclusions could be drawn regarding the effects on exercise performance of ingesting NaHCO₃.

In 1976, Sutton and colleagues found that compared to a control condition (221 s), alkalosis induced by ingestion of NaHCO₃ almost doubled the duration (356 s) subjects could cycle at 90% $\dot{V}O_2$max. Similar results were achieved during cycling at 95% $\dot{V}O_2$max in the same laboratory (Jones et al., 1977; Sutton et al., 1981) and also later in Japan (Iwaoko et al., 1988). Following Jones' laboratory study in 1977, field studies were carried out to ascertain the influence of exercise performance of differing durations and intensities. The initial field study conducted by Kinderman and colleagues in 1977 showed no significant influence of NaHCO₃ on a 400 m run. However, Gold-

TABLE 5-1. *(Continued)*

Duration	Distance	Dosage	Results
5–7 min	—	10 g	longer duration
4–7 min	—	20 g	longer duration
?	1.5 miles	3.5 g	no effect
3.6–5.9 min	—	0.3 g/kg	longer duration
2.5–7.5 min	—	0.3 g/kg	longer duration
60 min	400 m	190 mmol	no effect
2.5–7.5 min	—	0.3 g/kg	longer duration
~2 min	800 m	0.3 g/kg	faster time
30 sec	—	0.3 g/kg	no effect
60 sec	—	0.2 g/kg	longer duration on fifth bout
100 sec	—	0.2 g/kg	no effect on duration
1 min increments	—	0.3 g/kg	no effect
60 sec	—	0.36 g/kg	longer duration on fifth bout
—	800 m	0.3 g/kg	no effect
30 sec	—	0.3 g/kg	no effect
60–75 sec	—	0.3 g/kg	longer duration
60 sec	400 m	0.4 g/kg	faster time
120 sec	—	0.2 g/kg	no effect
120–180 sec	—	0.2 g/kg	longer duration

finch and associates (1988) found results that contradicted those of Kinderman et al. (1977) when they observed significant improvement of performance in a 400 m run under the influence of a $NaHCO_3$ load (56.9 s for $NaHCO_3$ vs 58.5 s for control). Perhaps the most convincing evidence of the ergogenic effects of $NaHCO_3$ loading on running performance was obtained by Wilkes and coworkers (1983). In their study, competitive varsity athletes ran significantly faster over 800 m following ingestion of $NaHCO_3$ (2:02.9 min) than with placebo (2:05.1 min) or under control conditions (2:05.9 min). However, in untrained university students, McKenzie and associates (1986) found no effects of $NaHCO_3$ on 800 m running performance.

In the 1980s, laboratory studies showed no effects of $NaHCO_3$ loading on maximal power output during progressive cycling (Kowalchuk et al., 1984), total work output during 30 s of maximal cycling (McCartney et al., 1983), total work during cycling at power outputs equivalent to 125% of $\dot{V}O_2$max (Katz et al., 1984), or total work during 2 min of maximal isokinetic cycling (Horswill et al., 1988). However, Bouissou et al. (1988), unlike Katz and coworkers

(1984), found that $NaHCO_3$ increased exercise duration to 75 s at power outputs equivalent to 125% $\dot{V}O_2$max compared with control conditions (62 s).

Since repeated bouts of heavy exercise have been shown to be associated with higher plasma [Lac^-] and [H^+] than single bouts of exercise (Hermansen & Osnes, 1972; McCartney et al., 1983), several laboratories (Costill et al., 1984; Parry-Billings & MacLaren, 1986; Wijnen et al., 1984) hypothesized that $NaHCO_3$ would enhance exercise performance in the final exercise bout of repeated intermittent exercise. In all these studies, the hypothesis was supported; performance during $NaHCO_3$ loading compared with control conditions was greatest in the final exercise bout.

Some contradictory results can be explained by the differing amounts of $NaHCO_3$ ingested. Horswill and colleagues (1988) attempted to determine the minimal performance-enhancing dose. Their maximum dose was 0.2 g/kg of body weight, and this failed to affect performance. Other studies that used doses of 0.3 g/kg found enhanced performance of high-intensity exercise lasting 1–6 min. The pre-400 m run $NaHCO_3$-loading studies of Kinderman and co-workers (1977), who found no performance enhancement using a dose of 0.2 g/kg body weight, are in contrast with those of Goldfinch and associates (1988), who found enhanced performance with a dose of 0.4 g/kg body weight. Similar findings occurred in the studies of Katz et al. (1984) and Bouissou et al. (1989) for the duration of performance at 125% $\dot{V}O_2$max. Bouissou and coworkers found significantly longer durations with a dosage of 0.3 g/kg, whereas Katz et al. saw no effect with a dosage of 0.2 g/kg. Thus, it appears that a dosage of at least 0.3 g/kg is ordinarily required to affect exercise performance.

No firm conclusion can be drawn regarding the effects of $NaHCO_3$ loading on exercise performance, but an hypothesis may be advanced on the basis of these studies. The $NaHCO_3$ has no effect during high-intensity exercise of 30 s duration or less, and activities that depend extensively upon oxidative metabolism are also not affected. However, it appears that $NaHCO_3$ will enhance the performance of both intense continuous exercise of 1–7.5 min duration and intense intermittent exercise, but the effect is highly dose-dependent.

EFFECTS OF $NaHCO_3$ ON EMG ACTIVITY AND PERCEIVED EXERTION

If $NaHCO_3$ improves performance during exercise, the concomitant changes in the electromyogram associated with fatigue and on the subjects' perception of effort should be lessened. Several studies

(Bouissou et al., 1989; Kostka & Cafarelli, 1982) have investigated the effects of induced alkalosis on EMG activity during exercise. Kostra and Cafarelli (1982) found that induced alkalosis had no effect on the integrated EMG at either 25% or 80% of $\dot{V}O_2$max performed for 15 min at each intensity, but at 80% $\dot{V}O_2$max, the integrated EMG increased linearly with time. A possible explanation for the similar electrical response to changes in extracellular [H^+] may be that increased motor unit recruitment and decreased firing frequency change reciprocally with time, resulting in no change in the integrated EMG. Bouissou and colleagues (1989) also found that alkalosis had no effect on the integrated EMG during cycling at an intensity of 125% $\dot{V}O_2$max, but alkalosis amplified the shift in the power spectrum toward lower frequencies. This shift was associated with fatigue; however, the mechanism for the shift is open to debate and has been reviewed elsewhere (De Luca, 1984). Even though several investigators have proposed that increased intramuscular [H^+] is responsible for the shift, no relationship has been found between intramuscular [H^+] and the frequency shift in the EMG. From these studies, it appears that alkalosis has no influence on the integrated EMG activity but amplifies the shift toward a lower frequency in the power spectrum caused by an as yet unknown mechanism.

When fatigue occurs, sensory processes are altered so that a constant work output requires more effort (Cafarelli, 1977; Cafarelli et al., 1977). In the study of Kostka and Cafarelli (1982), alkalosis during heavy exercise (80% $\dot{V}O_2$max) did not alter the sensation of effort. Robertson and colleagues (1986) found that during progressive cycling exercise, alkalosis did not alter the sensation of effort at lower work intensities; however, at 80% $\dot{V}O_2$max, the sensation of effort was lessened during alkalosis. Subsequently, Swank and Robertson (1989) found that alkalosis attenuated the sensation of effort of the legs, chest, and whole body during intermittent cycling exercise at 90% $\dot{V}O_2$max. Robertson et al. (1986) suggested that the decrease in extracellular [H^+] would result in a greater force-generating capacity in the muscle, possibly reducing the sensation of effort during the alkalotic state.

THE PHYSICOCHEMICAL CHANGES INDUCED BY NaHCO$_3$ LOADING

The main method of inducing alkalosis is to ingest gelatin capsules of NaHCO$_3$, usually with large quantities of fluid, over a 3-h period prior to exercising. Absorption of Na$^+$ into the plasma begins in the stomach as the acidic pH in the stomach dissolves the gelatin capsule. As the gastric fluid becomes neutral or alkalotic, some Na$^+$

is reabsorbed into the blood via active transport; however, the major site of Na^+ absorption is the small intestine. In addition to increasing plasma $[Na^+]$, the transfer of Na^+ leaves the gut relatively acid, leading to an increase of gut PCO_2 and to a diffusion of CO_2 into plasma; the net effect is an increase in plasma $[HCO_3^-]$ and a fall in $[H^+]$ (Feldman et al., 1984). In all the studies which used $NaHCO_3$ to induce alkalosis, a decrease in plasma $[H^+]$ and an increase in plasma $[HCO_3^-]$ relative to control conditions were observed. These changes have generally been assumed to be directly caused by the ingestion of $[HCO_3^-]$; however, as Stewart has emphasized (1981, 1983), several systems and fundamental laws govern $[H^+]$ and $[HCO_3^-]$ in aqueous solutions such as plasma and the cytosol of muscle; these considerations lead to the inference that plasma $[HCO_3^-]$ cannot be the result of HCO_3^- absorption by itself.

Strong electrolytes such as Na^+, K^+, Cl^- and La^-, which are completely or almost completely dissociated in solution, influence $[H^+]$ and $[HCO_3^-]$ through a strong ion difference (SID). The SID is the sum of all the strong-base cation concentrations (Eq/L) minus the sum of all the strong-acid anion concentrations. In biological solutions, the SID is almost always positive; to maintain electrical neutrality, the SID charge must be counterbalanced by the net negative charge contributed by $[OH^-]$ and $[H_+]$. This is illustrated by the following equation:

$$SID - [OH^-] + [H^+] = 0$$

Under a given set of conditions, the ion product of water, K'_w, is a constant, i.e., $[H^+] \times [OH^-] = K'_w$. Accordingly, if $[OH^-]$ increases to counteract a greater SID, $[H^+]$ must decrease; if SID decreases, $[H^+]$ must increase. Thus, the SID is a powerful determinant of $[H^+]$.

Weak electrolytes that are partially dissociated at physiological $[H^+]$ exert their influence through their total anion charge (A_{tot}) and their pKa. In plasma, the major weak electrolytes are plasma proteins; in muscle, they are proteins and phosphates. Carbon dioxide, through its interaction with water, also determines the concentration of $[H^+]$ and $[HCO_3^-]$. Thus, in this context, $[H^+]$ and $[HCO_3^-]$ are dependent variables and can change only through changes in PCO_2, SID and $[A_{tot}]$. Exchanges of $[H^+]$ and $[HCO_3^-]$ between body fluid compartments occur primarily through exchanges of strong ions and the movement of CO_2 down its partial pressure gradient by diffusion. Because of their large size and electrical charge, only minor exchanges of weak electrolytes occur between fluid compartments. Thus, during $NaHCO_3$ ingestion, changes in HCO_3^- will result mainly from increases in $[Na^+]$ and reductions in $[Cl^-]$ consequent to Cl^- excretion in urine with Na^+.

No data have been published regarding the physicochemical changes that occur in plasma and muscle following NaHCO$_3$ loading. Our laboratory has just completed a study to ascertain these changes in plasma following ingestion of 0.3 g of NaHCO$_3$/kg for 3 h prior to exercise (Figure 5-1). The [H$^+$] in arterial plasma decreases by 6 nEq/L, and the arterial plasma [HCO$_3^-$] increases by 7 mEq/L. The independent variables that determine the changes in [H$^+$] and [HCO$_3^-$] in plasma were also measured; no changes were observed in PCO$_2$ and [A$_{tot}$] (plasma proteins), but SID increased by 6.5 mEq/L. The increased SID of the arterial plasma was associated with a significant decrease in [Cl$^-$] and [K$^+$] by 7.0 and 0.5 mEq/L, respectively, with no change in [Na$^+$]. We conclude that the increase in [HCO$_3^-$] and decrease in [H$^+$] observed with oral ingestion of NaHCO$_3$ are not directly related to the addition of HCO$_3^-$ to the plasma, but rather to the resultant decrease in plasma [Cl$^-$].

The capsules of NaHCO$_3$ are taken over an 3-h period with large quantities of water (up to 1.5 L). This acute Na$^+$ and extracellular

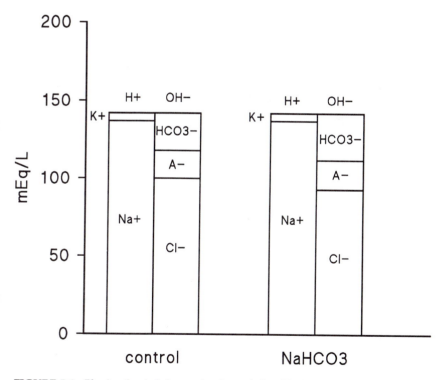

FIGURE 5-1. *Physico-chemical changes in plasma induced by ingestion of 0.3 g NaHCO$_3$/ kg body weight.*

volume overload results in natriuresis to precisely regulate extracellular fluid volume (Ballerman & Brenner, 1985; Bourgoignie et al., 1981). Since Na^+ transport into plasma along the nephron is electroneutral and driven by the Na^+/K^+ ATPase pump, chloride will remain in the renal tubule along with the sodium. The net effect is a precise regulation of arterial plasma $[Na^+]$ and extracellular fluid volume and a net loss of Cl^- from the plasma.

It is not known whether $NaHCO_3$-induced physicochemical changes in arterial blood influence extracellular $[H^+]$ or $[HCO_3^-]$ in human skeletal muscle. According to the in vivo skeletal muscle studies (Adler et al., 1965a; Adler et al., 1965b; Burnell, 1968; Heisler, 1975; Heisler & Piiper, 1972) that measured changes in intramuscular $[H^+]$ with induced extracellular metabolic alkalosis, intramuscular $[H^+]$ in human muscle would decrease by 18 nEq/L for every 9 nEq/L decrease in plasma $[H^+]$ induced by $NaHCO_3$ ingestion. These differences are explained by the different roles of PCO_2, SID, and A_{tot} in controlling H^+ in muscle and plasma (Figure 5-2).

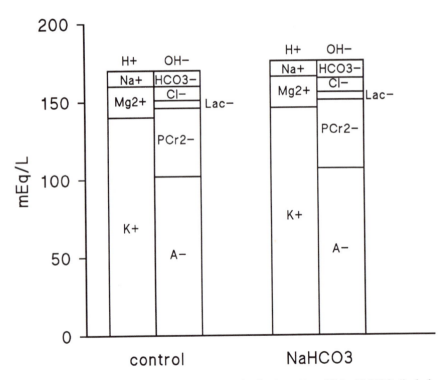

FIGURE 5-2. *Physico-chemical changes in muscle after ingestion of 0.3 g $NaHCO_3$/kg body weight.*

Based on the physicochemical properties, a reduction in intramuscular $[H^+]$ of this magnitude would be associated with an increase in intramuscular SID of 6 mEq/L, an increase in the dissociated form (A^-) of the $[A_{tot}]$ of 5 mEq/L, and an increase in intramuscular $[HCO_3^-]$ of 1 mEq/L. The increase in intramuscular SID can be accounted for by increases in intramuscular $[K^+]$ that occur with induced metabolic alkalosis either in vitro (Fenn & Cobb, 1934) or in vivo (Burnell et al., 1956).

The theoretical calculated changes which occur in intramuscular $[HCO_3^-]$ are consistent with data obtained with $NaHCO_3$ infusion in dogs (Burnell, 1968). In these studies, only a small percentage of the total HCO_3^- infused could be accounted for in the intracellular space, and the relatively small increase in intracellular $[HCO_3^-]$ has been attributed to the impermeability of the membrane to HCO_3^-. However, the changes in $[H^+]$ and $[HCO_3^-]$ in the plasma and muscle are not due to the impermeability of the muscle membrane to HCO_3^- but to the distribution of ions across the muscle membrane and the difference in physicochemical properties of each of these fluid compartments (Stewart, 1981).

Although recent studies of $NaHCO_3$ loading have focused on the effects of decreased intracellular $[H^+]$ and increased buffering on muscle performance, no attention has been paid to the potential effects of the physicochemical changes. Changes of strong ions in both plasma and muscle have long been known to be associated with fatigue processes in skeletal muscle (Boyle & Conway, 1941; Fenn, 1936). In order to maintain muscle function and force output, transmembrane ionic and chemical gradients must be maintained so as to maintain osmotic equilibration, membrane electrical potential, and acid-base homeostasis.

Recent studies (Kowalchuk et al., 1989) used sodium citrate rather than $NaHCO_3$ to induce alkalosis. They found no change in exercise performance compared to saline control following the same exercise protocol as the 1977 study of Jones and colleagues, despite similar changes in plasma $[H^+]$ and $[HCO_3^-]$. This suggests that the decreased $[H^+]$ and $[HCO_3^-]$ may not be the only relevant factors affecting muscle performance; the associated physicochemical changes induced by $NaHCO_3$ may also play a major part.

THE PHYSIOLOGICAL AND BIOCHEMICAL EFFECTS OF $NaHCO_3$ LOADING

The major emphasis of $NaHCO_3$ loading studies in humans has been to determine the $NaHCO_3$ effects on performance. Most studies have focused on the $[H^+]$ and $[HCO_3^-]$ induced in the plasma and on the changes that occur in [Lac⁻] in plasma, with little emphasis given to the biochemical or physiological mechanisms by which NaHCO₃ effects are exerted.

In all studies of alkalosis induced with NaHCO₃ ingestion, plasma or blood [Lac⁻] is higher during submaximal and maximal exercise compared with control conditions. The higher plasma [Lac⁻] observed following induced alkalosis could be due to enhanced glycolysis, increased Lac⁻ efflux from exercising muscle, or reduced uptake of Lac⁻ by other tissues.

Three human studies (Bouissou et al., 1988; Bouissou et al., 1989; Sutton et al., 1981) examined the effects of induced alkalosis on glycolysis and/or lactate accumulation in muscle. Bouissou et al. observed significantly greater Lac⁻ accumulation in muscle with alkalosis (32 mmol · kg⁻¹ wet weight) compared to control (17 mmol · kg⁻¹ wet weight); intramuscular [H⁺] was similar during both conditions, and the subjects exercised at 125% V̇O₂max. Sutton and colleagues exercised their subjects at 95% V̇O₂max; they found muscle [Lac⁻] concentrations were 14.7 and 17.1 mmol · kg⁻¹ wet weight during control and alkalosis conditions, respectively, with no differences in glycogen depletion between conditions, but this may be explained by the longer work duration in alkalosis. Even though these studies found increased [Lac⁻] in muscle and/or plasma, it is not possible to determine the effects of NaHCO₃ loading on glycolytic flux or lactate efflux from muscle.

Effects on Lactate Production

Spriet et al. (1986) studied the influence of extracellular metabolic alkalosis on metabolism and performance of perfused, isolated, rat hindlimb muscles during electrical stimulation by increasing [NaHCO₃] in the perfusate. This model serves as a closed metabolic system, enabling precise measurement of energy source utilization and of metabolites produced by muscle during electrical stimulation. No changes in initial tension development and fatigue were observed between control conditions and metabolic acidosis in this preparation. Compared to control, alkalosis had no significant effect on muscle glycogen utilization or total lactate production. However, despite the similar production of [Lac⁻] in the two conditions, there was a greater efflux and lower accumulation of [Lac⁻] in the muscle during alkalosis.

Effects on Lactate Efflux From Muscle

A positive relationship between extracellular [HCO₃⁻] and the efflux of [Lac⁻] from exercising muscle has been observed in isolated in situ muscles of dogs (Hirche et al., 1975; Steinhagen et al., 1976), in frog sartorius muscle (Mainwood et al., 1972; Mainwood & Lucier, 1972; Mainwood & Worsley-Brown, 1975; Seo, 1984), in isolated rat diaphragm (Mainwood & Cechetto, 1980), and in an isolated perfused rat hindlimb preparation (Spriet et al., 1985). These investigators attributed the increased efflux of [Lac$^-$] from exercising muscle to the increases in extracellular [HCO$_3^-$]. The influence of similar degrees of respiratory (decreased PCO$_2$) and metabolic (increased SID) alkalosis on the lactate efflux has been studied in the stimulated, isolated, perfused rat hindlimb preparation (Lindinger et al., 1990; Spriet et al., 1986). In these studies, compared to control, both alkalotic conditions increased Lac$^-$ efflux, but the effect was more pronounced during metabolic alkalosis than during respiratory alkalosis (Figure 5-3). Compared to control conditions, the Lac$^-$ efflux from muscle was increased by 0.21 uEq$\cdot$min$^{-1}\cdot$g^{-1} for a 10 nEq$\cdot$L decrease in perfusion [H$^+$] associated with respiratory alkalosis. During metabolic alkalosis for the same decrease in perfusion [H$^+$], a greater augmentation of lactate efflux was observed (0.475 uEq$\cdot$min$^{-1}\cdot$g^{-1}). These studies suggested that changes in extracellular strong ions exert a greater influence on [Lac$^-$] efflux than do changes in PCO$_2$. Although the previous studies (Hirche et al., 1975;

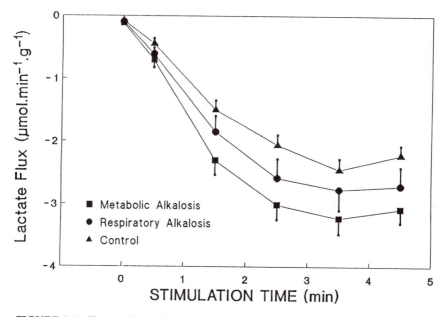

FIGURE 5-3. *The net efflux of lactate from perfused, isolated, rat hindlimb during 5 min of electrical stimulation under control, respiratory alkalosis, and metabolic alkalosis conditions.*

Mainwood & Worsley-Brown, 1975; Seo, 1984) have attributed the difference in Lac$^-$ efflux to differences in extracellular [HCO$_3^-$] acting directly, it seems possible that the strong ions that determine extracellular [HCO$_3^-$] and [H$^+$] may also influence Lac$^-$ efflux from exercising muscle.

The Lac$^-$ efflux across muscle membrane may be a process of simple or carrier-mediated diffusion (Juel, 1988a; Mason & Thomas, 1988; Putnam et al., 1986; Seo, 1984; Watt et al., 1988). The carrier-mediated diffusion of Lac$^-$ appears to be the predominant mechanism (Juel, 1988a; Mason & Thomas, 1988). Juel (1988a) suggested that approximately one-third of the total Lac$^-$ efflux can be accounted for by simple diffusion and the remainder is carrier-mediated. There is disagreement as to whether the carrier-mediated mechanism involves only an anionic monocarboxylate carrier (Juel, 1988a; Mason & Thomas, 1988) or also an anionic exchange mechanism (Putnam et al., 1986). The diffusion of Lac$^-$, whether through anionic channels (Woodbury & Miles, 1973) or through anionic channels plus the anionic monocarboxylate carrier mechanism (Mason & Thomas, 1988), appears to be inhibited by increasing [H$^+$] (Hutter & Warner, 1967). The anionic channel-mediated mechanism appears to be sensitive to changes in extra- and intracellular [Cl$^-$] and [Na$^+$]. Thus, the increased Lac$^-$ efflux during alkalosis in both animal and human studies may be accounted for by the direct effects of [H$^+$] on both transport mechanisms. However, the metabolic alkalosis induced by the changes in strong ions, i.e., Na$^+$ and Cl$^-$, may also increase Lac$^-$ efflux.

Effect of Potassium Homeostasis on Muscle Function

During high intensity exercise, with large accumulations of [Lac$^-$] and large depletions of phosphocreatine in contracting muscle, the efflux of [Lac$^-$] from the muscle is accompanied by a large efflux of K$^+$ and small influxes of Na$^+$, Cl$^-$, and water (Hermansen et al., 1984; Kowalchuk et al., 1988; Lindinger et al., 1987; Lindinger & Heigenhauser, 1988; Sjogaard, 1986; Sjogaard et al., 1985; Sjogaard & Saltin, 1982; Sreter, 1963). The large efflux of K$^+$ from muscle may be involved in maintaining intracellular osmolality and cell volume (Lauf, 1987) or may be important in maintaining intracellular ATP concentration (Castle & Haylett, 1987; Spruce et al., 1985). In addition, the large drop in intracellular [K$^+$] and the accumulation of [Lac$^-$] contribute equally to the decrease in the intracellular SID, resulting in an increased intracellular [H$^+$] (Kowalchuk et al., 1988; Lindinger & Heigenhauser, 1988).

There are several mechanisms by which an elevated extracellular [K$^+$] ([K$^+$]$_e$) and lower intracellular [K$^+$] ([K$^+$]$_i$) may be related to the fatigue process during heavy exercise. The observed increase in $[K^+]_e/[K^+]_i$ may inhibit excitation-contraction coupling and thus reduce the muscle's ability to produce tension. The increased $[K^+]_e/[K^+]_i$ reduces the resting membrane potential (Hodgkin & Horowicz, 1959), thus inactivating the fast inward Na^+ channels. This will lead to a lower amplitude of the action potential (Juel, 1986; Juel, 1988b). In addition, the lower $[K^+]_e/[K^+]_i$ will reduce the velocity of propagation of the action potential to the transverse tubule (Bigland-Ritchie et al., 1981). Both effects will lead to a smaller release of Ca^{++} from the sarcoplasmic reticulum. Increases in $[K^+]_e$ may result in reflex inhibition of motor neuron firing rates (Woods et al., 1987).

Compared to control, both respiratory (decreased PCO_2) and metabolic (increased SID) alkalotic conditions increased Lac^- efflux, decreased K^+ efflux, and reduced the increase in intracellular muscle water volume during stimulation in an isolated rat hindlimb preparation (Lindinger et al., 1990). Despite the same induced changes in plasma $[H^+]$, these decreases in potassium efflux were more pronounced during metabolic than respiratory alkalosis (Figure 5-4). The alkalosis induced by changes in plasma SID results in a greater ability of the muscle to maintain K^+, minimize increases in intracellular

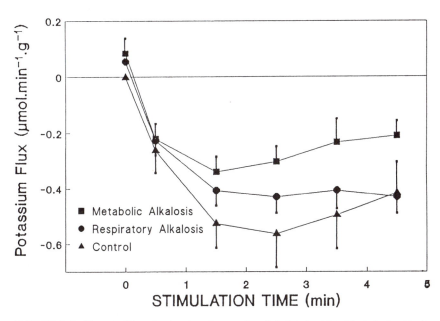

FIGURE 5-4. *The net efflux of potassium from perfused, isolated rat hindlimb during 5 min of electrical stimulation under control, respiratory alkalosis, and metabolic alkalosis conditions.*

[H^+], and maintain osmotic equilibrium across the muscle membrane. Thus, by decreasing K^+ efflux from exercising muscle, the ionic environment augments the effects of the decrease in extracellular [H^+] on the ability of muscle to maintain homeostasis.

Bouissou and colleagues (1989), in their study of humans, showed that intracellular [H^+] during alkalosis was similar to that during control conditions, but was accompanied by almost twice the accumulation of Lac^-. This suggests that the muscle's ability to maintain intracellular SID during alkalosis was enhanced. Based on the perfusion studies of Lindinger et al. (1990), a decrease in K^+ efflux from the muscle could explain the superior maintenance of intracellular [H^+] in the study of Bouissou et al. (1989). Thus, the ability to improve performance during heavy exercise may be related either to a lower intracellular [H^+] due to a higher intracellular [K^+] or to maintenance of the ratio of intracellular:extracellular potassium concentrations during alkalosis. In addition, the lower efflux of K^+ from muscle would result in a reduced stimulation of K^+ sensitive sensory nerve endings, leading to the lower perceived effort observed during alkalotic conditions (Robertson et al., 1986; Swank & Robertson, 1989).

Effects of Chloride on Muscle Function

The role of Cl^- in muscle function is controversial (Bretag, 1987). Exchange of Cl^- across the cell membrane plays an important role in [H^+] regulation in muscle (Aickin & Thomas, 1977). The muscle membrane has a high conductance for Cl^-, and the greatest part of this conductance is localized in the T-tubular system (Dulhunty, 1979). Because conductance of Cl^- and K^+ is high in the T-tubule, these ions are major determinants of the excitability of the T-tubule (Hodgkin & Horowicz, 1959). Reduction of extracellular [Cl^-] hyperpolarizes the muscle membrane (Dulhunty, 1979; Dulhunty, 1982; Aickin et al., 1989). Thus, in alkalosis, the lower extracellular [Cl^-], coupled with the lower [K^+]$_e$/[K^+]$_i$, would help to maintain membrane excitability in the T-tubule system.

In many of the in vivo studies that examined the influence of [H^+] or [HCO_3^-] on muscle function or lactate efflux, the results are difficult to interpret because other ions were commonly substituted for Cl^- to maintain osmotic pressure in the extracellular bathing media. In these studies, it was assumed that Cl^- was inert physiologically. However, Cl^- fluxes are important not only in acid-base homeostasis, but also in the maintenance of T-tubule excitability (Dulhunty, 1979). Caution must be exercised in interpreting the results of studies that used anion or cation substitutes for Cl^- to investigate other effects of [H^+] on muscle function; the effects of [H^+]

and [HCO_3^-] may be confused with those of Cl^- removal (Sharp & Thomas, 1981).

Two studies (Pannier et al., 1970; Renaud, 1989) used Lac^- substitution for Cl^- to examine the effect of extracellular [H^+] and [HCO_3^-] on muscle function. Muscle force was potentiated when Lac^- was substituted for Cl^-. In both studies, tension development was independent of both extracellular [H^+] and extracellular [HCO_3^-]. Although the mechanism by which Cl^- exerts its influence is unknown, it is apparent that consideration should be given to this when studying muscle function.

PRACTICAL IMPLICATIONS

Many substances used by athletes to enhance performance have been banned by athletic governing bodies such as International Olympic Committee and the Sport Medicine Council of Canada (1984). Although both laboratory and field studies have shown that alkalosis induced by $NaHCO_3$ ingestion significantly improved exercise performance that depends on glycolysis for ATP turnover, there is no ban on the use of $NaHCO_3$, and its use is difficult to detect. Although coaches and administrators of athletic teams are aware of the effects of ingesting $NaHCO_3$ to benefit althletic performance, the prevalence of its use is unknown. The use of any performance-enhancing agent clearly contravenes the current policies regarding doping.

Several authors (Gledhill, 1984; McKenzie, 1988; Wilkes et al., 1983) have suggested that it may be possible to detect and control the use of ingested $NaHCO_3$ by existing procedures, which include the collection of a urine specimen aerobically following the athletic event. In the studies performed by Wilkes and et al. (1983) and McKenzie (1988), $NaHCO_3$ (0.3 mg/kg) or a placebo were randomly assigned to subjects prior to running 800 m. Following the run, urine samples were collected aerobically, and urinary pH was determined. In both studies, urinary pH was significantly higher in those who had ingested $NaHCO_3$. In McKenzie's detailed study of 65 subjects, there was little overlap in the level of urinary pH between the two groups of subjects. No one who had ingested $NaHCO_3$ had a urinary pH of less than 6.8, whereas no one taking the placebo had a value greater than 7.0. McKenzie advocated using a urinary pH of 7.0 as an indicator of the use of $NaHCO_3$ loading; this would have detected 92% of the subjects who had done so in his study.

Generally, urine pH is acidic, but it can range from 4.5 to 8.2. Even though urinary pH in McKenzie's study (1988) suggested that a pH of 7.0 could be used as an indicator of $NaHCO_3$ loading, other factors can make the urine alkalotic and give a false positive test result (for review, see Charney & Feldman, 1989). These factors include vomiting, a vegetarian diet, a high carbohydrate diet, urinary infection, and a low glomerular filtration rate (Kiil, 1990). Thus, it would be almost impossible to detect confidently those who had loaded with $NaHCO_3$ for athletic competition.

It also appears that $NaHCO_3$ loading does not have any long-term side effects. In most of the studies cited, several subjects reported acute gastrointestinal distress such as nausea, diarrhea, and bloating. Taking the $NaHCO_3$ with a large amount of liquid will reduce these symptoms. If the $NaHCO_3$ enters the intestine as a hypotonic solution, most of it will be absorbed from the gut, with reduced adverse symptoms. In addition, we have found that greater alkalinization occurs with increased fluid intake.

Since ingestion of $NaHCO_3$ leads to a reduction in plasma $[K^+]$, cardiac arrhythmias could conceivably occur, but to date, there are no reported cardiac dysrhythmias with dosages up to 0.4 g/kg body weight, probably because plasma $[K^+]$ does not fall below 3 mEq/L.

CONSIDERATIONS FOR FUTURE RESEARCH

Even though field and laboratory studies have been conducted over the past 13 y, it may be that these results cannot be extrapolated to performance in elite athletes. It appears that a dose of 0.3 g $NaHCO_3$/kg body weight is necessary to have a beneficial effect on performance in high-intensity exercise of 1–7.5 min duration. However, the subjects of these studies were only moderately fit. In order to determine whether $NaHCO_3$-loading will enhance the performance of elite athletes, random double-blind trials should be conducted in this population. In addition, since glycolytic metabolism is important in exercise of up to 40 min duration (Jones et al., 1980), these trials should cover events lasting 45 s to 40 min.

It appears that the decreases in $[H^+]$ and $[HCO_3^-]$ in the plasma may not be the major contributors to the improved performance observed with $NaHCO_3$ loading but that changes which occur in fluid and strong ions in the intra- and extracellular fluid compartment may be of more importance. Studies should be conducted using a variety of alkalizing agents to ascertain the changes that occur in the physicochemical properties of both plasma and muscle and the subsequent effects on performance.

Previous studies conducted to determine the effects of $[HCO_3^-]$ and $[H^+]$ on muscle performance and their physiological and biological effects paid little attention to the alterations in independent variables by which these changes were brought about. The physicochemical characteristics of the extracellular fluid in the previous studies are not known. Thus, in future studies it will be important to establish the mechanism(s) by which $NaHCO_3^-$ exerts its effects in vivo and in vitro and, where possible, to obtain measurements of lactate and other strong ions (Na^+, K^+ and Cl^-) in plasma, muscle, and urine.

ACKNOWLEDGEMENTS

This work was funded by the Medical Research Council of Canada and the Heart and Stroke Foundation of Ontario. The research work of many graduate students, including J.M. Kowalchuk, M.I. Lindinger, N. McCartney, R.S. McKelvie, and L.L. Spriet provided major contributions to our understanding of acid-base homeostasis during exercise. Finally, we wish to thank R.B. Kreider, M. McKenna, and J.R. Sutton for their suggestions that improved this manuscript.

BIBLIOGRAPHY

Adler, S., A. Roy, and A.S. Relman (1965a). Intracellular acid-base regulation. I. The response of muscle cells to changes in CO_2 tension or extracellular bicarbonate concentration. *J. Clin. Invest.* 44:8–19.

Adler, S., A. Roy, and A.S. Relman (1965b). Intracellular acid-base regulation. II. The interaction between CO_2-tension and extracellular bicarbonate in the determination of muscle cell pH. *J. Clin. Invest.* 44:20–29.

Aickin, C.C., W.J. Betz, and G.L. Harris (1989). Intracellular chloride and the mechanism for its accumulation in rat lumbrical muscle. *J. Physiol. London* 411:437–455.

Aickin, C.C., and R.C. Thomas (1977). An investigation of the ionic mechanism of intracellular pH regulation in mouse soleus muscle fibres. *J. Physiol. London* 273:295–316.

Asmussen, E., W. Van Dobelin, and M. Nielson (1948). Blood lactate and oxygen debt after exhaustive work at different oxygen tensions. *Acta Physiol. Scand.* 15:57–62.

Ballerman, B.J. and B.M. Brenner (1985). Biologically active atrial peptides. *J. Clin. Invest.* 76:2041–2048.

Barr, D.P., H.E. Himwich, and R.P. Green (1923). Studies in the physiology of muscular exercise. I. Changes in acid-base equilibrium following short periods of vigorous muscular exercise. *J. Biol. Chem.* 55:495–523.

Bernard, C. (1859). De la matiere glycogene consideree comme condition de developpement de certains tissus, chez la foetus, avant l'apparition de la fonction glycogenique de foie. In: *Lecons sur le diabete.* Paris: J.-B. Balliere, 1877. (Extrait de *Compte Rend. des Seancs de l'Acad. des Sci.* 48, 1859.)

Berzelius, J. (1848). *Jahres-Bericht uber die Fortschritte der Chemie und Mineralogie,* vol. 27.

Bigland-Ritchie, B., F. Donovan, and C.S. Roussos (1981). Conduction velocity and EMG power spectrum changes in fatigue of sustained maximal efforts. *J. Appl. Physiol.* 51:1300–1305.

Bouissou, P., G. Defer, C.Y. Guezennec, P.Y. Estrade, and B. Serrurier (1988). Metabolic and blood catecholamine responses to exercise during alkalosis. *Med. Sci. Sports Exerc.* 20:228–232.

Bouissou, P., P.Y. Estrade, F. Goubel, C.Y. Guezennec, and B. Serrurier (1989). Surface EMG power spectrum and intramuscular pH in human vastus lateralis muscle during dynamic exercise. *J. Appl. Physiol.* 67: 1245–1249.

Bourgoignie, J.J., A.I. Jacob, A.L. Sallman, and J.P. Pennell (1981). Water, electrolyte and acid-base abnormalities in chronic renal failure. *Sem. Nephrol.* 1:91–111.

Boyle, P.J., and E.J. Conway (1941). Potassium accumulation in muscle and associated changes. *J. Physiol. London* 100:1–63.

Bretag, A.H. (1987). Muscle chloride channels. *Physiol. Rev.* 67: 618–724.

Burnell, J.M. (1968). In vivo response of muscle to changes in CO_2 tension or extracellular bicarbonate. *Am. J. Physiol.* 215:1376–1383.

Burnell, J.M., M.F. Vallamil, B.T. Uyeno, and B.H. Scribner (1956). The effect in humans of extracellular pH change on the relationship between serum potassium concentration and intracellular potassium. *J. Clin. Invest.* 35:935–939.

Cafarelli, E. (1977). Peripheral and central inputs to effort sense during cycling exercise. *Eur. J. Appl. Physiol. Occup. Physiol.* 37: 181–189.

Cafarelli, E., W.S. Cain, and J.C. Stevens (1977). Effort of dynamic exercise: influence of load, duration and task. *Ergonomics* 20: 147–158.

Castle, N.A., and D.G. Haylett (1987). Effect of channel blockers on potassium efflux from metabolically exhausted frog skeletal muscle. *J. Physiol. London* 383:31–43.

Charney, A.N., and G.M. Feldman (1989). Internal exchanges of hydrogen ions: gastrointestinal tract. In: D.W. Seldin and G. Giebisch (eds.) *The Regulation of Acid-Base Balance*. New York: Raven Press, pp. 89–105.

Chasiotis, D. (1983). The regulation of glycogen phosphorylase and glycogen breakdown in human skeletal muscle. *Acta Physiol. Scand. Suppl.* 518: 1–68.

Chasiotis, D., E. Hultman, and K. Sahlin (1983). Acidotic depression of cyclic AMP accumulation and phosphorylase *b* to *a* transformation in skeletal muscle of man. *J. Physiol. London* 335:197–204.

Cooke, R., K. Franks, G.B. Luciani, and E. Pate (1988). The inhibition of rabbit skeletal muscle contraction by hydrogen ions and phosphate. *J. Physiol. London* 395:77–97.

Costill, D.L., F. Verstappen, H. Kuipers, E. Jansson, and W. Fink (1984). Acid-base balance during repeated bouts of exercise: influence of HCO_3^-. *Int. J. Sports Med.* 5:228–231.

Danforth, W.H. (1965). Activation of glycolytic pathway in muscle. In: B. Chance, R.W. Estabrook, and J.R. Williamson (eds.) *Control of Energy Metabolism*. London: Academic Press, pp. 287–297.

Dawson, M.J., D.G. Gadian, and D.R. Wilkie (1978). Muscular fatigue investigated by phosphorus nuclear magnetic resonance. *Nature* 274:861–865.

De Luca, C. (1984). Myoelectrical manifestations of localized muscular fatigue in humans. *CRC Crit. Rev. Biomed. Eng.* 11:251–279.

Dennig, H., J.T. Talbott, H.T. Edwards, and D.B. Dill (1931). Effect of acidosis and alkalosis upon capacity for work. *J. Clin. Invest.* 9: 601–613.

Dobson, G.B., Y. Etsuo, and P.W. Hochachka (1986). Phosphofructokinase control in muscle: nature and reversal of pH-dependent ATP inhibition. *Am. J. Physiol.* 250:R71-R76.

Donaldson, S.K.B., L. Hermansen, and L. Bolles (1978). Differential direct effects of H^+ on Ca^{2+}-activated force of skinned fibers from the soleus, cardiac and adductor magnus muscles of rabbits. *Pfluegers Arch.* 376:55–65.

DuBois-Reymond, E. (1849). Cited in Lieben, F. (1935). *Geschichte der physiologischen Chemie*. Leipzig and Wien: Franz Duticke.

Dulhunty, A.F. (1978). The dependence of membrane potential on extracellular chloride concentration in mammalian skeletal muscle. *J. Physiol. London* 276:67–82.

Dulhunty, A.F. (1979). Distribution of potassium and chloride permeability over the surface and t-tubule membranes of mammalian skeletal muscle. *J. Membrane Biol.* 45:293–310.

Dulhunty, A.F. (1982). Effects of membrane potential on mechanical activation in skeletal muscle. *J. Gen. Physiol.* 79:233–251.

Fabiato, A., and F. Fabiato (1978). Effects of pH on the myofilaments and the sarcoplasmic reticulum of skinned cells from cardiac and skeletal muscles. *J. Physiol. London* 276:233–255.

Feldman, G.M., M.A. Arnold, and A.N. Charney (1984). On the mechanism of luminal CO_2 generation during jejunal bicarbonate absorption. *Am. J. Physiol.* 246:G687-G694.

Fenn, W.O. (1936). Electrolytes in muscle. *Physiol. Rev.* 16:450–487.

Fenn, W.O., and D.M. Cobb (1934). The potassium equilibrium in muscle. *J. Gen. Physiol.* 17:629–656.

Fuchs, F., Y. Reddy, and F.N. Briggs (1970). The interaction of cations with the calcium-binding site of troponin. *Biochim. Biophys. Acta* 221:407–409.

Gledhill, N. (1984). Bicarbonate ingestion and anaerobic performance. *Sports Med.* 1:177–180.

Goldfinch, J., L. McNaughton, and P. Davies (1988). Induced metabolic alkalosis and its effects on 400-m racing time. *Eur. J. Appl. Physiol.* 57:45–48.

Heisler, N. (1975). Intracellular pH of isolated rat diaphragm muscle with metabolic and respiratory changes of extracellular pH. *Respir. Physiol.* 23:243–255.

Heisler, N., and J. Piiper (1972). Determination of intracellular buffering properties in rat diaphragm muscle. *Am. J. Physiol.* 222:747–753.

Hermansen, L., and J.B. Osnes (1972). Blood and muscle pH after maximal exercise in man. *J. Appl. Physiol.* 32:304–308.

Hermansen, L., A. Orheim, and O. Sejersted (1984). Metabolic acidosis and changes in water and electrolyte balance in relation to fatigue during maximal exercise of short duration. *Int. J. Sports Med.* 5 (Suppl.):110–115.

Hill, A.V. and H. Lupton (1923). Muscular exercise, lactic acid and the supply and utilization of oxygen. *Quart. J. Med.* 16:135–171.

Hirche, H., V. Hornbach, H.D. Langohr, U. Wacher, and J. Busse (1975). Lactic acid permeation rate in working gastrocnemii of dogs during metabolic alkalosis and acidosis. *Pfluegers Arch.* 356:209–222.

Hodgkin, A.L., and P. Horowicz (1959). Movements of Na and K in single muscle fibres. *J. Physiol. London* 145:405–432.

Horswill, C.A., D.L. Costill, W.J. Fink, M.G. Flynn, J.P. Kirwan, J.B. Mitchell, and J.A. Houmard (1988). Influence of sodium bicarbonate on sprint performance: relationship to dosage. *Med. Sci. Sports Exerc.* 20:566–569.

Hutter, O.F., and A.E. Warner (1967). The pH sensitivity of the chloride conductance of frog skeletal muscle. *J. Physiol. London* 189:403–425.

Iwaoka, K., H. Hatta, Y. Atomi, and M. Miyashita (1988). Lactate, respiratory compensation thresholds and distance running performance in runners of both sexes. *Int. J. Sports Med.* 9:306–309.

Iwaoka, K., S. Okagawa, Y. Mutoh, and M. Miyashita (1989). Effects of bicarbonate ingestion on the respiratory compensation threshold and maximal exercise performance. *Jap. J. Physiol.* 39:255–265.

Jervell, O. (1928). Investigation of the concentration of lactic acid in blood and urine. *Acta Med. Scand.* 24 (Suppl.):1–135.

Johnson, W.R., and D.H. Black (1953). Comparison of effects of certain blood alkalinizers and glucose upon competitive endurance performance. *J. Appl. Physiol.* 5:577–578.

Jones, N.L., G.J.F. Heigenhauser, A. Kuksis, C.G. Matsos, J.R. Sutton, and C.J. Toews (1980). Fat metabolism in heavy exercise. *Clin. Sci.* 59:469–478.

Jones, N.L., J.R. Sutton, R. Taylor, and C.J. Toews (1977). Effect of pH on cardiorespiratory and metabolic responses to exercise. *J. Appl. Physiol.* 43:959–964.

Juel, C. (1986). Potassium and sodium shifts during in vitro isometric muscle contraction, and the time course of the ion-gradient recovery. *Pfluegers Arch.* 406:458–463.

Juel, C. (1988a). Intracellular pH recovery and lactate efflux in mouse soleus muscles stimulated in vitro: the involvement of sodium/proton exchange and a lactate carrier. *Acta Physiol. Scand.* 132:363–371.

Juel, C. (1988b). Muscle action potential propagation velocity changes during activity. *Muscle Nerve* 11:714–719.

Katz, A., D.L. Costill, D.S. King, M. Hargreaves, and W.J. Fink (1984). Maximal exercise tolerance after induced alkalosis. *Int. J. Sports Med.* 5:107–110.

Kiil, F. (1990). The paradox of renal bicarbonate reabsorption. *News Physiol. Sci.* 5:13–17.

Kindermann, W., J. Keul, and G. Huber (1977). Physical exercise after induced alkalosis (bicarbonate or tris-buffer). *Eur. J. Appl. Physiol.* 37:197–204.

Kostka, C.E., and E. Cafarelli (1982). Effect of pH on sensation and vastus lateralis electromyogram during cycling exercise. *J. Appl. Physiol.* 52:1181–1185.

Kowalchuk, J.M., G.J.F. Heigenhauser, M.I. Lindinger, J.R. Sutton and N.L. Jones (1988). Factors influencing hydrogen ion concentration in muscle after intense exercise. *J. Appl. Physiol.* 65:2080–2089.

Kowalchuk, J.M., G.J.F. Heigenhauser, and N.L. Jones (1984). Effect of pH on metabolic and cardiorespiratory responses during progressive exercise. *J. Appl. Physiol.* 57:1558–1563.

Kowalchuk, J.M., S.A. Maltais, K. Yamaji, and R.L. Hughson (1989). The effect of citrate loading on exercise performance, acid-base balance and metabolism. *Eur. J. Appl. Physiol.* 58:858–864.

Krebs, H. (1964). Gluconeogenesis. *Proc. R. Soc. London, Series B.* 159:545–564.

Lauf, P.K. (1987). Physiology and biophysics of chloride and cation cotransport. *Fed. Proc.* 46:2377–2394.

Lindinger, M.I., and G.J.F. Heigenhauser (1988). Skeletal muscle ion fluxes in the stimulated, perfused rat hindlimb. *Am. J. Physiol.* 254:R117-R126.

Lindinger, M.I., G.J.F. Heigenhauser, and L.L. Spriet (1987). Effects of intense swimming and tetanic electrical stimulation on skeletal muscle ions and metabolites. *J. Appl. Physiol.* 63:2331–2339.

Lindinger, M.I., G.J.F. Heigenhauser, and L.L. Spriet (1990). Effects of alkalosis on skeletal muscle lactate and ion fluxes. *Can. J. Physiol. Pharmacol.* 68: 820–829.

Mainwood, G.W., and D. Cechetto (1980). The effect of bicarbonate concentration on fatigue and recovery in isolated rat diaphragm. *Can. J. Physiol. Pharmacol.* 58:624–632.

Mainwood, G.W., and G.E. Lucier (1972). Fatigue and recovery in isolated frog sartorius muscles: the effects of bicarbonate concentration and associated potassium loss. *Can. J. Physiol. Pharmacol.* 50: 132–142.

Mainwood, G.W., and P. Worsley-Brown (1975). The effects of extracellular pH and buffer concentration on the efflux of lactate from frog sartorius muscle. *J. Physiol. London* 250:1–22.

Mainwood, G.W., P. Worsley-Brown, and R.A. Patterson (1972). The metabolic changes in frog sartorius muscles during recovery from fatigue at different external bicarbonate concentrations. *Can. J. Physiol. Pharmacol.* 50:143–155.

Margaria, R., H.T. Edwards, and D.B. Dill (1933). The possible mechanisms of contracting and paying the oxygen debt and the role of lactic acid in muscular contraction. *Am. J. Physiol.* 106:689–715.

Mason, M.J., and R.C. Thomas (1988). A microelectrode study of the mechanisms of L-lactate entry into and release from frog sartorius muscle. *J. Physiol. London* 400:459–479.

McCartney, N., G.J.F. Heigenhauser, and N.L. Jones (1983). Effects of pH on maximal power output and fatigue during short-term dynamic exercise. *J Appl. Physiol.* 55:225–229.

McCartney, N., L.L. Spriet, G.J.F. Heigenhauser, J.M. Kowalchuk, J.R. Sutton and N.L. Jones (1985). Muscle power and metabolism in maximal intermittent exercise. *J. Appl. Physiol.* 60:1164–1169.

McKenzie,D.C. (1988). Changes in urinary pH following bicarbonate loading. *Can. J. Sports Sci.* 13: 254–256.

McKenzie, D.C., K.D. Coutts, D.R. Stirling, H.H. Hoeben, and G. Kuzara (1986). Maximal work production following two levels of artificially induced metabolic alkalosis. *J. Sport Sci.* 4:35–38.

Meyerhof, O. (1920a). Ueber die Beziehung des Milchsaure zur Warmebildung und Arbeitsleistung des Muskels in der Anaerobiose. *Pfluegers Arch.* 182:232.

Meyerhof, O. (1920b). Kohlehydrat- und Milchsaure-umsatz im Froschmuskel. *Pfluegers Arch.* 185:11.

Nakamaru, Y., and A. Schwartz (1972). The influence of hydrogen ion concentration on calcium binding and release by skeletal muscle sarcoplasmic reticulum. *J. Gen. Physiol.* 59:22–32.

Nasse, O. (1877). Bemerkungen zur Physiologie der Kohlehydrate. *Pfluegers Arch.* 14:473.

Nosek, T.M., K.Y. Fender, and R.E. Godt (1987). It is diprotonated inorganic phosphate that depresses force in skinned skeletal muscle fibers. *Science* 236:191–193.

Pannier, J., J. Weyne, and I. Leusen (1970). Effects of pCO_2, bicarbonate and lactate on the isometric contraction of isolated soleus muscle of the rat. *Pfluegers Arch.* 320:120–131.

Parnas, J.K. and R. Wagner (1914). Ueber den Kohlehydratumsatz isolierber Amphibienmuskelin und uber die Beziehungen zwischen Kohlehydratschwund und Milchsaurebildung im Muskel. *Biochem. Z.* 61:387.

Parry-Billings, M. and D.P.M. MacLaren (1986). The effect of sodium bicarbonate and sodium citrate ingestion on anaerobic power during intermittent exercise. *Eur. J. Appl. Physiol.* 55: 524–529.

Putnam, R.W., A. Roos, and T.J. Wilding (1986). Properties of the intracellular pH-regulating systems of frog skeletal muscle. *J. Physiol. London* 381:205–219.

Ranke, J. (1865). *Tetanus*. Leipzig: Engelmann.

Renaud, J.M. (1989). The effect of lactate on intracellular pH and force recovery of fatigued sartorius muscles of the frog, rana pipiens. *J. Physiol. London* 416:31–47.

Robertson, R.J., J.E. Falkel, A.L. Drash, A.M. Swank, K.F. Metz, S.A. Spungen, and J.R. LeBoeuf (1986). Effect of blood pH on peripheral and central signals of perceived exertion. *Med. Sci. Sports Exerc.* 18:114–122.

Seo, Y. (1984). Effects of extracellular pH on lactate efflux from frog sartorius muscle. *Am. J. Physiol.* 247:C175–C181.

Sharp, A.P. and R.C. Thomas (1981). The effects of chloride substitution on intracellular pH in crab muscle. *J. Physiol. London* 312:71–80.

Sjogaard, G. (1986). Water and electrolytes during exercise and their relation to muscle fatigue. *Acta Physiol. Scand.* 128 (Suppl. 556):129–136.

Sjogaard, G., R.P. Adams, and B. Saltin (1985). Water and ion shifts in skeletal muscle of humans with intense dynamic knee extension. *Am. J. Physiol.* 248:R190-R196.

Sjogaard, G., and B. Saltin (1982). Extra- and intracellular water spaces in muscle of man at rest and with dynamic exercise. *Am. J. Physiol.* 243:R271-R280.

Sport Medicine Council of Canada (1984). *Doping Control: Educational Presentation*. Ottawa: Government of Canada, Fitness and Amateur Sport.

Spriet, L.L., M.I. Lindinger, G.J.F. Heigenhauser, and N.L. Jones (1986). Effects of alkalosis on skeletal muscle metabolism and performance during exercise. *Am. J. Physiol.* 251: R833-R839.

Spriet, L.L., M.I. Lindinger, R.S. McKelvie, G.J.F. Heigenhauser, and N.L. Jones (1989). Muscle glycogenolysis and H^+ concentration during maximal intermittent cycling. *J. Appl. Physiol.* 66:8–13.

Spriet, L.L., C.G. Matsos, S.J. Peters, G.J.F. Heigenhauser, and N.L. Jones (1985). Effects of acidosis on rat muscle metabolism and performanace during heavy exercise. *Am. J. Physiol.* 248:C337-C347.

Spriet, L.L., K. Soderlund, M. Bergstrom, and E. Hultman (1987). Skeletal muscle glycogenolysis, glycolysis, and pH during electrical stimulation in men. *J. Appl. Physiol.* 62: 616–621.

Spruce, A.E., N.B. Standen, and P.R. Stanfield (1985). Voltage-dependent ATP-sensitive potassium channels of skeletal muscle membrane. *Nature London* 316:736–738.

Sreter, F.A. (1963). Cell water, sodium, and potassium in stimulated red and white mammalian muscles. *Am. J. Physiol.* 205:1295–1298.

Steinhagen, C., H.J. Hirche, H.W. Nestle, U. Bovenkamp, and I. Hosselmann (1976). The interstitial pH of the working gastrocnemius muscle of the dog. *Pfluegers Arch.* 367:151–156.

Stewart, P.A. (1981). *How to Understand Acid-Base: A Quantitative Acid-Base Primer for Biology and Medicine.* New York: Elsevier-North Holland.

Stewart, P.A. (1983). Modern quantitative acid-base chemistry. *Can. J. Physiol. Pharmacol.* 61:1444–1461.

Sutton, J.R., N.L. Jones, and C.J. Toews (1976). Growth hormone secretion in acid-base alterations at rest and during exercise. *Clin. Sci.* 50: 241–247.

Sutton, J.R., N.L. Jones, and C.J. Toews (1981). Effect of pH on muscle glycolysis during exercise. *Clin. Sci.* 61:331–338.

Swank, A., and R.J. Robertson (1989). Effect of induced alkalosis on perception of exertion during intermittent exercise. *J. Appl. Physiol.* 67:1862–1867.

Trivedi, B., and W.H. Danforth (1966). Effect of pH on the kinetics of frog muscle phosphofructokinase. *J. Biol. Chem.* 241:4110–4112.

Watt, P.W., P.A. MacLennan, H.S. Hundal, C.M. Kuret, and M.J. Rennie (1988). L(+)-lactate transport in perfused rat skeletal muscle: kinetic characteristics and sensitivity to pH and transport inhibitors. *Biochim. Biophys. Acta* 944:213–222.

Wijnen, S., F. Verstappen, and H. Kuipers (1984). The influence of intravenous NaHCO$_3^-$ administration on interval exercise: acid-base balance and endurance. *Int. J. Sports Med.* 5:130–132.

Wilkes, D., N. Gledhill, and R. Smyth (1983). Effect of acute induced metabolic acidosis on 800-m racing time. *Med. Sci. Sports Exerc.* 15:277–280.

Wilson, J.R., K.K. McCully, D.M. Mancini, B. Boden, and B. Chance (1988). Relationship of muscular fatigue to pH and diprotonated Pi in humans: a P-NMR study. *J. Appl. Physiol.* 64:2333–2339.

Woodbury, J.W., and P.R. Miles (1973). Anion conductance of frog muscle membranes: one channel, two kinds of pH dependence. *J. Gen. Physiol.* 62:324–353.

Woods, J.J., F. Furbusch, and B. Bigland-Ritchie (1987). Evidence for a fatigue-induced reflex inhibition of motoneuron firing rates. *J. Neurophysiol.* 58:125–137.

DISCUSSION

COSTILL: Our experience is that a very large amount of sodium citrate must be consumed to induce any of the changes seen with a much smaller dosage of sodium bicarbonate.

HEIGENHAUSER: I agree with you.

COSTILL: Do you know of any studies that have been successful in producing performance advantages using sodium citrate?

HEIGENHAUSER: I don't. Some studies have, unfortunately, used sodium chloride as a placebo; I don't think sodium chloride is a valid placebo because it results in a diuresis with a loss in the urine of both sodium and chloride. But a little bit more of the sodium than chloride is lost in the urine, and the subjects end up being slightly acidotic.

SPRIET: Given the gastrointestinal problems, how practical is it to use bicarbonate loading in athletics?

HEIGENHAUSER: If capsules are used, they must dissolve in the stomach. Capsules that dissolve in the small intestine will create problems. Also, enough water has to be ingested to assure that the sodium bicarbonate hits the intestines in an isotonic state. If it is hypertonic, adverse effects will result. I think slow infusion is the best way, to tell you the truth.

ROBERTSON: In our experiments, we had no problem at all. We found that the administration of the capsules is best accomplished 2 h before exercise. Most of the previous studies used 3 h, and I'm not sure why, unless that happens to be the time course of the peak shift in pH following administration of ammonium chloride, which was the reciprocal treatment in the early paradigms.

We found that the peak alkalotic shift in pH came 2 h prior to the exercise performance. We gave all of the capsules within a 15 min period and had no diarrhea problem. Many of the studies have spread the bicarbonate ingestion out, almost right up until performance was initiated. I think there may have been problems with that. Furthermore, the peak alkalotic shift probably occurred in many of these studies well into the exercise or even after the exercise was concluded.

HEIGENHAUSER: I agree with you. Generally, we stopped about an hour before exercise. I think the real key to the problem is to give a lot of water with the capsules. If you can do that and get an increase in the urine output, you're better off—rather than loading and having an increase in the sodium within the plasma.

ROBERTSON: Jones and Sutton suggested that the improvements they showed in performance of high-intensity exercise were a function of changes in metabolism as a result of induced alkalosis. They used lactic acid changes as a marker for glycolytic energy yield. You've cast some doubt on that concept for human studies. Is that correct?

HEIGENHAUSER: Yes. They were one of the few groups that used plasma lactate concentrations rather than blood lactate concentrations. Their lactate concentrations were quite a bit higher than those in most of the studies. Also, the distribution of lactate across the RBC is different under alkalotic conditions compared to acidotic and control conditions; that is a confounding factor in trying to interpret plasma lactates.

Another confounding issue is the variation in time to exhaustion with the various treatments. Conclusions about the rates of glycolysis are very difficult because of that. There is a study with exercise at 125% $\dot{V}O_2$max that found that the muscle lactate concentration under the alkalotic condition was almost double that under the placebo condition. Despite the fact that there was such a large change in the lactate concentrations, the muscle pH values under the two conditions were identical. If potassium were being maintained within the muscle under alkalosis, the retention of the cation could have maintained the intracellular pH, despite the almost doubled lactate concentration. Some good studies have to be done looking at the metabolic events in human subjects to ascertain what is really happening with glycolysis.

Another question to be answered is: With this short exercise duration, how quickly can the lactate move from the intracellular to the extracellular spaces? According to the animal studies, this process seems to be speeded up.

We have also studied the uptake of lactate between alkalotic and acidotic conditions, and it appears that acidosis enhances the uptake of lactate into inactive tissue, whereas alkalosis reduces it. So part of the increased plasma lactate under alkalosis could be due to a slower rate at which lactate is being taken up into inactive muscle and oxidized.

The enzyme that seems to be critical to bicarbonate loading effects on glycolysis is pyruvic dehydrogenase (PDH). The PDH reaction is a phosphatase reaction; an increase in hydrogen ion might activate PDH and allow for faster removal of lactate via the Krebs cycle. In this way you might regulate the acidosis in the muscle by metabolizing glycolytic intermediates more rapidly.

EICHNER: Are you satisfied that most of the clinical studies had adequate controls for possible plasma volume differences?

HEIGENHAUSER: We did not look at the plasma volume per se, but we looked at the plasma proteins and at the relationship between hematocrit and hemoglobin; we found no differences between the alkalosis and control conditions.

COYLE: As I understand it, you are suggesting that it is the loss of chloride in the urine that is largely responsible for the effects of sodium bicarbonate loading on plasma pH?

HEIGENHAUSER: Eventually, yes. But the primary effect is the excretion of sodium, because sodium is acted on by the sodium-potassium pump. When sodium enters the lumen of the kidney, there has to be an anion that accompanies it, and that anion is chloride. With sodium bicarbonate loading, the CO_2 goes from the gut into the blood and is eventually exhaled at the mouth. So essentially, all you're doing is giving sodium. But as the fluid volume loading is detected by the right atrium, you get a natriuretic effect. This causes the sodium to be excreted by the kidney, and water is excreted with it. But an anion has to move as well, so chloride is also excreted. As a result, you get a decrease of chloride within the plasma, and this results in the alkalosis, not the increases in plasma sodium.

COYLE: If sodium loss in urine is prevented by the limited kidney blood flow and urine formation during strenuous exercise, would you expect that the bicarbonate would have less of an erogenic effect?

HEIGENHAUSER: Yes, but that is speculation only.

On another matter, Bodil Nielsen showed that if sodium bicarbonate rather than sodium chloride is given as a fluid replacement, temperature can be maintained better in the exercising rat. Therefore, one might speculate that sodium bicarbonate infusions to increase fluid volume might aid temperature regulation and perhaps performance during long-term events.

CLARKSON: What's the effect of alkalosis on lactate transport in the heart?

HEIGENHAUSER: I haven't studied that literature, but the transport of lactate across membranes appears to be highly dependent upon the hydrogen ion concentration. An increased hydrogen ion concentration in the extracellular fluid will enhance the movement of lactate into the intracellular space.

CLARKSON: So wouldn't that facilitate the performance of the heart muscle, since it relies on lactate as an energy source during exercise?

HEIGENHAUSER: That could be. The heart can utilize lactate very effectively.

SHERMAN: In the types of activities that these protocols usually employ, i.e., very high intensity exercise for a relatively short duration, it is my impression there is a large influx of water into the intracellular space.

HEIGENHAUSER: I wouldn't say into the intracellular space but rather out of the vascular space. Very little is going to the intracellular space. Most of the fluid is going into the interstitial space.

SHERMAN: Does that imply that the muscle analyses should be done on freeze-dried samples as opposed to wet samples?

HEIGENHAUSER: Most of our analyses were done on freeze-dried muscle. But in the rat hindlimb study, we did not put in an extracellular marker. There was less movement of water into the muscle during the alkalotic conditions in most of our experiments. Also, there was less during the metabolic alkalosis than during respiratory alkalosis. With alkalosis, the lactate concentrations were lower in the muscle. This suggests better osmoregulation in alkalotic conditions, and that could be very important to maintain homeostasis.

GREGG: The plasma lactate data suggest that the accumulation of lactate is due to a decrease in uptake by tissues other than working muscle. That is an interesting idea because the premise of your early studies was that maybe glycolysis was running at a faster rate with a higher energy turnover. Higher energy turnover makes a lot of sense to me for its potential to enhance performance. Everything we've been told before today implied a greater substrate availability or energy enhancement. Now, suddenly you're telling us that we have an ergogenic aid that has nothing to do with energy enhancement. In fact, it is decreasing lactate removal by inactive tissues. How can I get an ergogenic effect with something that does not affect energy turnover?

HEIGENHAUSER: The energy turnover is affected in inactive tissue rather than active tissue.

GREGG: If that is true, then the skeletal muscle lactate efflux is the same. Your lactate data support the idea that there is no change in glycolysis, i.e., no change in energy production.

HEIGENHAUSER: That is true in the rat hind limb. But we did that experiment wrong. We should have used chloride rather than sodium, and I think the results would have been different.

GREGG: So there would be higher lactate efflux and greater glycogen breakdown?

HEIGENHAUSER: There would also be more work done by the muscle during that period of time. You've got to look at the electrolyte and fluid data to get a handle on what is happening with performance and metabolism. It is clear now—at least in my mind—that metabolism does not appear to be the limiting factor in performance. The limiting factor appears to be in the excitation-contraction coupling. The release of calcium from the sarcoplasmic reticulum could be the limiting factor, rather than the utilization of substrate. I think if you can drive the muscle, the substrate will be there. ATP does not seem to be limiting.

GREGG: So by changing the electrolytes, the calcium release mechanism can be changed?

HEIGENHAUSER: You've got to maintain the membrane potential. By maintaining the intracellular potassium concentrations, you can maintain the membrane potential. Chloride also helps in maintaining the membrane potential, so if you can maintain a lower extracellular chloride concentration, you can maintain or stabilize the T-tubule membrane potential.

SPRIET: I agree with George's analysis, especially in brief, high-power exercise, where it has long been suggested that increases in hydrogen ion down-regulate phosphorylase and phosphofructokinase. The majority of the recent studies suggest that the muscle is well set-up to keep those enzymes active at a very low pH. My thinking has changed over the last five years. The electrolyte changes probably don't exert their primary effect on provision of ATP.

HEIGENHAUSER: There is strong evidence that there are positive modulators that can override the adverse effects of hydrogen ions on these rate-limiting enzymes.

CONLEE: If that is true, why would we not see a broader spectrum of the effects of bicarbonate loading, rather than there being such a narrow range of performance that is affected?

HEIGENHAUSER: The only study that has looked at performance longer than 6 min was a rather poorly done study by Black and Johnson. We've got to look at events up to 50 min in duration because in such events, lactate concentrations in plasma are about 11–

12 mM. We also need to study the effect of bicarbonate loading on factors such as temperature regulation.

CONLEE: It seems to me that any electrolyte changes that affect calcium release in muscle would affect all types of exercise.

HEIGENHAUSER: I think the electrolyte profile is very important. Some of the rate-limiting enzymes within glycolysis are very sensitive to changes in the ratios between sodium and potassium. We're getting changes of 30 mM potassium within the muscle and small increases in sodium. These effects in the test tube have been shown to inactivate some of the enzymes. Therefore, enzyme inhibition is not only a pH effect, but also an effect of changes in the various electrolytes. It is clear that a change in chloride, for example, does have an effect, and most of the studies in acid-base regulation have blatantly changed the chloride concentration and assumed that chloride is inert. Chloride is not inert.

TERJUNG: You're setting up a straw man when you imply that on the basis of cuvette-determined conditions, we can assume an influence of hydrogen ions or electrolytes on the rate of glycolysis within the muscle cell during intense exercise. In fact, such an influence hasn't been shown in animals or humans. That is, hydrogen ion and other ionic changes haven't been shown to inhibit glycolytic flux. This flux is very high, even when the pH in the muscle is down to 6.3. Yet, in the cuvette, such changes in ions show an effect on PFK so, even though the adverse impact should be there according to the test tube data, it isn't present in the intact organism.

HEIGENHAUSER: Not in vivo, it is not there. That is what I have tried to indicate—that pH is not that important. It is the calcium link that is most likely important. But it is very difficult to say what is the primary factor that results in fatigue in this type of exercise. I think you've got to have an open mind and say that it is probably multifactorial. You can look at variables that are related to fatigue, but whether they, indeed, cause fatigue is a different story.

ROBERTSON: Our experiments looked at performance times of up to 10.5 min and showed a positive effect of bicarbonate on performance. You indicate that the upper limit is 7.5 min, and we've extended a little bit beyond that.

TERJUNG: It seems to me that there might be some effects on microvascular responses to exercise when modifying the pH with a base load. For example, I think that you could have a redistribution of blood flow in the microvasculature that could have an impact on ion exchange rates across cell membranes. Such changes might account for the water changes.

HEIGENHAUSER: That's possible; the microcirculation might be affected.

6

Blood Doping and Oxygen Transport

Lawrence L. Spriet, Ph.D.

INTRODUCTION

Blood doping has attracted considerable interest in the past two decades due to its potential to increase maximal oxygen uptake ($\dot{V}O_2$max) and improve endurance performance. An individual is blood doped by removing a certain volume of blood, storing the red blood cells (RBCs) in frozen form, and reinfusing the RBCs in a saline solution at a later date after normal RBC levels in the body have been restored. The intent is to increase the number of RBCs per unit volume of blood, deliver more oxygen (O_2) to the working tissues, and thereby increase $\dot{V}O_2$max and aerobic endurance performance. This technique has also been referred to as blood boosting, blood packing, and induced erythrocythemia.

An essential prerequisite for testing the efficacy of blood doping

213

is to produce a significant increase in the concentration of RBCs in the blood expressed either as the number of RBCs per volume of blood or as the hematocrit (Hct), i.e., the percent of a given volume of blood that consists of RBCs. The increase in Hct is associated with a concomitant increase in the concentration of hemoglobin ([Hb]), the protein responsible for carrying O_2 in the blood. Generally, blood doping produces similar increases in Hct and [Hb]. Throughout this chapter, [Hb] is reported to denote the increase in the number of RBCs per unit volume of blood, and Hct is reported only in the absence of [Hb] data.

In the blood doped state, a significant increase in [Hb] increases the arterial O_2 content (CaO_2) of the blood. If the cardiac output during maximal exercise (Q_{max}) is unaltered or increased, systemic O_2 transport will increase (Q_{max} x CaO_2). As a result, more O_2 will be delivered to the working muscles, and the potential for a greater O_2 uptake exists. Any increase in the $\dot{V}O_2$max means that a given submaximal power output requires a smaller percentage of the new $\dot{V}O_2$max. If the performance task requires exercise to exhaustion during an incremental test or at a given submaximal power output, the lower relative intensity should result in a prolonged exercise time. In a competitive race where the fastest time wins, the individual is able to exercise at a higher absolute power output (and O_2 uptake) and race time should decrease. The ability to complete the above exercise tasks is used as a measure of aerobic endurance performance throughout the chapter.

In order for an increased [Hb] to produce an increase in $\dot{V}O_2$max, many assumptions must be met. They include: 1) that Q_{max} is not decreased following blood doping, 2) that the percent distribution of Q_{max} to the working muscles is not decreased, and 3) that the exercising muscles possess the oxidative capacity to use the additional O_2 that is delivered.

The scientific community has studied blood doping to determine if a physiological basis for enhanced $\dot{V}O_2$max and endurance performance exists and for the basic information it contributes to understanding the factors that limit $\dot{V}O_2$max in the normocythemic individual (normal [Hb]). The transport of O_2 from the atmosphere to the working muscles during intense exercise is a complex process, involving numerous physiological systems. If blood doping increases $\dot{V}O_2$max, it suggests that systemic O_2 transport normally limits maximal oxygen uptake. If no increase in $\dot{V}O_2$max results, O_2 transport is not limiting, and the limitation to performance may lie in the muscle's local circulation or ability to utilize O_2. It is a distinct possibility that the predominant factor limiting $\dot{V}O_2$max may differ between individuals of varying genetic and environmental (e.g., training) status.

The demonstration that blood doping does increase $\dot{V}O_2max$ and endurance performance also led to experiments examining its potential ergogenic effects in a variety of exercise situations in different environments, most notably at altitude and in high ambient temperatures.

The interest in blood doping in athletic circles has stemmed mainly from rumors of its use in the Olympiads of 1972, 1976, 1984, and 1988 and in numerous world championships. The endurance sports implicated include distance running, cycling, cross-country skiing, and the biathlon. Accusations of blood doping have been leveled at athletes from several nations. However, documentation or confessions of blood doping in actual competitions have been rare because attempts to identify users of this technique have rarely been made at major international competitions. Notable exceptions to the absence of individuals who have acknowledged participation in blood doping were members of the men's cycling team and the administering physician who represented the USA at the 1984 Olympics. These individuals freely confessed to having employed blood doping to improve cycling endurance performance. As a direct result of this occurrence, the International Olympic Committee added blood doping to the list of banned agents. However, research attempts to develop detection methods have been largely unsuccessful.

The purpose of this chapter is to chronologically review the blood doping research with particular emphasis on the changes in $\dot{V}O_2max$, endurance performance, O_2 transport, and selected additional central circulatory variables (blood volume, Q_{max}, and CaO_2) during intense aerobic exercise. Several of the concepts examined in this chapter have been previously reviewed (Gledhill, 1982, 1985; Sawka & Young, 1989), and readers are encouraged to also consult these excellent papers. The present review focuses mainly on blood doping experiments performed at sea level and normal ambient temperatures (20–30°C). For a more detailed examination of blood doping experiments at high altitude and in high ambient temperatures, readers are asked to consult Robertson et al. (1982, 1988) and Sawka and Young (1989).

EARLY ATTEMPTS AT BLOOD DOPING

The first study of blood doping examined whether exercise tolerance to hypoxia could be improved by four infusions of 500 mL of donor whole blood over 4 d (Pace et al., 1947). The homologous transfusion of 2 L of matched donor blood in five naval volunteers increased resting Hct by 26% (46.2 to 58.3). The tolerance of the subjects to hypoxia, assessed by the heart rate (HR) response to submaximal exercise at simulated altitudes, was improved. The same exercise HR, before and after transfusion, was attained at altitudes of 3,139 and 4,724 m, respectively. This study is unique for two reasons: 1) all future blood doping studies used the subject's own blood (autologous) and not matched donor blood (homologous) for reinfusion, and 2) the authors were successful in achieving a significant postreinfusion increase in Hct. It would be approximately 30 years before blood doping studies were again successful in achieving what they set out to accomplish, i.e., a significant increase in Hct, [Hb], and O_2 carrying capacity. Without an increase in [Hb], there will not be a resultant increase in maximal O_2 transport (Q_{max} x CaO_2) unless the reinfusion of blood increases blood volume and Q_{max} is increased through an increase in stroke volume (SV). Unfortunately, a series of studies from 1960 to 1979 was largely unsuccessful in increasing [Hb] and therefore unable to properly examine the effects of induced erythrocythemia on VO_2max and endurance performance.

With autologous reinfusion, the removed blood must be stored according to clinically accepted standards from the time of withdrawl to reinfusion. In most early studies, blood was routinely refrigerated at 4°C, but storage time by this method is limited to 3 weeks in North America. Several problems arise when refrigerated blood must be reinfused following a 3-week storage period. Red blood cells continue to age and degenerate during refrigeration storage, and 15–20% are lost prior to reinfusion (Valeri, 1976). Additional RBCs are lost during handling, and many become fragile during storage and are hemolyzed following reinfusion (Valeri, 1976). Therefore, the result of refrigeration storage is that only 60% of the withdrawn cells are viable following reinfusion. Consequently, the reinfusion of RBCs from 1 unit of blood (1 unit = ~450 mL whole blood) within 3 weeks of withdrawl produced minimal increases in [Hb] (0.7–2.6%) over pre-phlebotomy values (Bell et al., 1976; Frye & Ruhling, 1977; Gullbring et al., 1960; Pate et al., 1979; Videman & Rytomaa, 1977; Williams et al., 1973). Therefore, it is not surprising that studies using these procedures did not observe increases in VO_2max or endurance performance.

If two or more units of blood are withdrawn and stored, more viable RBCs are available for reinfusion. However, as Gledhill et al. (1978) demonstrated, the reestablishment of normal [Hb] requires 5–6 weeks following the removal of two units of blood in active healthy males. For trained endurance runners, up to 10 weeks were required to restore normal [Hb] following the removal of two units of blood (Buick et al., 1980). Therefore, forced reinfusion of refrigerated RBCs after only 3 weeks occurs at a time when [Hb] has not returned to normal levels.

Robinson et al. (1966) reinfused two units of whole blood following 2 weeks of refrigeration; they increased Hct from 41.7 to 43.7% but reported no increase in $\dot{V}O_2$max when compared to pre-reinfusion values. Von Rost et al. (1975) reported that a 2.7% increase in Hct (~1 Hct unit) following the reinfusion of two units of refrigerated blood increased $\dot{V}O_2$max by 9% and performance by 37%. Ekblom et al. (1972) waited 4 weeks before reinfusing two units of refrigerated blood and increased [Hb] by 2.1% and $\dot{V}O_2$max by 5.5%. Endurance performance, assessed by a treadmill run designed to exhaust the subject in ~5 min, increased by 15.6%. The reinfusion of three units of blood increased [Hb] by a small 1.3%. Surprisingly, endurance performance increased by 25% despite no change in $\dot{V}O_2$max (Ekblom et al., 1972). A later study reinfused two units of blood following 5 weeks of refrigeration and produced a 4.5% increase in [Hb] and an 8% increase in $\dot{V}Q$max (Ekblom et al., 1976).

Although the reinfusion of two to three units of refrigerated blood increased the number of viable RBCs delivered, the reinfusions occurred when Hb concentrations were not fully recovered, resulting in small [Hb] increases of 1.3–4.5% above normal. Consequently, it is difficult to reconcile the large increases in $\dot{V}O_2$max reported by Von Rost et al. (1975) and Ekblom et al. (1972) with the small increases in [Hb] observed in these investigations. Calculations of the increase in O_2 transport (Q_{max} x CaO_2) resulting from 2.1–2.7% increases in [Hb], assuming a constant Q_{max}, suggest that the measured increases in $\dot{V}O_2$max were double the expected amount. In a subsequent study, Q_{max} was directly measured with the dye-dilution technique and was unchanged following the reinfusion of two units of blood (Ekblom et al., 1976). The calculated O_2 transport following reinfusion in this study increased by ~140 mL/min, whereas the measured $\dot{V}O_2$max increased by 340 mL/min. This suggested that increased O_2 extraction was responsible for the unexpectedly large increase in $\dot{V}O_2$max following blood doping. However, the data from these studies have been questioned on methodological grounds. Pre-reinfusion $\dot{V}O_2$max testing was not done, and double-blind procedures were not employed. The inability to reproduce these results with the reinfusion of three units of blood casts further doubt on the validity of the findings (Ekblom et al., 1972). A possible explanation is that the reported control $\dot{V}O_2$max values performed at the outset of the studies were, in fact, submaximal.

In summary, blood doping studies prior to 1980 were largely

unsuccessful in their attempts to test the hypothesis that an elevated [Hb] and hence an increased CaO_2 enhanced $\dot{V}O_2$max and endurance performance. The major reason was an inability to significantly alter the independent variable, [Hb] or CaO_2, following reinfusion! Contributing to this problem was the use of insufficient RBC volumes, RBC loss associated with the refrigeration storage method, reinfusion of RBCs before pre-phlebotomy or normal [Hb] was re-established, and the lack of well controlled experimental designs.

CONTEMPOPARY BLOOD DOPING EXPERIMENTS

Effects on $\dot{V}O_2$max and Endurance Performance

Attempts to examine the ergogenic effects of blood doping since 1980 are categorized as those that employed the freeze-preserve method to store RBCs. Without fail, these studies have achieved substantial increases in [Hb]. With the freezing technique, RBCs can be stored indefinitely, and cell loss due to handling and fragility is minimized (Valeri, 1976). The indefinite storage time permits the reinfusion to be made after verifying that normocythemia in the subject has been re-established. Gledhill (1982) has thoroughly reviewed the importance of the freeze preservation technique in blood doping. It should be noted that one study is included in this section where three units of blood were stored by refrigeration, because reinfusion did produce a 4.2% increase in [Hb] (Berglund & Hemmingsson, 1987). Table 6–1 summarizes the major findings of these investigations in a manner similar to that in the report of Gledhill (1982) for studies prior to 1981.

Buick et al. (1980) were the first to conclusively demonstrate that a significant increase in [Hb] elevated $\dot{V}O_2$max and enhanced endurance performance in highly trained elite distance runners. In a cross-over, double-blind design involving two groups of subjects, measurements of $\dot{V}O_2$max and endurance performance at $\sim$95% $\dot{V}O_2$max were made prior to phlebotomy and following: 1) restoration of normocythemia, 2) a sham saline reinfusion, 3) reinfusion of two units of freeze-preserved blood, and 4) restoration of normocythemia. There were no differences in [Hb] in the pre-phlebotomy, normocythemic, and sham conditions. Following the reinfusion of two units of blood, [Hb] increased from 15.1 to 16.4 g/dL at rest and from 15.7 to 16.7 g/dL during intense running (Figure 6–1). $\dot{V}O_2$max increased from 5.11 to 5.37 L/min, and treadmill run time at $\sim$95% of the normocythemic $\dot{V}O_2$max increased from 7.20 to 9.65 min (Figure 6–1).

The authors concluded that the elevated [Hb] increased O_2

TABLE 6-1. *Summary of Blood Doping Studies Using Freeze Preserved RBCs.*

Author (year)	Units Reinfused[1]	Time of Test[2]	[Hb] vs. Control[3]	$\dot{V}O_2$max versus Control[3]	End Cap. versus Control[3]
Williams et al. (1978)	1	2 h	+2.7%		+5.1%
		7 d	3.3%		+4.3%
Cottrell (1979) (Abstract)	1		—	~+2%[4]	—
Buick et al. (1980)	2	1 d	+8.0%*	+5.1%*	+34%*
		7 d	+9.3%*	+4.5%*	+20%*
Williams et al. (1981)	2	1–2 d	+7.6%*		+2.4%*
Goforth et al. (1982, Abstract)	2	?	?	+11.2%	+2.6%
Robertson et al. (1982)	4	1 d	+27.8%*	+12.8%*	+15.8%*
Thomson et al. (1982, 1983)	2	1–3 d	+11.6%*	+11.4%*	—
Robertson et al. (1984, 1988)[5]	2	2 d	+15.8%*	+10.0%*	+23%*
		8 d	+10.9%*	+10.4%*	+26%*
		14 d		+7.9%*	+19%*
Spriet et al. (1986)	1	2–7 d	+8.2%*	+0.4%	—
	2	2–7 d	+9.5%*	+4.0%	—
	3	2–7 d	+10.1%*	+6.8%*	—
Sawka et al., (1987a)	2	3 d	—	+11.1%*	
Muza et al. (1987)	3–5	10 d	+11.8%*	+8.2%*	
Celsing et al. (1987)	2	1 d	+5%*[6]	+7.4%*	
Brien & Simon (1987)	3[7]	5 d	+4.2%		~+3.5%*
Berglund & Hemmingsson (1987)	2	3 h	+2.3%		+5.3%*
		14 d			+3.1%*
Sawka et al. (1988)	2	3 d	+6.1%	+5.2%	—
Brien et al.(1989)	2	2 d	+7.3%*	+10.3%*	+0.9%*

[1] 1 unit equals the RBCs from 1 unit of whole blood (~450 ml)
[2] time from reinfusion to testing
[3] control refers to normocythemia before phlebotomy and/or before reinfusion
[4] calculated from submaximal HR
[5] female subjects
[6] increase in Hct
[7] RBCs stored with refrigeration technique
* significantly increased from control values, P<0.05

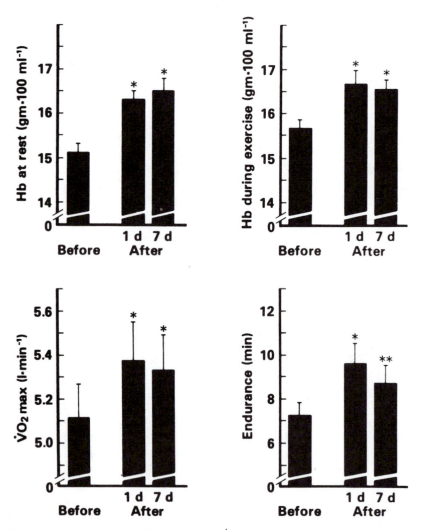

FIGURE 6-1. *Hemoglobin (Hb) concentration, $\dot{V}O_2max$, and aerobic endurance performance before and after autologous reinfusion of two units of freeze-preserved blood. X ± SE, n = 11; 1 d and 7 d signify 1 and 7 days after reinfusion. Asterisk indicates values significantly different from pre-reinfusion value (*, P<0.01; **, P<0.05). The data have been redrawn with permission from Buick et al. (1980).*

transport and ultimately O_2 delivery to the contracting muscles and afforded the increase in $\dot{V}O_2max$. Assuming a constant arterial Hb-O_2 saturation and a constant Q_{max} of 30 L/min, approximately 330 mL of additional O_2 was delivered to the muscles each minute. Of this, 260 mL were extracted. The increase in $\dot{V}O_2max$ following reinfusion also suggested that central O_2 transport limited $\dot{V}O_2$max during normocythemia in these elite endurance runners. It should also be restated that the use of the freeze preservation technique for storing RBCs was instrumental in achieving the 8% increase in [Hb] and the ability to test the hypothesis that increased CaO_2 and O_2 transport would increase $\dot{V}O_2$max.

Prior to the report by Buick et al. (1980), Williams et al. (1978) published a carefully controlled study examining the ergogenic effects of blood withdrawl and reinfusion using the freezing technique. However, only one unit of blood was reinfused 3 weeks following phlebotomy, and [Hb] increased by only 3.3%. Time to exhaustion in a progressive treadmill run was increased by a nonsignificant 4.1%, and $\dot{V}O_2$max was not measured. These findings conflicted with those of Ekblom et al. (1972), who reported significant increases in $\dot{V}O_2$max and run time to exhaustion at a maximal power output with increases in [Hb] of 1.3–2.1%. However, the results of Williams et al. (1978) should be given stonger consideration than those of Ekblom et al. because Williams et al. controlled for training status of the subjects, employed a control group, and used a double-blind experimental procedure. In support of the Williams et al. (1978) study, experiments by Cottrell (1979) and Spriet et al. (1986) reported no significant increase in $\dot{V}O_2$max following the reinfusion of one unit of freeze preserved blood.

Subsequent blood doping studies have consistently reported a post-reinfusion increase in $\dot{V}O_2$max and/or improved endurance performance when the RBC freeze preservation technique was employed. Williams et al. (1981) reported a 7% increase in [Hb] and decreased 5-mile times in 12 well-trained runners following the reinfusion of two units of blood. Mean treadmill run time decreased from 30:10 to 29:26 (min:s) for an improvement of 2.4%, and most of the improvement occurred in the final 2 miles. The study employed a double-blind cross-over design, and each subject served as his own control with a sham reinfusion of two units of saline.

Three additional blood doping studies were published in 1982 (Goforth et al., 1982; Robertson et al., 1982; Thomson et al., 1982). Goforth et al. (1982) reported that the reinfusion of two units of blood increased $\dot{V}O_2$max from 4.10 to 4.56 L/min and decreased 3-mile run time by 23.7 s in six trained distance runners. A sham reinfusion had no effect on run time. Robertson et al. (1982) reinfused five well-trained mountain climbers with four units of blood and reported a 28% increase in resting [Hb] (13.80 to 17.63 g/dL) 24 h following the reinfusion. The $\dot{V}O_2$max increased from 3.28 to 3.70 L/min, and total run time during a multistage treadmill test increased from 793 to 918 s. Thomson et al. (1982) reinfused two units of blood into four untrained subjects and increased [Hb] from 14.7 to 16.4 g/dL and $\dot{V}O_2$max from 4.0 to 4.5 L/min. In an additional paper from the same study, subjects ran at the same percentage (~67%) of their pre- and post-reinfusion $\dot{V}O_2$max values for 90 min and completed 13% more work in the reinfused condition (Thomson et al., 1983).

Robertson et al. (1984) were the first to demonstrate that blood doping had a significant ergogenic effect in women. The reinfusion of two units of blood into nine active women increased [Hb] from 12.7 g/dL to 14.7, 14.7, and 14.3 g/dL, 2, 8, and 14 d after reinfusion, respectively. The $\dot{V}O_2$max was increased by 8–10%, and time to exhaustion during a progressive cycling test was increased by 19–26% on the three post-reinfusion test days.

In a study primarily designed to examine central circulatory dymanics, Spriet et al. (1986) sequentially reinfused three units of blood into four highly trained elite endurance runners. The reinfusion of one unit had no effect on $\dot{V}O_2$max during treadmill running. The second unit increased resting [Hb] from 14.7 to 15.8 g/dL and increased $\dot{V}O_2$max from 5.04 to 5.24 L/min. Although each subject increased his $\dot{V}O_2$max, the small sample size prevented statistical significance. The reinfusion of a third unit of blood increased $\dot{V}O_2$max in three out of four subjects to a mean value of 5.38 L/min, which was significantly greater than the pre-reinfusion (5.04 L/min) value. Celsing et al. (1987) also examined the effect of sequential reinfusions on $\dot{V}O_2$max. Five units of blood were removed once per week for 5 weeks. When [Hb] had returned to pre-phlebotomy levels, each subject received three to five reinfusions of one unit of blood in a 12–14 d period. Following three to five reinfusions, [Hb] increased from 15.2 to 17.0 g/dL, and $\dot{V}O_2$max rose from 4.36 to 4.68 L/min. The responses to the intermediate reinfusions were not reported in tabular format and appeared only in a figure. However, it appeared that subsequent to the initial reinfusion, [Hb] and $\dot{V}O_2$max increased linearly with sequential reinfusions.

Sawka et al. (1987a, 1988) published two investigations examining the thermoregulatory effects of blood doping during exercise in the heat. In these studies they measured treadmill $\dot{V}O_2$max in a comfortable environment (20°C) before and after reinfusion. The reinfusion of two units of blood increased [Hb] by 10% and increased $\dot{V}O_2$max from 4.28 to 4.75 L/min in six fit, heat-unacclimated men. In five trained and heat-acclimated men, $\dot{V}O_2$max increased from 4.26 to 4.48 L/min. The latter finding was not significant due to the small sample size.

Between 1987 and 1989, three studies were published which examined the effects of blood doping on athletic performance in field settings. Berglund and Hemmingsson (1987) reinfused three units of blood into well-trained cross-country skiers and reported 5.3 and 3.1% improvements in 15 km race times, 3 h and 14 d post-reinfusion, respectively. Unfortunately, the RBCs were stored by refrigeration, and the corresponding increases in [Hb] were only 4.2 and 2.3%. Brien and Simon (1987) increased the resting Hct of well trained runners from ~42 to ~47% via the reinfusion of two units of blood. Mean 10 km run time was significantly improved by 69 s from a control mean of ~33 min. Brien et al. (1989) also examined the effects of blood doping on 1500 m run time on a track in four well trained runners. The reinfusion of two units of blood increased resting [Hb] from 15.1 to 16.2 g/dL and $\dot{V}O_2$max from 4.08 to 4.50 L/min. Race time decreased significantly from 4:19.5 to 4:15.0 (min:s).

Sawka et al. (1987b) examined the relationship between the reinfusion of two units of blood and $\dot{V}O_2$max from four existing blood doping studies involving 30 subjects. Their analysis indicated that almost all subjects (29 of 30) will increase their $\dot{V}O_2$max after reinfusion. In addition, the individual data showed no relationship between the [Hb] and $\dot{V}O_2$max after reinfusion. They argued that individuals may respond differently to blood reinfusion for a variety of physiological reasons. They also suggested that subjects with $\dot{V}O_2$max values of 50–65 mL O_2 .kg^{-1} .min^{-1} may have the largest increase in $\dot{V}O_2$max with blood doping. However, the relationship was not convincing and did not include all of the existing literature data. However, it does appear that this type of analysis warrants further examination.

An attempt to summarize the effects of blood doping on running performance in competitive race situations (1500 m to 10 km) appears in Figure 6–2. The data from four studies that reinfused two units of blood are summarized. The cumulative post-reinfusion improvement in run time increases as a function of the distance run. The improvements in run time that can be expected following blood doping at 2, 6, and 10 km are approximately 7, 30, and 68 s.

The overwhelming conclusion from these studies is that $\dot{V}O_2$max and exercise endurance performance are enhanced by blood doping. Generally, when the post-reinfusion [Hb] increase is greater than 4–6%, $\dot{V}O_2$max and aerobic endurance performance will be improved. The physiological mechanism primarily responsible for these improvements is thought to be an increased CaO_2 and O_2 transport during maximal exercise. This assumes that no major changes occurred in central circulatory parameters, such as blood volume and Q_{max}, and that the proportion of Q_{max} distributed to the exercising muscle is not compromised.

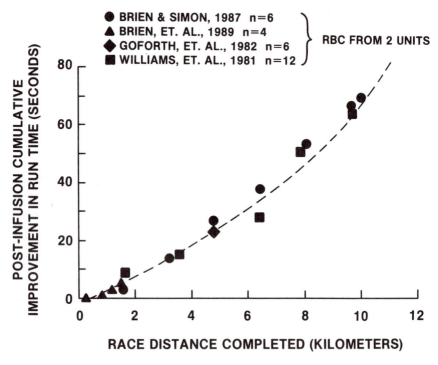

FIGURE 6-2. *The cumulative improvement in run time following the reinfusion of 2 units of freeze-preserved blood as a function of race distance completed. The data are from the four studies indicated, and the figure is courtesy of M.N. Sawka.*

Effects on the Central Circulation

The discussion of central circulatory changes with blood doping will be limited to those studies which have demonstrated an increase in [Hb]. These studies are summarized in Table 6–2. During the blood doping procedure, RBCs are normally reinfused following reconstitution with a volume of saline so that the Hct of the solution is 50–70%. Because the reinfusion is complete in less than 1 h, the blood volume should be acutely expanded. This has led to the suggestion that Q_{max} may be augmented through enhanced venous return. If right atrial pressure, atrial filling, ventricular filling, and, ultimately, end-diastolic volume are increased during maximal exercise, SV and Q_{max} may also be augmented. For a given CaO_2, an increased Q_{max} would also contribute to an increase in O_2 transport.

It has also been suggested that the elevated blood viscosity that accompanies increases in Hct may result in a reduction of the heart's ability to pump blood during maximal exercise. If Q_{max} is reduced, it may counteract the increases in CaO_2, leaving O_2 transport unchanged or reduced following blood doping.

Blood Volume. It is generally stated that acute increases or decreases in blood volume (BV) are quickly compensated for by appropriate changes in plasma volume so that BV is returned to normal levels within a few hours (Gregerson & Dawson, 1959). Because most blood doping studies reinfused RBCs at a Hct of 50%, any increase in Hct or [Hb] after reinfusion must reflect reductions in plasma volume, as normal BV is restored. Therefore, if measurements of [Hb], VO_2max and performance are made at least 24 h after reinfusion, they should reflect a situation where BV is not significantly altered from pre-reinfusion levels.

The few attempts made to estimate or measure BV before and after blood doping suggest that BV is not altered or increased by a modest amount (5%) by this procedure (Table 6–2). Resting BV, estimated by the principle of mass balance, increased by a non-significant 2.7–4.8%, 1–7 d following the reinfusion of two units of blood (Buick et al., 1980; Spriet et al., 1986). Reinfusion of a third unit increased BV an additional 2.7% (Spriet et al., 1986). The increases in BV corresponded to the mass of the added RBCs, suggesting that plasma volume (PV) was unaltered. However, it must be remembered that these calculations assume a 100% RBC survival rate and that the volume of individual RBCs is unchanged following blood doping.

Studies that measured total *in vivo* RBC volume directly and then calculated BV from Hct values reported 0–2.4% increases in BV at rest and during maximal exercise (Celsing et al., 1987; Ekblom et al., 1976). Sawka et al. (1987a) also reported no change in blood volume at rest 3 d following the reinfusion of two units of blood in heat-unacclimated subjects. Direct measurements of RBC volume and plasma volume revealed an increase in total RBC volume and a decrease in PV. In heat-acclimated subjects, BV was increased significantly (5.3%) 24 h following the reinfusion of two units of blood (Sawka et al., 1988).

In a related study, Kanstrup and Ekblom (1984) manipulated [Hb] and BV experimentally and measured VO_2max and endurance performance during seven different combinations of BV and [Hb]. Unfortunately, no combination matched the blood doping situation of normovolemic erythrocythemia. The closest combination had a BV that was 4–5% higher and a [Hb] that was 2–4% higher than control conditions. With this combination, VO_2max and endurance performance were increased by 6 and 31%, respectively.

In conclusion, it is unlikely that BV changes contribute signifi-

TABLE 6-2. *Summary of Measured and Estimated Central Circulatory Changes Following Blood Doping.*

Author, year	CaO_2[1] (mL O_2/dL)	Q_{max}[2] (L/min)	Increase in O_2 transport[3] (mL O_2/min)			Change in VO_2max (mL/min)	BV (L)
			meas. Q	calc. 30 L	Q 25 L		
Robinson, 1966	—	21–22	?	—		+1.4%	?[4]
Ekblom et al. (1976)	19.94 / 20.77	28.7 / 28.3	4860 / 5000 / +140			+340	5.2 / 5.2
Buick et al. (1980)	20.41 / 21.71	30/25 / "		5210 / 5540 / +330	4340 / 4610 / +270	+260	4.99 / 5.23[5] / 5.16[6]
Robertson et al. (1982)	19.04[7] / 24.33	22.78[8] / 22.78	3690 / 4710 / +1020			+420	—
Thomson et al. (1982)	19.0 / 21.0	23.4 / 25.9	3820 / 4620 / +800			+450	—
Robertson et al. (1984)	16.52[7] / 19.11	17.7 / 17.4	2480 / 3830 / +350			+240	—
Spriet et al. (1986) 2 units of blood	19.6 / 21.7	28.2 / 29.8	4650 / 5370 / +720			+200	5.38 / 5.53

Study	CaO_2[1]	VO_2 max[2]	BV	Q_{max}	O_2 transport[3]	% increase	CaO_2
Spriet et al. (1986) 3 units of blood	21.7 / 22.2	29.8 / 33.3	5370 / 6080 / +710			+140	5.53 / 5.68
Celsing et al. (1987)	19.78[7] / 22.10	30/25 "		5040 / 5640 / +600	4200 / 4700 / +500	+360	5.41 / 5.54
Sawka et al. (1987a)	18.07[7] / 19.89	30/25 "		4610 / 5070 / +460	3840 / 4230 / +390	+470	5.75 / 5.71
Sawka et al. (1988)	19.37[7] / 20.54	30/25 "		4940 / 5240 / +300	4120 / 4370 / +250	+220	5.35 / 5.65

For CaO_2, Q_{max}, O_2 transport, and blood volume (BV), the top value is normocythemia before reinfusion, and bottom value is erythrocythemia after reinfusion. All data were recorded during maximal exercise or calculated from maximal exercise data unless otherwise noted.

[1] CaO_2, directly measured or calculated from measured [Hb] x 1.34 mL O_2/g Hb x 97% Hb-O_2 saturation in pre- and post-reinfusion conditions.
[2] measured Q at 85–100% VO_2 max or estimated at 30 and 25 L/min
[3] O_2 delivery calculated as Q_{max} x CaO_2 x 0.85 (assuming 85% of Q_{max} was distributed to working muscles in both conditions).
[4] increase in blood volume not documented
[5] blood volume 2 d after reinfusion
[6] blood volume 7 d after reinfusion
[7] exercise [Hb] unavailable; CaO_2 calculated from resting [Hb]
[8] Q estimated by authors

cantly to alterations in Q_{max} following blood doping in most trained individuals. The exception to this is in heat-acclimated subjects. Further experiments are needed with these subjects to determine if the elevated BV affects Q during maximal exercise.

Maximal Cardiac Output and O_2 Transport. Robinson et al. (1966) were the first to measure central circulatory parameters during a blood doping-like situation. The infusion of 1.0–1.2 L of blood into six men increased Hct acutely by 4.8% (41.7 to 43.7) and elevated blood volume by an undetermined amount. The $\dot{V}O_2$max and Q_{max} during running were unchanged at ~3.2 and 21–22 L/min, but central venous pressure increased from 1.2 to 8.6 mm Hg following reinfusion (Table 6–2).

A summary of more recent attempts to measure central circulatory parameters also appears in Table 6–2. Ekblom et al. (1976) reported that a 4.2% increase in [Hb] had no effect on Q_{max} (28.7 to 28.3 L/min) determined by dye-dilution during cycle ergometer exercise. Thomson et al. (1982) measured no change in Q (CO_2 rebreathing) before and after reinfusion in subjects who ran at several intensities up to 85% $\dot{V}O_2$max. Predicted Q values for power outputs between 85 and 100% $\dot{V}O_2$max were also unaffected by blood doping. Maximal Q (CO_2 rebreathing) was unchanged at ~17–18 L/min in female subjects who exercised on a cycle ergometer before and after reinfusion of two units of blood (Robertson et al., 1984). In a study of graded erythrocythemia during treadmill running, Q was measured with the dye-dilution technique at 91% pre-reinfusion $\dot{V}O_2$max following the reinfusion of two and three units of blood (Spriet et al., 1986). The reinfusion of two units had no significant effect on Q (28.2 to 29.8 L/min) or SV (164 to 181 mL) (Figure 6–3). Following reinfusion of a third unit, Q increased non-significantly to 33.3 L/min, and SV increased significantly to 207 mL. Cardiac output was also measured at 100 and 110% of pre-reinfusion $\dot{V}O_2$max, but the large increases following erythrocythemia suggested that a problem with the dye-dilution technique existed during running tests at maximal workloads (Spriet et al., 1980).

The conclusion based on this small amount of work is that Q_{max} is most likely unchanged or increased only slightly by blood doping. Because maximal heart rate (HR) is unaffected, SV remains constant or slightly increased. The relevance of this finding is that concern over the potential negative effects of blood doping-induced increases in blood viscosity on the heart are unfounded. Q_{max} is not compromised during this procedure, and a stable Q_{max} means that increases in O_2 transport following blood doping are mainly a function of increased CaO_2. It must be noted, however, that measure-

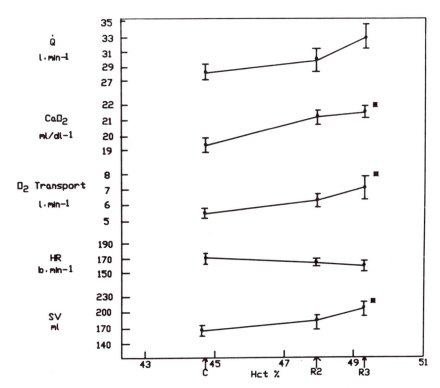

FIGURE 6-3. *Central circulatory responses to running at 91% of the control (pre-reinfusion) $\dot{V}O_2max$ versus hematocrit (Hct) in the control (C) condition and following the reinfusion of two (R2) and three (R3) units of freeze-preserved blood. X ± SE, n = 4. Q = cardiac output; CaO_2 = arterial O_2 content; HR = heart rate; SV = stroke volume. O_2 transport and SV were calculated. *Asterisk signifies value that is significantly different from control, P<0.05. The data are reproduced with permission from Spriet et al. (1986).*

ments of Q during maximal or supramaximal exercise are difficult to perform, and the relatively large error (10%) of all techniques used to measure Q in heavy exercise may mask small changes that occur following blood doping.

An attempt to calculate the theoretical increases in O_2 transport that occurred following blood doping appears in Table 6–2. Maximal exercise data and directly measured CaO_2 and Q_{max} data were used when available. When measured data were not available, CaO_2 was calculated from [Hb], assuming 1.34 mL O_2/g Hb and a Hb-O_2 saturation of 97% before and after reinfusion. This also assumed that O_2 offloading was unaffected by reinfusion. These assumptions seem reasonable because the percent Hb-O_2 saturation was unchanged following the reinfusion of up to three units (Ekblom et al., 1976;

Gledhill et al., 1980), and numerous investigators have reported no post-reinfusion changes in 2,3-diphosphoglycerate concentration and the partial pressure of O_2 required for 50% Hb-O_2 saturation (Brien & Simon, 1987; Buick et al., 1980; Ekblom et al., 1976; Robertson et al., 1984; Sawka et al., 1987a; Williams et al., 1981). Two separate calculations of O_2 transport were made that assumed the same Q_{max} before and after reinfusion; one set of calculations used a Q of 25 L/min and one used Q = 30 L/min. It was also assumed that 85% of Q_{max} was distributed to the working muscles in both pre- and post-reinfusion conditions.

In the studies that measured Q at 85–100% $\dot{V}O_2$max, O_2 transport increased by 350–800 mL/min while increases in $\dot{V}O_2$max were only 140–450 mL/min (Robertson et al., 1984; Spriet et al., 1986; Thomson et al., 1982). This finding is important to the understanding of the factors that limit $\dot{V}O_2$max and raises the following possibilities. The fact that $\dot{V}O_2$max did increase with increased O_2 transport implicates the central circulation as an important limiting factor during normocythemia. However, if all of the extra O_2 transport is actually delivered to the working muscles, it suggests that the metabolic potential of the muscle to extract and use O_2 is a limiting factor during blood doping. On the other hand, if a greater proportion of Q is directed away from exercising muscle following reinfusion, the increase in O_2 delivery may match the actual increase in $\dot{V}O_2$max. The conclusion would then be that the limiting factor for $\dot{V}O_2$max still lies with the central circulation in the erythrocythemic condition. Support for the latter postulate comes from studies reporting increases in $\dot{V}O_2$max with sequential reinfusions of RBCs (Celsing et al., 1987; Spriet et al., 1986). In one study where CaO_2 and Q were measured, O_2 transport increased by 700 mL/min following the reinfusion of two units of blood and by the same amount following a third unit (Spriet et al. 1986). Corresponding $\dot{V}O_2$max increases were 200 and 140 mL/min. However, only the total $\dot{V}O_2$max increase of 340 mL/min was statistically significant because this invasive study employed only four subjects. If the increase in O_2 delivery is well matched to the increase in $\dot{V}O_2$max, explanations are required for why more of the increase in O_2 transport is not directed to working muscle, but to other tissues of the body during maximal exercise.

The only exception to the above findings is the work of Ekblom et al. (1976), who reported a 340 mL/min increase in $\dot{V}O_2$max, despite O_2 transport increases of only 140 mL/min. A lower mixed venous O_2 content and increased O_2 extraction could account for this discrepancy. However, Thomson et al. (1982) reported no change in directly measured femoral venous O_2 content during running following a 12% increase in [Hb] and a 450 mL/min increase in $\dot{V}O_2$max. These data suggest that the increase in $\dot{V}O_2$max following blood doping is a function of the increased CaO_2. Because of the previously cited methodolgical problems with the Ekblom et al. (1976) study, it seems possible that the control $\dot{V}O_2$max data were in fact submaximal. This would result in overestimated increases in $\dot{V}O_2$max following blood doping.

However, when examining the studies in which Q_{max} was not measured, but assumed to be constant at 25 or 30 L/min in both pre-and post-reinfusion conditions, the mismatch between increases in O_2 transport and $\dot{V}O_2$max is less apparent. The calculations from the work of Robertson et al. (1982; Q = 22.78 L/min, as estimated by the authors) and Celsing et al. (1987) do suggest a larger increase in O_2 transport than $\dot{V}O_2$max (Table 6–2). Conversely, the studies of Buick et al. (1980) and Sawka et al. (1987a, 1988), at a Q_{max} of 25 or 30 L/min, suggest that the increase in $\dot{V}O_2$max was reasonably matched to the increase in O_2 transport.

The questions of whether all the extra O_2 transported during blood doping is delivered to the working muscles and where the limiting factor lies during this condition cannot be resolved with existing data. Further study directed at measurements of local blood flow in working muscles and non-working tissues following blood doping are required. These studies should include individuals with a wide range of aerobic fitness and training levels.

Optimal Hct for O_2 Transport. There has been considerable discussion in the blood doping literature regarding the optimal Hct for O_2 transport (Buick et al., 1980; Robertson et al., 1982, 1984; Spriet et al., 1986). Does a Hct exist where the combination of CaO_2 and Q_{max} results in an optimal O_2 transport to the periphery? The interest in this topic has arisen largely from studies in resting and submaximally exercising dogs, in whom Hct has been varied from normal values of 40–45% (Crowell & Smith, 1967; Murray et al., 1962; Richardson & Guyton, 1959; Weisse et al., 1964). Under resting conditions, decreases in Hct to as low as 20% produced increases in Q, and increases in Hct up to 80% produced reductions in Q. These findings were attributed to changes in the viscosity of the blood. Oxygen transport, the product of Q and CaO_2, was the greatest or "optimal" when the Hct was in the normal range of 40–45%. However, one study reported an increase in the optimal Hct from 30–40% at rest to 50–60% during rhythmic isotonic exercise in dog muscle (Gaehtgens et al., 1979).

In blood doping studies involving human subjects, interest has centered around viscosity changes in the 45–55% Hct range. There is a positive linear relationship between Hct and viscosity up to a Hct of approximately 60%. The increases in viscosity in this Hct range are comparatively small. However, an exponential relationship exists between Hct and viscosity when Hct exceeds 60% (Stone et al. 1968). Therefore, as all investigations involving humans examined Hcts below 60%, viscosity increases should not be as critical as those described in dog experiments where Hcts exceeded 60%. Buick et al. (1980) reported that the optimal Hct for maximally exercising humans was in excess of 45%, and Robertson et al. (1982) concluded from their experiments that it fell between 43 and 55%. The sequential reinfusion experiments of Spriet et al. (1986) and Celsing et al. (1987), where $\dot{V}O_2$max increased when maximal exercise Hcts reached mean values of 50.5% and 51.8%, support this suggestion. Celsing et al. (1987) concluded that, regardless of an individual's initial [Hb], the increase in CaO_2 with blood doping overrides the effect of increased viscosity up to individual Hct values of 55% ([Hb] = 20 g/dL).

It appears that the investigations in which resting dogs were used have little relevance when defining the optimal Hct for O_2 transport in maximally exercising humans. In addition, changes in blood vessel diameter, blood flow, internal body temperature, and distribution of BV during exercise are all factors that make extrapolations from resting data inappropriate (Buick et al. 1980). It should also be noted that comparisons of *in vivo* and *in vitro* blood viscosity measurements suggest that *in vitro* measurements overestimate blood viscosity in the vascular bed (Djojosugito et al. 1970; Gustafsson et al. 1980). Consequently, it is reasonable to expect that the small increases in Hct and viscosity that occur with blood doping are not sufficient to compromise Q_{max} in healthy individuals.

Additional Benefits of Blood Doping

Blood doping also affects submaximal exercise performance. When $\dot{V}O_2$max is increased following blood doping, a given absolute power output represents a lower percentage of the new $\dot{V}O_2$max, or a lower relative power output. For example, in the study by Spriet et al. (1986), the power output representing 91% of the pre-reinfusion $\dot{V}O_2$max was only 87 and 85% of the new $\dot{V}O_2$max values following the reinfusion of two and three units of blood, respectively. Consequently, many investigations have reported unchanged $\dot{V}O_2$, lower HR and BP, lower venous and arterial lactate (La) concentrations, and higher venous and arterial pH values at a standardized submaximal power output following blood doping (Buick et al., 1980; Celsing et al., 1987; Ekblom et al., 1976; Pace et al., 1947; Robertson et al., 1982, 1984, 1988; Spriet et al., 1986).

As discussed by Buick et al. (1980) and Robertson et al. (1984), the post-reinfusion increase in CaO_2 and widening of the arterio-venous O_2 difference caused a reduction in Q at a given submaximal $\dot{V}O_2$. The decreased Q was a function of a decreased HR, as SV is generally constant at a HR above 120 beats/min (Rowell, 1969). The decreased post-reinfusion [La] at power outputs of 70–90% $\dot{V}O_2$max was attributed to a decreased proportion of energy required or resulting from anaerobic sources, because the new power output required a lower percentage of the new $\dot{V}O_2$max. The decrease in La production significantly improved the arterial and venous acid-base status at a standard power output (Buick et al., 1980; Spriet et al., 1986). Enhanced buffering capacity of the arterial blood resulting from the elevated [Hb] may also contribute to the improved arterial acid-base status (Buick et al., 1980). Blood doping also improves the ability to thermoregulate, which may result in less blood flow to the skin and more to the working muscles during exercise to exhaustion at a standard submaximal power output (Sawka et al., 1987, 1988). In summary, the lower relative power output, greater blood buffering, and improved thermoregulation may all contribute to the prolonged time to exhaustion during exercise at a standard submaximal power output (Buick et al., 1980) and to the decreased time required to run a given distance (Williams et al., 1981; Brien & Simon, 1987).

Subject Safety

Of obvious concern during the blood doping procedure is the safety of subjects. As clearly stated in the American College of Sports Medicine (1987) position stand on blood doping, transfusions of all types carry medical risks. Transfusions with homologous blood are associated with several potential medical risks, e.g., hepatitis and acquired immune deficiency syndrome (AIDS), and should be avoided. Homologous transfusions are typically not employed for scientific purposes. However, because training does not have to be compromised by blood withdrawals, homologous transfusions in competitive athletes do occur. The transfusion of cyclists in the 1984 Olympics with blood from family members is a known example. Autologous reinfusions, performed with the proper medical supervision, substantially reduce the medical risks. It should also be noted that reinfusions producing Hct values during exercise above 55% have not been carefully studied and may produce viscosity-related problems.

Concern has been expressed over the possibility that cardiovascular function may be compromised at some level of blood doping. An earlier section established that Q is unaffected or possibly increased slightly during maximal exercise following blood doping.

Spriet et al. (1986) recorded modified lead II electrocardiograms during maximal treadmill running in four elite runners before and after reinfusion of two and three units of blood. No evidence of abnormalities or myocardial ischemia was found. If the small increases in blood viscosity associated with blood doping were significant, increases in arterial blood pressure (BP) would be expected. However, direct measurements of arterial BP during maximal running were also unchanged by the sequential blood reinfusions. Systolic BP during submaximal running (91% of pre-reinfusion $\dot{V}O_2$max) was reduced following blood doping. However, this power output represented only 87 and 85% of the new $\dot{V}O_2$max after reinfusions of two and three units of blood, respectively. Ekblom et al. (1976) also stated that direct BP measurements were unchanged during maximal running in well trained men following a 4.2% increase in [Hb], but presented no supporting data.

Robertson et al. (1984) reported no changes in ausculatory BP responses during maximal cycling in active females following the reinfusion of two units of blood. Systolic BP was significantly reduced during submaximal work representing 70% of the pre-reinfusion $\dot{V}O_2$max. Celsing et al. (1987) reinfused three to five units of blood into well trained males and found no change in asculatory BP during submaximal running.

It should also be noted that well trained mountain climbers ran to exhaustion without incident after the reinfusion of four units of blood (Robertson et al. 1982). The well trained subjects in the study by Celsing et al. (1987) also ran to exhaustion without clinical complications. Some of the subjects in the latter study were purposely chosen to represent the high end of normal Hb (20 g/dl) and Hct (55%) values. During exercise, the subjects in these two studies had the highest post-reinfusion Hcts reported in the literature.

There is no conclusive evidence to suggest that the cardiovascular system is compromised following the reinfusion of three to five units of freeze-preserved autologous blood in healthy, active, trained, or well trained elite subjects where Hct values reached 55% during maximal exercise. The above statement applies to laboratory and normal environmental settings and may not apply to individuals experiencing environmental extremes such as hot ambient temperatures, high altitude exposure, and dehydration; in these conditions, decreases in PV may increase Hct and viscosity further.

SUGGESTIONS FOR FUTURE RESEARCH

The study of blood doping has been valuable to the understanding of factors limiting $\dot{V}O_2$max. Most research suggests that the ability of the central circulation to deliver O_2 to the working muscles sets the upper limit for $\dot{V}O_2$. Most of this work has been done with healthy, active, trained, or well trained elite endurance athletes or subjects. It would be of interest to subject a group of sedentary individuals to blood doping to determine if the local blood flow or aerobic capacity of sedentary muscles limits $\dot{V}O_2$max. If this were the case, and blood doping did not increase $\dot{V}O_2$max, would aerobic training shift the limitation to the central circulation?

Several investigators have reported that elite endurance athletes experience arterial O_2 desaturation during maximal exercise (Dempsey et al., 1984; Rowell et al., 1964; Williams et al., 1986). A recent study suggests that pulmonary gas exchange may contribute to the limitation of $\dot{V}O_2$max in athletes who experience reductions in Hb-O_2 saturation during exercise at sea level (Powers et al., 1989). Blood doping could be used to test this postulation by examining the role of the central circulation in limiting $\dot{V}O_2$max in these subjects. If the respiratory system does limit $\dot{V}O_2$max in this population of athletes, blood doping should be less effective in increasing $\dot{V}O_2$max than it is in a group that does not desaturate.

One aspect of blood doping requiring further research is the effect of reinfusion on local muscle blood flow. Is all of the extra measured or calculated O_2 that is transported following reinfusion actually delivered to the working muscles? Experiments to address this question require the isolation of a working muscle group in the intact human being, where arterial and venous blood can be sampled and blood flow can be measured during intense exercise. Measurements of local muscle CaO_2, CvO_2, $\dot{V}O_2$, and blood flow coupled with whole body $\dot{V}O_2$max and Q_{max} should answer the above question and determine whether regional hemodynamic or metabolic factors are limiting for $\dot{V}O_2$max during erythrocythemia. A suitable model for this work has been described by Andersen et al. (1985). With this model, only the muscles that extend the lower leg about the knee are exercised; femoral arterial and venous catheters permit blood sampling and the measurement of blood flow, and cardiorespiratory measurements at the mouth can be made simultaneously.

There is some controversy regarding the length of time that the ergogenic effect of blood doping lasts. In the original blood doping study by Buick et al. (1980), 16 weeks were required to attain normal Hb values following the reinfusion of two units of blood. This time period was similar to the average 120 d life span of a RBC. Surprisingly, while run time to exhaustion had returned to pre-reinfusion values following 16 weeks, $\dot{V}O_2$max remained significantly elevated in 11 highly trained endurance runners. The authors suggested that training at a higher than normal intensity during the erythrocythemic period may have produced an increase in Q_{max}. An increase in Q_{max} of only 1.5 L/min would be needed to account for the increases in O_2 transport and $\dot{V}O_2max$. If this did occur, it needs to be clearly understood why there was no corresponding increase in endurance time. A potential problem may have been subject motivation following 22 weeks of participation in the study. Further investigations are required to answer these questions, as few studies have examined [Hb] beyond 2–4 weeks after reinfusion.

PRACTICAL CONSIDERATIONS

Blood Doping and Ethical Considerations

It is clear that the International Olympic Committee's definition of doping applies to blood doping, and the procedure is therefore banned from use in competition (American College of Sports Medicine, 1987; Dugal & Bertrand, 1976). Unfortunately, as will be discussed in a later section, no reliable method for the detection of blood doping exists. Factors such as training status, altitude acclimation, hydration status, and normal individual differences all contribute to a broad range of [Hb] in a group of athletes. Athletes with lower [Hb] may feel that blood doping is an acceptable method to compensate for these differences or inequalities. For example, Celsing et al. (1987) purposely chose to study subjects that had either very high or very low resting Hb values. They reported a [Hb] range of 12.3–17.8 g/dL in a group of male athletes that were all well trained. In addition, Clement et al. (1977) measured Hb levels of 18 g/dL in some endurance athletes at the 1976 Olympics who were not suspected of blood doping. Subjects involved in blood doping experiments often have mean Hb levels of 14–16 g/dL and experience post-reinfusion increases to only 15–17 g/dL. An additional problem for athletes is that intense training produces an increase in BV (Convertino et al., 1980; Green et al., 1984), which dilutes the Hb and leaves the endurance trained athletes with a lower [Hb] than the normal population (Clement et al., 1977).

Another reason why blood doping may be used as an ergogenic aid is that some athletes believe it produces results similar to those experienced during altitude acclimation, a procedure that is not banned in athletic competitions. A typical altitude acclimation scheme would be for well trained endurance athletes who normally reside at sea level to sojourn to a higher altitude. The lower barometric pressure and partial pressure for O_2 is reported to produce an increased [Hb] in a matter of days to weeks (Lenfant & Sullivan, 1971). If the athlete trains at altitude, where $\dot{V}O_2max$ and endurance performance are reduced (Faulkner et al., 1968), detraining will occur. This detraining can be avoided by transportation to sea level for 1–2 h each day for training sessions or by training at altitude in an O_2 enriched environment (Balke et al., 1976). If these procedures are followed and the athlete returns to sea level with an increased [Hb], $\dot{V}O_2$max and endurance performance may be increased. It follows that the much less expensive but outlawed blood doping procedure may be seen by athletes as an attractive alternative for improving endurance performance. The fault in the above logic is the fact that the early [Hb] changes during altitude exposure are due to reductions in PV and not to rapid synthesis of extra RBCs, because total red cell volume is unchanged (Alexander et al., 1967; Surks et al. 1966).

Detection of Blood Doping During Competitions

At present, there is no effective method to detect blood doping in athletes. Attempts to devise potential methods for the detection of blood doping are confounded by the factors responsible for the wide range in [Hb]: training status, altitude acclimation, hydration status, and normal variations in [Hb] (American College of Sports Medicine, 1987). Until a reliable and accurate method to test for blood doping appears, the governing bodies of sport must rely on the integrity of athletes, coaches, and medical personnel to comply with the ban on this procedure.

Berglund et al. (1987, 1989) have recently reported attempts to correlate various hematologic parameters to the use of blood doping. In their initial study, RBCs were stored via refrigeration for 4 weeks prior to reinfusion (Berglund et al., 1987). Subjects performed a 15 km cross-country ski race 3 h following the reinfusion. Serum erythropoietin concentration decreased to 60% of control values 24 h after reinfusion and remained at this level for 4 weeks. Serum iron and bilirubin concentrations increased transiently by ~3-fold on the day of the reinfusion and returned to control levels following 1 d. Unfortunately, the increases in iron and bilirubin were related to the fragility of RBCs following 4 weeks of refrigeration. The authors attempted to devise an algorithm that would detect blood doping and result in no false positives. Their attempt was only 50% successful (3/6 blood doped subjects were detected), but an equally serious problem was the relevance of this work to blood doping when freeze-preserved RBCs are used.

In the second study by Berglund et al. (1989), the freeze-preserved RBCs from three units of blood were reinfused into eight men and four women, producing 11.5 and 18.4% increases in [Hb], respectively. Serum erythropoietin concentration increased by 50%

5 h after reinfusion, decreased to 66% of control values 1 d following the reinfusion, and remained low for 4 weeks after reinfusion. Again, an algorithm based on an increase in [Hb] and a decrease in erythropoietin was used to predict blood doping. The success rate was 75% one week after reinfusion and 25% after two weeks. The authors emphasized that the value of the algorithm to predict blood doping in a given individual was questionable. Its use would also require pre- and post-competition blood samples and could be confounded by recent altitude training, because little is known regarding the time course of erythropoietin normalization after exposure to altitude.

Because of the difficulty in devising a detection method for blood doping, the most realistic approach may be to require repeated [Hb] measurements from endurance athletes in the 120 d preceeding large international competitions such as the Olympics and World Championships. Measurements would be required at approximately two-week intervals, and both sojourns to altitudes higher than the residence altitude and exposure to hypoxia would be banned during this time. However, this might force all elite endurance athletes to permanently reside at altitude. It is interesting to note that several cross-country skiers on the World Cup circuit have volunteered for regular blood sampling in an attempt to prove they do not use blood doping and to convince other skiers to submit to the same testing.

Erythropoietin: A New Blood Doping Technique?

Red blood cell production in the bone marrow is mediated by erythropoietin (EPO), a hormone produced in the kidneys. Anemia and hypoxia increase the production of EPO, and clinical polycythemic states and hypertransfusion decrease its production. Human EPO is now being produced commercially with a recombinant DNA technique. The recombinant EPO was approved for clinical use in Canada and the United States in 1989. Administration of the artificially produced EPO has been shown to increase RBC production in patients with renal insufficiency and in autologous blood donors (Eschbach et al., 1987; Goodnough et al., 1988). Treatment with EPO also increased the exercise capacity of patients with renal disease (Mayer et al., 1988). It appears that artificial EPO will prove beneficial to all patients suffering from anemia.

Recent evidence suggests that injections of EPO are now being used in athletic circles in an attempt to enhance performance in elite endurance athletes (Cowart, 1989). Ekblom (1989) examined the effects of EPO injections on hematologic and performance variables in active subjects. Small doses of EPO were given to 15 subjects over a 7-week period. In the experimental group, [Hb] increased by 30%, endurance performance increased by at least 10% in all cases, and maximal aerobic power increased in parallel to the [Hb] increase. The International Olympic Committee recently banned the use of artificial EPO from competition. However, the detection of this practice alone or in combination with blood doping will be difficult because the body also produces the hormone, and it has a short half-life.

SUMMARY AND CONCLUSIONS

Recent research on the ergogenic effects of blood doping has clearly demonstrated that the procedure increases $\dot{V}O_2$max and improves aerobic endurance performance. Early controversy regarding the ergogenic properties of blood doping was a function of the difficulty in achieving significant increases in [Hb]. If two (or more) units of blood are withdrawn from an individual and the RBCs are freeze-preserved for at least 6 weeks, the subsequent autologous reinfusion of the stored RBCs produces a significant 6–15% increase in [Hb]. Post-reinfusion $\dot{V}O_2$max is routinely increased by 4–11%, run time for a given distance is shortened, and exercise time during an incremental exercise test or at a given submaximal power output is prolonged.

The physiological basis for the ergogenic effect of blood doping is the increase in arterial blood O_2 content (CaO_2) or carrying capacity. Blood volume and maximal cardiac output are generally unchanged following blood doping; thus, the increase in O_2 transport (Q_{max} x CaO_2) is primarily a function of the increased CaO_2. An undetermined amount of the extra O_2 that is transported is actually delivered to and extracted by the working muscles. The evidence suggests that the central circulation limits $\dot{V}O_2$max during normocythemia. The limiting factor during erythrocythemia has not been clearly identified, but sequential reinfusion experiments suggest that the oxidative potential of the muscle is not exceeded, even after the reinfusion of up to five units of blood.

The blood doping procedure does not compromise the cardiovascular system up to a maximal exercise Hct of 55% in controlled laboratory environments. No reliable method for detecting blood doping presently exists, even though this procedure is banned from use during athletic competitions.

The author strongly agrees with the American College of Sports Medicine position stand on the use of blood doping during athletic competitions (American College of Sports Medicine, 1987). It states that blood doping is an ergogenic aid and that its use is unethical and unjustifiable. However, clinically controlled autologous RBC reinfusion experiments are valid and contribute significantly to scientific inquiry regarding human cardiovascular, hematologic, and metabolic responses during exercise. Of interest to those who wish to further improve their aerobic endurance is the fact that humans have not evolved to the status of the horse. The horse is capable of physiologically blood doping itself during maximal exercise by releasing RBCs stored in the spleen into the circulation (Thomas & Fregin, 1981).

BIBLIOGRAPHY

Alexander, J.K., L.H. Hartley, M. Modelski, and R.F. Grover (1967). Reduction of stroke volume during exercise in man following ascent to 3,100 m altitude. *J. Appl. Physiol.* 23:849–858.
American College of Sports Medicine (1987). Position stand on blood doping as an ergogenic aid. *Med. Sci. Sports Exerc.* 19:540–542.
Andersen, P., R.P. Adams, G. Sjogaard, A. Thorboe, and B. Saltin (1985). Dynamic knee extension as a model for the study of an isolated exercising muscle in humans. *J. Appl. Physiol.* 59:1647–1653.
Balke, B., J.T. Daniels, and J.A. Faulkner (1976). Training for maximum performance at altitude. In: R. Margaria (ed.) *Exercise at Altitude.* Milan: Excerpta Medica Foundation, pp. 179–186.
Bell, R.D., R.T. Card, M.A. Johnson, T.A. Cunningham, and F. Baker (1976). Blood doping and athletic performance. *Aust. J. Sports Med.* 8:133–139.
Berglund, B., P. Hemmingsson, and G. Birgegard (1987). Detection of autologous blood transfusions in cross-country skiers. *Int. J. Sports Med.* 8:66–70.
Berglund, B., and P. Hemmingsson (1987). Effect of reinfusion of autologous blood on exercise performance in cross-country skiers. *Int. J. Sports Med.* 8:231–233.
Berglund, B., G. Birgegard, L. Wide, and P. Pihlstedt (1989). Effects of blood transfusions on some hematological variables in endurance athletes. *Med. Sci. Sports Exerc.* 21:637–642.
Brien, A.J., and T.L. Simon (1987). The effect of red blood cell reinfusion on 10-km race time. *J. Amer. Med. Assoc.* 257:2761–2765.
Brien, A.J., R.J. Harris, and T.L. Simon (1989). The effects of an autologous infusion of 400 mL red blood cells on selected hematological parameters and 1,500 m race time in highly trained runners. *Bahrain Med. Bull.* 11:6–16.
Buick, F.J., N. Gledhill, A.B. Froese, L. Spriet, and E.C. Meyers (1980). Effect of induced erythrocythemia on aerobic work capacity. *J. Appl. Physiol.* 48:636–642.
Celsing, F., J. Svedenhag, P. Pihlstedt, and B. Ekblom (1987). Effects of anemia and stepwise-induced polycythemia on aerobic power in individuals with high and low hemoglobin concentrations. *Acta Physiol. Scand.* 129:47–57.
Clement, D.B., R.C. Asmundson, and C.W. Medhurst (1977). Hemoglobin values: Comparative survey of the 1976 Canadian Olympic team. *J. Can. Med. Assoc.* 117:614–616.
Convertino, V.A., J.E. Greenleaf, and E.M. Bernhauer (1980). Role of thermal and exercise factors in the mechanism of hypervolemia. *J. Appl. Physiol.* 48:657–664.
Cottrell, R. (1979). British army tests blood boosting. *Phys. Sportsmed.* 7:14–16.
Cowart, V.S. (1989). Erythropoietin: A dangerous new form of blood doping? *Phys. Sportsmed.* 17:115–118.
Crowell, J.W., and E.E. Smith (1967). Determinant of the optimal hematocrit. *J. Appl. Physiol.* 22:501–504.
Dempsey, J., P. Hansen, and K. Henderson (1984). Exercise-induced hypoxemia in healthy persons at sea level. *J. Physiol. Lond.* 255:161–175.
Djojosugito, A.M., B. Folkow, B. Oberg, and S.W. White (1970). A comparison of blood viscosity measured in vitro and in a vascular bed. *Acta Physiol. Scand.* 78:70–84.
Dugal, R., and M. Bertrand (1976). Doping. In: *IOC Medical Commission Handbook* Montreal: Comite Orginisateur des Jeux Olympiques, pp.1–31.
Ekblom, B., A.N. Goldbarg, and B. Gullbring (1972). Response to exercise after blood loss and reinfusion. *J. Appl. Physiol.* 40:175–180.
Ekblom, B., G. Wilson, and P.-O. Astrand (1976). Central circulation during exercise after venesection and reinfusion of red blood cells. *J. Appl. Physiol.* 40:379–383.
Ekblom, B. (1989). Effects of iron deficiency, variation in hemoglobin concentration and erythropoietin injections on physical performance and relevant physiological parameters. *Proceedings of First I.O.C. World Congress on Sport Sciences* pp. 9–11.

Eschbach, J.W., J.C. Egrie, M.E. Downing, J.K. Browne, and J.W. Adamson (1987). Correction of the anemia of end-stage renal disease with recombinant human erythropoietin. Results of a combined phase I and II clinical trial. *N. Eng. J. Med.* 316:73–78.

Faulkner, J.A., J. Kollias, C.B. Favour, E. Buskirk, and B. Balke (1968). Maximum aerobic capacity and running performance at altitude. *J. Appl. Physiol.* 24:685–691.

Frye, A.J., and R.O. Ruhling (1977). RBC reinfusion, exercise, hemoconcentration, and $\dot{V}O_2$. *Med. Sci. Sports* 9:69. (Abstract).

Gaehtgens, P., F. Kreutz, and K.H. Albrecht (1979). Optimal hematocrit for canine skeletal muscle during rhythmic isotonic exercise. *Europ. J. Appl. Physiol.* 41:27–39.

Gledhill, N., F.J. Buick, A.B. Froese, L. Spriet, and E.C. Meyers (1978). An optimal method of storing blood for blood boosting *Med. Sci. Sports* 10:40. (Abstract).

Gledhill, N., L.L. Spriet, A.B. Froese, D.L. Wilkes, and E.C. Meyers (1980). Acid-base status with induced erythrocythemia and its influence on arterial oxygenation during heavy exercise. *Med. Sci. Sports Exerc.* 12:122. (Abstract).

Gledhill, N. (1982). Blood doping and related issues: a brief review. *Med. Sci. Sports Exerc.* 14:183–189.

Gledhill, N. (1985). The influence of altered blood volume and oxygen transport capacity on aerobic performance. In: R.L. Terjung (ed) *Exerc. Sport Sci. Rev.* New York: MacMillan, pp. 75–93.

Goforth, H.W., N.L. Campbell, J.A. Hogdon, and A.A. Sucec (1982). Hematologic parameters of trained distance runners following induced erythrocythemia. *Med. Sci. Sports Exerc.* 14:174. (Abstract).

Goodnough, L.T., S. Rudnick, T. Price et al. (1988). Erythropoietin therapy in autologous blood donors. *Blood* 72(Suppl. 1):138a. (Abstract).

Green, H.J., J.A. Thomson, M.E. Ball, R.L. Hughson, M.E. Houston, and M.T. Sharratt (1984). Alterations in blood volume following short-term supramaximal exercise. *J. Appl. Physiol.* 456:145–149.

Gregerson, M.I., and R.A. Dawson (1959). Blood volume. *Physiol. Rev.* 39:307–342.

Gullbring, B., A. Holmgren, T. Sjostrand, and T. Strandell (1960). The effect of blood volume variations on the pulse ratio in supine and upright positions during exercise. *Acta Physiol. Scand.* 50:62–71.

Gustafsson, L., L. Appelgren, and E. Myrvold (1980). The effect of polycythemia on blood flow in working and nonworking skeletal muscle. *Acta Physiol. Scand.* 109:143–148.

Kanstrup, I.-L., and B. Ekblom (1984). Blood volume and hemoglobin concentration as determinants of maximal aerobic power. *Med. Sci. Sports Exerc.* 16:256–262.

Lenfant, C., and K. Sullivan (1971). Adaptation to altitude. *New Eng. J. Med.* 264:1298–1309.

Mayer, G., J. Thum, and E.M. Cada (1988). Working capacity is increased following recombinant human erythropoietin treatment. *Kidney Int.* 34:525–528.

Murray, J.F., P. Gold, and B.L. Johnson (1962). Systemic oxygen transport in induced normovolemic anemia and polycythemia. *Am. J. Physiol.* 203:720–724.

Muza, S.R., M.N. Sawka, A.J. Young, R.C. Dennis, R.R. Gonzalez, J.W. Martin, and C.R. Valeri (1987). Elite special forces: physiological description and ergogenic influence of blood reinfusion. *Aviat. Space Environ. Med.* 58:1001–1004.

Pace, N., E.I. Lozner, W.V. Consolazio, G.C. Pitts, and L.J. Pecora (1947). The increase in hypoxia tolerance of normal man accompanying the polycythemia induced by transfusion of erythrocytes. *Am. J. Physiol.* 148:152–163.

Pate, R.R., J. McFarland, J. Van Wyck, and J. Okocha (1979). Effects of blood reinfusion on endurance performance in female distance runners. *Med. Sci. Sports* 11:97. (Abstract).

Powers, S.K., J. Lawler, J.A. Dempsey, S. Dodd, and G. Landry (1989). Effects of incomplete pulmonary gas exchange on $\dot{V}O_2max$. *J. Appl. Physiol.* 66:2491–2495.

Richardson, T.Q., and A.C. Guyton (1959). Effects of polycythemia and anemia on cardiac output and other circulatory factors. *Am. J. Physiol.* 197:1167–1170.

Robertson, R.J., R. Gilcher, K.F. Metz, G.S. Skrinar, T.G. Allison, H.T. Bahnson, R.A. Abbott, R. Becker, and J.E. Falkel (1982). Effect of induced erythrocythemia on hypoxia tolerance during physical exercise. *J. Appl. Physiol.* 53:490–495.

Robertson, R.J., R. Gilcher, K.F. Metz, C.J. Casperson, T.G. Allison, R.A. Abbott, G.S. Skrinar, J.R. Krause, and P.A. Nixon (1984). Hemoglobin concentration and aerobic work capacity in women following induced erythrocythemia. *J. Appl. Physiol.* 57:568–575.

Robertson, R.J., R. Gilcher, K.F. Metz, C.J. Casperson, T.G. Allison, R.A. Abbott, G.S. Skrinar, J.R. Krause, and P.A. Nixon (1988) Effect of simulated altitude erythrocythemia in women on hemoglobin flow rate during exercise. *J. Appl. Physiol.* 64:1644–1649.

Robinson, B.F., S.E. Epstein, R.L. Kahler, and E. Braunwald (1966). Circulatory effects of acute expansion of blood volume: studies during maximal exercise and at rest. *Circ. Res.* 19:26–32.

Rowell, L.B., H.L. Taylor, Y. Wang, and W.S. Carlson (1964). Saturation of arterial blood with oxygen during maximal exercise. *J. Appl. Physiol.* 19:284–286.

Rowell, L.B. (1969). Circulation. *Med. Sci. Sports* 1:15–22.

Sawka, M.N., R.C. Dennis, R.R. Gonzalez, A.J. Young, S.R. Muza, J.W. Martin, C.B. Wenger, R.P. Francesconi, K.B. Pandolf, and C.R. Valeri (1987a). Influence of polycythemia on blood volume and thermoregulation during heat-stress. *J. Appl. Physiol.* 62:912–918.

Sawka, M.N., A.J. Young, M.R. Muza, R.R. Gonzalez, and K.B. Pandolf (1987b). Erythrocyte reinfusion and maximal aerobic power: an examination of modifying factors. *J. Am. Med. Assoc.* 257:1496–1499.

Sawka, M.N., R.R. Gonzalez, A.J. Young, S.R. Muza, K.B. Pandolf, W.A. Latzka, R.C. Dennis, and C.R. Valeri (1988). Polycythemia and hydration: effects on thermoregulation and blood volume during exercise-heat stress. *Amer. J. Physiol.* 255:R456-R463.

Sawka, M.N., and A.J. Young (1989). Acute polycythemia and human performance during exercise and exposure to extreme environments. In: K.B. Pandolf (ed.) *Exerc. Sport Sci. Rev.* Baltimore:Williams and Wilkins, pp. 265–294.

Spriet, L.L., N. Gledhill, A.B. Froese, D.L. Wilkes, and E.C. Meyers (1980). The effect of induced erythrocythemia on central circulation and oxygen transport during maximal exercise. *Med. Sci. Sports Exerc.* 12:122. (Abstract).

Spriet, L.L., N. Gledhill, A.B. Froese, and D.L. Wilkes (1986). Effect of graded erythrocythemia on cardiovascular and metabolic response to exercise. *J. Appl. Physiol.* 61:1942–1948.

Stone, H.O., H.K. Thompson, and K. Schmidt-Nielsen (1968). Influence of erythrocytes on blood viscosity. *Am. J. Physiol.* 214:913–918.

Surks, M.I., K.S.K. Chin, and L.O. Matoush (1966). Alterations in body composition in man after acute exposure to high altitude. *J. Appl. Physiol.* 21:1741–1746.

Thomas, D.P., and G.F. Fregin (1981). Cardiorespiratory and metabolic responses to treadmill exercise in the horse. *J. Appl. Physiol.* 50:864–868.

Thomson, J.M., J.A. Stone, A.D. Ginsburg, and P. Hamilton (1982). O_2 transport during exercise following blood reinfusion. *J. Appl. Physiol.* 53:1213–1219.

Thomson, J.M., J.A. Stone, A.D. Ginsburg, and P. Hamilton (1983). The effects of blood reinfusion during prolonged heavy exercise. *Can. J. Appl. Sport Sci.* 8:72–78.

Valeri, C.R. (1976). *Blood Banking and the Use of Frozen Blood Products.* Cleveland: CRC Press.

Videman, T., and T. Rytomaa (1977). Effect of blood removal and auto-transfusion on heart rate response to a submaximal workload. *J. Sports Med. Phys. Fitness* 17:387–390.

Von Rost, R., W. Hollmann, H. Liesen, and D. Schulten (1975). Uber den Einfluss einer Erythrozyten-Retransfusion auf die kardio-pulmonale Leistungsfahigkeit. *Sportarzt Sportmedizin* 26:137–144.

Weisse, A.B., F.M. Carlton, H. Kuida, and H.H. Hecht (1964). Hemodynamic effects of normovolemic polycythemia in dogs at rest and during exercise. *Am. J. Physiol.* 207:1361–1366.

Williams, J., S. Powers, and K. Stuart (1986). Hemoglobin desaturation in highly trained athletes during heavy exercise. *Med. Sci. Sports Exerc.* 18:168–173.

Williams, M.H., A.R. Goodwin, R. Perkins, and J. Bocrie (1973). Effect of blood reinjection upon endurance capacity and heart rate. *Med. Sci. Sports* 5:181–186.

Williams, M.H., M. Lindhjem, and R. Schuster (1978). The effect of blood infusion upon endurance capacity and ratings of perceived exertion. *Med. Sci. Sports* 10:113–118.

Williams, M.H., S. Wesseldine, T. Somma, and R. Schuster (1981). The effect of induced erythrocythemia upon 5-mile treadmill run time. *Med. Sci. Sports Exerc.* 13:169–175.

DISCUSSION

ROBERTSON: There is apparently a gender specific response to blood doping. There have been comparatively few studies done with females, but in those studies, two units of autologous blood reinfusion actually produced a change in both performance and maximal oxygen uptake similar to what we see in males after infusion of three to four units of blood. I think that's strictly a matter of differences in total blood volume between males and females. Secondly, we really need more information about the rate of decay in hemoglobin concentration and all the associated ergogenic effects following blood doping. Most of the evidence indicates that once reinfusion of two or more units of blood takes place, hemoglobin concentration and all of the associated oxygen transport and delivery functions remain stable for about 14 days. Later, there is some fairly predictable decay that seems to follow the half life of the red cell. But there are few studies that follow this decay and the subsequent abatement of performance from 14 d all the way out to 120 d. We need to know at what point that performance drop-off is significant.

SPRIET: In the Buick study, we examined subjects for 120 d, week by week, to see when they did come back to normal, and we were very surprised to see that it took almost the same length of time as the life span of a red blood cell. The implication was that maybe even five or six weeks down the road from the blood doping, these people were experiencing benefits, perhaps both in training and actual competition. There is no doubt that this has to be addressed further.

COYLE: What is the evidence that altitude training, or endurance training at sea level for that matter, does indeed increase red cell mass? To my knowledge, there is no direct evidence of that.

SPRIET: Dr. Sawka has pointed out that it takes a long time before you actually get altitude-induced increases in red cell mass. Part of the confusion is that while you may see increases in hemoglobin concentration rather quickly, that is mainly an effect of a loss of plasma volume. It might take a month or six weeks to get a true increase in red cell mass. The problem with a prolonged stay at altitude is that athletes find it difficult to train at high intensity at a reduced barometric pressure. A way to get around that would be to either bring them back down to sea level every day to train or to put them in an oxygen-enriched environment in which they could attain the intensity of training that would maintain their fitness. But one of the problems to bringing them back down to altitude is that they still may be working with the reduced blood volume because of the altitude-induced decrease in plasma volume.

COYLE: But your assumption is that 4–6 weeks of training will eventually increase red cell volume?

SPRIET: Well, it is not really the training that we are assuming is doing it. It is just living in that hypoxic environment that stimulates the red cell mass.

COYLE: But even living at high altitude, to my knowledge, hasn't been shown conclusively to increase red cell volume. Long-term residents at high altitude, in fact, do have an increased red cell mass. When people live at altitude and come down to sea level, they generally show a reduction in fitness; even if they train, they don't show an improvement at altitude or back at sea level. Another approach would be to have people live at sea level and take them up intermittently to high altitude. It has been shown that when subjects went up and then came back down intermittently, they kept getting repeated spikes of erythropoietin. After about 12 d at sea level, the erythropoietin returns to normal. So what you might be able to do is live at sea level, do some mountain training at altitude once or twice a day, and come back down. In this way you avoid the nutritional problems of living at altitude, and you also may get a stimulus for increased erythropoietin. There has been some suggestion that the Germans may be doing that with some altitude chamber training.

BUTTERFIELD: In a study at Pike's Peak we found an increase in red blood cell mass in adequately nourished people in about three weeks.

SAWKA: Blood doping, by increasing oxygen carrying capacity of the blood, may produce a better distribution of a given cardiac output. Also, if a better blood distribution to various tissues leads to an improved ability to thermoregulate in certain situations, that means that for a given blood volume, you may have less blood in the skin and more in the central circulation.

I think that we agree that in a sterile laboratory situation, blood doping can be used safely. However, in practical terms we are talking about a free running athlete, and under these conditions, it may not be safe.

Finally, there is a great deal of individual variability in responses to blood doping. If you give a group of subjects several units of red blood cells, you can increase hemoglobin by 10% and improve maximal oxygen uptake. But there is considerable variability in the $\dot{V}O_2$max data. For example, if you look at the individual values for hemoglobin and plot them against the changes in maximal oxygen uptake for the same individuals, although the mean values for the group may show a 10% increase in hemoglobin and a 10% improvement in $\dot{V}O_2$max, the individual values show no relationship between change in hemoglobin and change in $\dot{V}O_2$max.

SPRIET: There is no doubt that after blood doping, a given work load represents a lower percentage of the new $\dot{V}O_2$max, and I think that probably is the major factor accounting for improved endurance at given workload. But I can't discount the fact that there are other factors that may contribute to that enhanced performance. For example, hemoglobin in the blood may contribute to buffering of ion fluctuations. Furthermore, it may be that you are able to thermoregulate better in the blood doped situation, which means that you can distribute more of your cardiac output to the tissues that need it. That is an important point with respect to understanding what happens during endurance. But I think the most critical effect is that athletes are working at a lower percentage of their new $\dot{V}O_2$max after blood doping. I agree that it is important to look at individual data, but when you measure a change in hemoglobin following doping and a change in $\dot{V}O_2$max, I am not surprised that there is a large variability because the change in hemoglobin doesn't necessarily tell you anything about the extra oxygen that may have been delivered to that individual.

SAWKA: That's the point. Each individual within a group may be improving in a different manner.

HEIGENHAUSER: One of the basic assumptions of red blood cell doping is that O_2 delivery is limiting to muscle. There are arguments pro and con for that. The increases in maximal O_2 uptake could also be due to changes in red blood cells that alter the ability of the muscle to do work so the muscle is able to increase its oxygen uptake. The red blood cell is not inert; it contributes to osmoregulation, acid base regulation, and transport of CO_2. If you increase the environmental oxygen concentration, you get effects similar to those you get by increasing the RBC mass. You can get about 10–15% increase in oxygen uptake, despite the fact that you are not changing the hematocrit.

SPRIET: One of the big limitations with these central circulatory measurements is that they can't tell you what might be happening at the cellular level. They can't even tell you whether or not the extra oxygen has been delivered, although the data suggest that some of it has been delivered. So, there is no question that better measurements at the cellular level should be made.

HEIGENHAUSER: I also want to comment on the effects of exposure to altitude. This exposure causes alterations within the muscle itself. Therefore, not only do you get the increased oxygen delivery, but you also get changes in blood flow dynamics and changes in metabolic function. I think the study that was done at Pike's Peak this year really showed dramatic effects on metabolism as the subjects came down to sea level. They had both things going for them: changes in red blood cell mass plus enzymatic adaptations in the muscle that could be of an added benefit to the increases in oxygen delivery.

SPRIET: That is a good point. Adaptations, whether in respiration, central circulation, peripheral circulation, or muscle metabolism, could all potentially lead to enhanced performance in certain individuals.

EICHNER: Certainly there is no doubt that if erythropoietin goes high enough, red cell mass increases, and it can work rather quickly. When erythropoietin was given to normals in preparation for releasing the hormone on the market, the mean hematocrit was up within two weeks from 42 to 49, and two of the subjects were closer to 55. They were phlebotomized because of concern about clots and strokes. In response to Ed Coyle's question regarding altitude, I think it is indisputable that if erythropoietin goes high enough, red cell mass will go up. Secondly, there is accumulating evidence that exercise, at least in the upright posture—skiing, cycling, running—causes bursts of erythropoietin. Whether these increases are enough to have any effect is still questionable, but I think it is reasonable to expect that in time training might cause an increase in red cell mass.

What I am really worried about is the abuse of erythropoietin by athletes. I am not so worried about somebody starting competition with a hematocrit of 50 but about somebody starting with a hematocrit of 60, 70, or even 80—which is theoretically possible if someone uses too much erythropoietin. If a runner starts a hot weather marathon at a hematocrit of 55, he may finish the race at a hematocrit of 65 if he gets dehydrated. There was an admission by one of the physicians at the ACSM conference in Salt Lake City, that he knew three cyclist using erythropoietin. As most of you know, there have been 15 deaths that may be related to erythropoietin use in cyclists in Holland in the last three years. I think the use of erythropoietin is going to eventually obviate blood boosting by autologous transfusion because using erythropoietin is an easy way to blood dope.

SPRIET: I couldn't agree with you more. The only information I could find on erythropoietin was a newspaper article that described Bjorn Ekblom's erythropoietin study, which he seems to have done with very good controls. The results are incredible. They gave "low doses" of erythropoietin for seven weeks to 15 randomly chosen recreational athletes, and 15 controls received a placebo. According to this article, in seven weeks hemoglobin concentration was increased by almost one-third, and every one of these athletes increased his endurance performance by at least 10%.

POWERS: The assumption here is that the ergogenic potential in blood doping is a widening of the A-V O_2 difference. We have only one paper to go on, and that is a paper by Thomson et al. (1982), who measured femoral venous O_2 content and showed that blood doping increased the A-V O_2 difference. As far as commenting on what is happening at the cellular level, it is very difficult for me to do that. Very puzzling, of course, is why in the femoral venous outflow there is any oxygen at all if, in fact, the oxygen delivery is the problem. A lot of people believe that it is simply mismatching between where the red blood cells are and where the cells that can utilize the oxygen are. Or, possibly, the red blood cell passes through the muscle too fast and doesn't have the time to completely unload its oxygen.

WILMORE: I am very intrigued by the data in the Buick study after 7 d, where there is a discrepancy between $\dot{V}O_2$max changes and performance changes. I am very eager to hear an explanation of that.

SPRIET: That study obviously provided us with quite a few questions as to what was going on because the athletes did not bring their hemoglobin concentration back down to normal until about 17 or 18 weeks following the study. I have to backtrack slightly and mention that in the study the subjects were divided into two groups— six in one group and five in another. The first group received the sham infusion first and then the reinfusion. The trouble with doing it the opposite way, which is what the other group did, i.e., blood reinfusion first and then the sham, is you have to make a decision as to whether to give the sham soon after the reinfusion when the hemoglobin concentration is still up, or to allow the hemoglobin concentration to come all the way back to normal before giving the sham. This was a problem that we didn't anticipate because we thought the hemoglobin concentration would come down fairly quickly. We made the decision to wait until the hemoglobin was normalized before giving the sham reinfusion, which, of course, meant that we ended up waiting 16–17 weeks. In those subjects tested 16–17 weeks later, $\dot{V}O_2$max was still elevated, and yet their endurance time was not. As far as a good explanation for that, we really don't have any. The one we put forth in the paper is rather weak. That was that the subjects had been involved in the study 10–12 weeks longer than we had promised them, and we thought that possibly they were not pushing themselves as hard on the treadmill. But I don't believe that because these people are very good at going to the exhaustion end-point time and time again. If that finding is reproducible, it has some interesting ramifications for what benefit you might expect from this type of manipulation with respect to training.

HEIGENHAUSER: One of the things you've also got to look at is the age of the red blood cell and the changing function of the red blood cell with aging. You primarily examined the hemoglobin concentrations but did not look at the other functions of the red blood cell, which could have changed during that period of time. In this regard, erythropoietin might be advantageous because the red cells would be younger and have better function.

ROBERTSON: There is one point I think might reconcile the difference in opinion between George Heigenhauser and Jack Wilmore with respect to the Buick study, where $\dot{V}O_2$max remained elevated and endurance performance declined at the end of the 120 d. There may be a dissociation between oxygen-carrying capacity and buffering capacity of the red cell as a function of aging. The role that the added red cell mass may play in buffering and its effect on performance is glossed over in the blood doping literature.

Another point that bears on the central versus peripheral issue is that there is a fairly large number of studies that show more oxygen being delivered in the doped state than is taken up. There are two conclusions that seem to be offered. One is that in the doped state there are peripheral factors that seem to predominate in limiting maximal oxygen uptake. The other is one that bothers me a little bit, and that is a prevailing hypothesis that, somehow or other, this added oxygen is shunted away from active tissue and resides in some metabolically inactive pool. It has to be metabolically inactive, or it would show up in the total body oxygen uptake, which it doesn't. Well, that seems to be a fairly convenient scapegoat for explaining something in the literature that is quite inconsistent.

SPRIET: The sequential reinfusion studies showing further increases in $\dot{V}O_2$max with more and more reinfusions suggest to me that what is being delivered to the muscle is being used because otherwise I have a hard time rationalizing why a third unit, a fourth unit, and a fifth unit of blood will produce further increases in $\dot{V}O_2$max. It may be more complicated than delivery. It may be that in some situations you're pushing blood through cells that are already taking up as much oxygen as they can, and the limiting factors in those cells is something metabolic, whereas other cells can still take up some of the oxygen. I think it is extremely complicated, and I don't know that we can do much more than we've done with these central measurements. What we've done is set the stage for a lot of peripheral studies to try to answer some of these questions about blood doping.

7

Anabolic/Androgenic Steroids and Growth Hormone

John A. Lombardo, M.D.

Robert C. Hickson, Ph.D.

David R. Lamb, Ph.D.

INTRODUCTION

Because athletic prowess has long been associated with large skeletal muscles, leanness, aggressive behavior, and other masculine characteristics, it is only natural that athletes have sought to improve their athletic performance by eating foods and ingesting or injecting substances thought to increase muscle mass or otherwise enhance masculinity. Anabolic/androgenic steroids and growth hormone are two of these substances. Both of these types of hormones can have dramatic effects on muscle mass under certain conditions, and both have been associated with mild to moderate adverse effects that are common, and with severe, even life-threatening, adverse effects that are quite rare. Both substances are banned by sports governing bodies, and their nonmedical use is considered unethical and illegal in many nations. Nevertheless, reports continue to accumulate that athletes and non-athletes, both young and old, male and female, are abusing these substances in increasing numbers.

The purpose of this chapter is to review the evidence pertinent to the rationale for use of these drugs, the prevalence of their use, their ergogenicity, and their adverse side effects.

ANABOLIC/ANDROGENIC STEROIDS

Background

According to Forbes (1947), the masculinizing properties of the male reproductive system have been reported since the 18th century. Androsterone and dehydroandrosterone were isolated from male urine in 1931, and androsterone was first synthesized in 1934. This led to the commercial production of androsterone and testosterone. Testosterone was isolated from bull testes in 1935 and found to be much more potent than androsterone (Newerla, 1943).

Testosterone, the building block from which anabolic steroids are developed, is a steroid hormone that has two common classifications for its general actions:

1) An androgenic (masculinizing) effect, e.g., deepening of the voice, growth of body and facial hair, development of sexual organs, etc.
2) An anabolic (tissue building) effect that stimulates the development of muscle mass and enhancement of long bone growth.

These anabolic and androgenic effects are not completely separable because the cell receptor sites appear to be the same; hence, steroid hormones similar in structure to testosterone are designated as anabolic/androgenic hormones (Kochakian, 1976).

Kochakian (1935) and Kochakian and Murlin (1935) had demonstrated that castration caused a negative nitrogen balance (loss of tissue protein) in dogs. This was slightly alleviated with the injection of an extract of human male urine. With the commercial availability of testosterone, Kochakian (1937) proved the protein anabolic action of the masculinizing sex hormones (androgens) in animals. Kenyon and his associates (1938) demonstrated similar anabolic effects of androgens in humans. Kochakian's contribution to the field of protein metabolism and the anabolic action of androgens is recognized as the key which opened the door not only to the clinical applications of androgens but also to their use for performance enhancement (Wright, 1978). Simonson et al. (1944) studied the effects of methyl testosterone on six men, 48–67 years of age, who complained of excessive fatigability or loss of working capacity. Significant steroid-associated increases were found in strength of back muscles in four of the six subjects. Support was thus given for Boje's (1939) belief in the enhancement of physical performance by reproductive hormones.

Bodybuilders reportedly were using testosterone in the late 1940s and 1950s (Wright, 1978), but the reports of Soviet use of androgens in weightlifting in 1954 and subsequent experimentation by Dr. John Ziegler and U.S.A. weightlifters are credited with the initiation of widespread androgen use by athletes (Starr, 1981; Todd, 1987; Wade, 1972). In 1958, the synthetic androgen, methandrostenolone (Dianabol[R]), the first "anabolic steroid," was released, and the anabolic/androgenic steroid era in sports had its birth.

Incidence of Steroid Use

There are two sources of information regarding incidence of use of anabolic/androgenic steroids in athletics. One is the results of drug testing of various groups; these results document the number of individuals who have metabolites of these drugs measured in their urine by various tests (Table 7-1). The second source of information is surveys administered to various groups (Tables 7-2, 7-3, 7-4). Estimates of incidence of drug use obtained by either method are believed to be low (Yesalis et al., 1989). The surveys are not believed to be confidential by the athletes, and this leads to improper information. The number of positive drug tests simply measures the incidence of positive urine tests at a single point in time, the day of the test, and not the incidence of use during the training period.

This is especially true for testing at the time of an event, e.g., the Olympics, because anabolic/androgenic steroids are drugs used during training and not for the event itself.

Ergogenic Effects

The use of anabolic/androgenic steroids has been reported (Tables 7-1 through 7-4) in various types of athletes, e.g., weightlifters, bodybuilders, throwers (javelin, discus, hammer, and shotput), track and field participants, football players, swimmers, sprinters, and middle and long distance runners in track. Another group of users of these drugs is those individuals for whom physical appearance is so important that they use anabolic/androgenic steroids so that they can "look good."

The benefits desired by these anabolic/androgenic steroid users include:

1. Alteration in body composition (increase in lean mass and reduced fat)
2. Increase in strength
3. Increase in endurance
4. Reduction in recovery time from intense workouts (thereby allowing more frequent and/or higher intensity workouts)
5. Enhancement of athletic performance

TABLE 7-1. *Anabolic Steroid Use Based on Announced Drug Testing**

Year	Drug Testing Site	Test Results	% Positive
1976	Olympic Games (Montreal)	8 positives 275 analyses	2.9%
1980	Olympic Games (Moscow)	0 positives 1500 analyses	0.0%
1983	Pan American Games (Caracas)	15 positives 825 analyses	1.8%
1984	Olympic Games (Los Angeles)	17 positives 1510 analyses	1.1%
	(10 'sanctioned' positives; 17 positives)**		
1986– 1987	NCAA Championships and Bowl Games	26 positives 3360 analyses	0.8%
1987	US Olympic Festival (Greensboro)	6 positives 628 analyses	0.9%
1987– 1988	NCAA Championships and Bowl Games	9 positives 2385 analyses	0.4%
1988	Olympic Games (Seoul)	30 positives 1500 analyses	2.0%
	(10 'sanctioned' positives; 30 positives)**		

* From: Yesalis, C.E., J.E. Wright, J.A. Lombardo (1989).
** For the past two Summer Olympiads, the number of laboratory 'positives' has exceeded the number of athletes sanctioned (see, for example, Catlin et al., 1987). No satisfactory explanation is available.

TABLE 7-2. *Self-reported anabolic steroid use among high school students*

Investigator and year	Site and study population	Number of subjects	AS Use rate	Response rate
Newman (1986)	Michigan—11 school districts, 8, 10, 12 grades	5029	8th 10th 12th Total 3% 2% 2% 3% M F 5% 1%	NR
		1426 (seniors only)		
Buckley, et al. (1988)	24 states, 46 high schools 12 grade males	3403	M 6.6%	50%
Johnson et al.(1989)	Arkansas—6 schools 11th grade	1775	M F T 11% 0.5% 5.7%	99.5%
McLain (1989)	Ilinois—one school	2075	M F T 6.7% 1.7% 4.1%	98%
Windsor & Dumitru (1989)	Texas—5 schools	901	M F T 5.0% 1.4% 3.0%	89%

* Not reported
From: Yesalis, C.E., Wright, J.E., Lombardo, J.A. Anabolic—Androgenic Steroids: a synthesis of existing data and recommendations for future research. *Clinical Sports Medicine* 1 (3); 109–134, 1989.

TABLE 7-3. *Self-reported anabolic steroid use among collegiate students*

Investigator and year	Site and study population	Number of subjects	AS use rate	Response rate
Dezelsky et al. (1985)	Five universities 1970, 73,76,80,84	4171	15% athletes (1970) 20% athletes (1976–84) 1% nonathletes (1984)	NR*
Anderson & McKeag (1985)	Intercollegiate athletes at 11 universities	2100	9% football 5% Div I athletes 4% men's basketball and track 1% women's swimming	72%
Anderson & McKeag (1989)	Intercollegiate athletes at 11 universities	2300	M F 6.4% 1% 10% football 5% Division I & II athletes 4% Division II athletes 5% men's track and field 1% women's swimming, track and field, softball	78%
Pope et al. (1988)	Three universities	1010 males 147 varsity athletes	2% 9.4%	30%

* Not reported

From: Yesalis, C.E., Wright, J.E., Lombardo, J.A. Anabolic—Androgenic Steroids: a synthesis of existing data and recommendations for future research. *Clinical Sports Medicine* 1 (3): 109–134, 1989.

TABLE 7-4. *Self-reported anabolic steroid use among athletes*

Investigator and year	Site and study population	Number of subjects	AS use rate	Response rate
Ljungqvist, 1975	Elite Swedish track and field athletes	99	31% 75% throwers 0% middle and long distance runners	69%
Frankle et al. 1984	Weight lifters in three gymnasiums	250	44%	NR*
Newman 1987	Elite women athletes in over 15 sports	271	3%	59%
Yesalis et al. 1988	Elite powerlifters	45 ques 20 phone	33.3% 55%	74%

* Not reported

From: Yesalis, C.E., Wright, J.E., Lombardo, J.A. Anabolic—Androgenic Steroids: a synthesis of existing data and recommendations for future research. *Clinical Sports Medicine* 1 (3); 109–134, 1989.

To evaluate the benefit of anabolic/androgenic steroids in these areas, two sources of information are available. One is the scientific literature, which is fraught with contradiction and confusion, and the other is the more consistent but often questionable anecdotal evidence given by athletes and other steroid users.

Effects in Laboratory and Domestic Farm Animals. There is consistency in the results of the animal studies regarding the use of anabolic steroids. Normal male animals have consistently shown no increase in body weight or improvement in performance after anabolic/androgenic steroid treatment (Hickson et al., 1976; Richardson, 1977; Young et al., 1977). The problems with the application of these results to humans are the types of exercise (running on a treadmill and swimming vs. progressive resistance exercise) and the uncertainty in the simulation of the psychological effects of competitive drive of the human in the animal.

However, castrated male rats (Kochakian & Endahl, 1959; Heitzman, 1976), normal female rats (Exner et al., 1973; Hervey & Hutchinson, 1973), steers (Heitzman, 1976), and castrated male poultry (Nesheim, 1976) consistently exhibited significant increases in nitrogen retention and lean body mass after treatment with androgenic/anabolic steroids.

Effects in Human Beings.

Aerobic Capacity and Endurance. Because anabolic steroids stimulate the bone marrow to produce red blood cells (erythropoiesis), it has been hypothesized that steroid administration could increase the oxygen-carrying capacity of the blood and thereby improve maximal oxygen uptake ($\dot{V}O_2$max) and aerobic endurance performance. There have been reported increases in indirect measures of aerobic

ANABOLIC/ANDROGENIC STEROIDS **255**

capacity ($\dot{V}O_2$max) with anabolic/androgenic steroids in males in some studies (Albrecht & Albrecht, 1969; Johnson & O'Shea, 1969; Keul et al., 1976). But there also have been reports of no increase in aerobic capacity with steroid use (Johnson et al., 1972; Fahey & Brown, 1973; Johnson et al., 1975; Hervey et al., 1976).

Because tests of $\dot{V}O_2$max (and especially tests that do not directly measure $\dot{V}O_2$max) are not necessarily good predictors of endurance performance, it is unclear what effect steroid use has on such performance. It would be interesting to observe the effects of steroids on a direct measure of aerobic endurance performance. However, because the effects of steroids on red blood cell production in normal men are relatively small, there are only weak rationales for hypothesizing a beneficial effect of steroids on endurance performance, due to this mechanism.

Body Composition. Athletes believe that anabolic/androgenic steroid use will increase lean body mass and decrease the amount of body fat. Are these beliefs supported by the experimental studies? Unfortunately, the variations in subjects, methods, and materials confound the interpretation of the results of these studies. Griggs et al. (1989), using pharmacologic doses of testosterone enanthate (3 mg/kg weekly), reported significant increases in muscle protein synthesis in normal non-exercising men. However, they found no significant increase in muscle fiber diameter despite significant increases in body weight. Crist et al. (1983) studied the effects of a low dose of steroids for three weeks on the body composition of experienced weight trainers, who consumed supplemental protein. Crist et al. (1983) used underwater weighing and found no increase in lean body mass. Hervey et al. (1981) studied experienced weightlifters for six weeks with no dietary controls but with 100 mg methandrosterolone daily. They found significant increases in lean body mass by underwater weighing, skinfolds, and anthropometric measurements. Similar results were found by Hervey et al. (1976) in an earlier study, differing only in the choice of subjects (inexperienced weightlifters).

Table 7-5 compares these and other studies on the effects of anabolic/androgenic steroids on lean body mass. Fowler et al. (1965), Fahey and Brown (1973), Golding et al. (1974), Stromme et al. (1974), and Crist et al. (1983) reported no significant change in lean body mass with the use of anabolic/androgenic steroids. But O'Shea (1971), Johnson et al. (1972), Ward (1973), Stamford and Moffatt (1974), Hervey et al. (1976, 1981), Loughton and Ruhling (1977), and Alen et al. (1984) all found significant increases in lean body mass. Interestingly, only Golding et al. (1974) and Crist et al. (1983) found no increases in lean body mass with experienced weight trainers, and only Hervey et al. (1976) found significant lean body mass increases with inexperienced weightlifters.

In summary, although there are contradictory data in the literature in regards to the effect of anabolic/androgenic steroids on lean body mass, the majority of the evidence suggests that there is often a positive effect of steroid administration on lean body mass. Accordingly, the American College of Sports Medicine (1987) has concluded that "... anabolic/androgenic steroids, in the presence of an adequate diet, can contribute to increases in body weight, often in the lean mass compartment."

Strength Performance. Athletes also believe that there is an enhancement in strength when anabolic steroids are used in conjunction with progressive resistance exercises. When one examines the scientific literature, contradictory results are once again found.

Stamford and Moffatt (1974) found significant increases in strength in their study of prisoners who were experienced weight trainers and who were given supplemental protein with a low dosage of anabolic/androgenic steroids. On the other hand, Crist et al. (1983) found no significant increases in strength under similar conditions. The short duration of the treatment period (3 weeks) and the dosage of drug (100 mg nandrolone decanoate/week), which was much less than that used by athletes, are notable criticisms of the study by Crist et al.

About one-half of the research reports have shown no significant increase in strength with the use of anabolic/androgenic steroids (Fowler et al., 1965; Fahey & Brown, 1973; Golding et al., 1974; Stromme et al., 1974; Hervey et al., 1976; Loughton & Ruhling, 1977; Crist et al., 1983). Other studies have shown significant increases in strength (O'Shea, 1971; Ward, 1973; Stamford & Moffatt, 1974; Hervey et al., 1981; Alen et al., 1984). As a whole, this research does not give overwhelming support for the presence or absence of an ergogenic effect of anabolic/androgenic steroids on strength.

The contradiction is well illustrated by comparing two studies by the same laboratory (Hervey et al., 1976; Hervey et al., 1981; Table 7-6). These similar studies both employed a cross-over design with a six-week treatment of drug or placebo, a five- or six-week wash-out period, and a six-week treatment on the opposite condition. Both studies used the dosage most closely resembling the amount used by many of the athletes who abuse anabolic/androgenic steroids, but they still showed differences in the effects of steroids on strength. The major difference between the two studies was the weight-lifting experience of the subjects. Because many variables affect maximal strength performance, it is extremely difficult to detect statistically significant effects of any experimental

TABLE 7-5. *Anabolic Steroid Effects on Body Mass and Strength*

Study	Golding et al. (1974)	Stromme et al. (1974)	Hervey et al. (1974)	Hervey et al. (1976)	Ward (1973)	Fahey & Brown (1973)	Stamford & Moffatt (1974)	Crist et al. (1983)	Loughton & Ruhling (1977)	Fowler et al. (1965)	O'Shea (1971)	Alen et al. (1984)
Duration (wks)	12	8	6 ×3	6 ×3	5	9	8	3 ×3	7	16	4	24
Intensity	Mod → Heavy	Mod → Heavy	Mod → Heavy	Mod → Heavy	Heavy	Light → Mod		Heavy → Heavy	Mod → Heavy	Light	Mod → Heavy	Heavy
Frequency	4	3	–	–	3?	3	3	–	6	5	3	6
Drug/ Dosage	? 10 ?	Mes 75–100	Met 100	Met 100	Met 10	Nand 1/kg wk	Met 10	Nand test 100/wk	Met 10	Met 20	Met 10	Var
Diet	← Prot	← Prot	–	–	–	–	← Prot	← Prot	← Prot	–	← Prot	Adeq Prot
Exp/ Inexp	Exp	Inexp?	Exp	Inexp	Exp	Inexp	Exp	Exp	Exp? Inexp	Inexp	Exp	Exp
WT/LBM	– SF	– Ant	+ UW SF Ant	+ UW SF Ant	+ UW	– UW	+ Ant	– UW	+ BWT	– SF Ant	+ SF	+ SF
Strength	–	–	–	–	+	–	+		–	+	+	+

Legend: Durat (weeks) = duration; Intens. = Intensity; Mod = Moderate; Freq. = Frequency of workouts (days) Met: methandrosteneolone; Nand = Nandrolone; Prot = protein; Exp = experienced weight trainer; Inexp = Inexperience weight trainer; WT = weight, LBM = lean body mass; SF = skinfolds; Ant = anthropometric; UW = underwater weighing; BWT = body weight

From: Lombardo, J. Ergogenic Effects of Anabolic-Androgenic Steroids. National Institute of Drug Abuse Monograph (in press).

TABLE 7-6. *Comparison of two studies by Hervey et al. (1976, 1981).*

	1976	1981
Methandrostenolone Dose	100 mg/d	100 mg/d
Subject Number & Source	N = 11	N = 7
	Physical Education	Experienced
	Majors	Weightlifters
Body Weight Effects	Increase	Increase
Fat Free Mass Effects	Increase	Increase
Strength Effects	No Change	Increase

treatment. Therefore, because many studies do report a positive effect of steroid administration on strength performance, the American College of Sports Medicine (1987) has concluded that "the gains in muscular strength achieved through high intensity exercise and proper diet can be increased by the use of anabolic/androgenic steroids in some individuals."

Reasons for Discrepant Effects Reported on Strength. Control of independent variables such as diet, weight-training experience, and drug dosage has been inconsistent in the experimental studies on the ergogenic effects on anabolic/androgenic steroids. Lamb (1984) concluded that there is no systematic pattern in the variables to explain the differences in steroid effects on strength. Wright (1978) and Yesalis et al. (1989) proposed a number of potential explanations for the confusing results (Table 7-7).

The resistance-training experience of the subjects is hypothesized to be a factor because early strength gains by inexperienced weight trainers will be largely due to early development of neuromuscular skill and strength in completing the lifts. The effect of administration of anabolic/androgenic steroids in novice lifters will thus be small and probably insignificant. However, when steroids are used by an experienced weight trainer who typically makes very small strength gains per training cycle, the drug-enhanced effect on strength can be statistically significant (Wright, 1978; Yesalis et al., 1989). However, there are reports of insignificant drug effects on experienced lifters (Crist et al., 1983; Golding et al., 1974).

The dosage of the drug is another variable often mentioned as potentially confounding in the interpretation of results of steroid treatment on strength. The low dosage found to be ergogenically effective by Ward (1973) and O'Shea (1971) is much less than the dose used by athletes. Accordingly, low dosages probably do not account totally for an absence of reported ergogenic effects of steroids on strength.

Intensity of training is another important variable that could conceivably affect the outcome of steroid use on strength. Unfor-

TABLE 7-7. *Reasons for a Lack of Consensus on Anabolic Steroid Effects on Health and Performance Variables in Human Subjects**

Subjects	The number of subjects, their experience in weight training, and their physical condition at the start of the study varied.
Diet	Most diets were not controlled or recorded.
Training programs	Volumes and intensities varied.
Testing programs	Strength often not measured in the training mode. Body composition often assessed from skinfold estimates. Health effects often mismeasured (not organ specific) or not measured.
Drugs	Variable. Few have reported on athletes self-administering multiple drugs.
Study	Some crossover, some single blind, some double blind, some not blind, some without controls.
Drug mechanism	Unknown and varying degrees of anabolic, anticatabolic, and motivational effects, depending upon the circumstances.
Dosages	Variable. Only two studies administered dosages approximating those currently used by competing athletes.
Length of study	Variable and generally short; very few have reported on prolonged training and anabolic steroid self-administration.
Placebo effect	Well documented for most drugs; yet most data suggest that athletes can readily detect anabolic steroid administration, making it virtually impossible to conduct blind studies.
Data interpretation	Variable, dependent upon the background and experience (scientific, clinical, athletic, administrative), general perspective and goals of interpreters.
Legal and ethical	Preclude design and execution of well-controlled studies using doses and patterns of administration of drugs with unknown long term effects in healthy volunteers in a manner comparable to those of many current anabolic steroid users.

* From: Yesalis et al. (1989).

tunately, it is difficult to determine weight-training intensity in some reports. Most experiments fall into a "moderate to moderately heavy" range of intensity (Golding et al., 1974; Stromme et al., 1974; Hervey et al., 1976; O'Shea, 1971; Hervey et al., 1981). Fahey and Brown (1973) and Fowler et al. (1965), had low-intensity training. Only Ward (1973), Stamford and Moffatt (1974), and Alen et al. (1984) used very high-intensity training.

These explanations (Table 7-7) represent reasonable hypotheses to explain some of the different results of studies that evaluated the effects of anabolic steroids on strength, but the hypotheses have not been adequately tested in well-controlled studies.

Effects of Steroid Use in Women and Children. No scientific experiments have been performed on the ergogenic effects of anabolic/ androgenic steroids in women and children. It is considered especially unethical to perform such studies in women and children because of the virilizing side effects of these drugs. However, based on the results of studies on castrated male animals (Kochakian & Endahl, 1959; Heitzman, 1976) and on normal female animals, (Exner et al., 1973; Hervey & Hutchinson, 1973; Heitzman, 1976; Nesheim, 1976), one could expect a positive effect of steroids on lean body mass in women and children, who have lower endogenous levels of testosterone than adult males. Such expections, at least for women, are born out by observations of extreme muscular development in many of those women bodybuilders who admit to steroid use.

Mechanism of Ergogenic Action of Anabolic Steroids. Ligand binding to specific cytoplasmic or nuclear receptor molecules initiates the steroid hormone actions within cells. The steroid receptor complex then undergoes activation or transformation. Activation results in a conformational change and an increased ability for some receptors to translocate to the nuclei and to bind to specific DNA regions on hormone-responsive proteins (Schmidt & Litwack, 1982). Hormone receptor binding appears to have a central regulatory role in the actions of steroids. For example, with the use of the glucocorticoid antagonist RU 38486, which binds to the glucocorticoid receptor, Konagaya et al. (1986) were able to demonstrate attenuation of the skeletal muscle atrophy associated with glucocorticoid administration.

Based on the presence of androgen receptors, skeletal muscles can be considered androgen responsive (Snochowski et al. 1981). The in vitro binding studies of Saartok et al. (1984) have shown that a number of androgenic/anabolic steroids have affinity for the androgen receptor. This finding argues against the existence of a separate anabolic steroid receptor. However, several of the tested anabolic steroids had very low relative binding affinity. Such steroids may have alternate actions such as influencing enzymatic activation involved in metabolizing anabolic and catabolic hormones or displacing other steroids from the testosterone-estradiol binding globulin (TeBG) within the circulation (Saartok et al., 1984). Consequently, there is the possibility of direct anabolic steroid effects on muscle, particularly through the androgen receptor.

However, the ability of anabolic steroids to exert their effects through this mechanism has been questioned (Wilson, 1988). The low androgen receptor binding capacity and low binding affinity for androgens by skeletal muscle (Hickson et al., 1983), when considered with normally high circulating hormone levels of men, suggest that the receptor is at near ligand saturation under most conditions. Therefore, for anabolic steroids to operate through the androgen receptor, it would likely be necessary that they have very high anabolic potency, high affinity for the receptor, and be administered in pharmacological amounts in order to obtain occupancy of the receptor.

It is possible that androgens could accelerate muscle growth by increasing the secretion or activity of other growth promoting substances such as growth hormone and insulin-like growth factors. There is some evidence for an androgen effect on growth hormone secretion in adult hypogonadal men (Liu et al., 1987). Also, in one study on boys with impaired growth and/or development, administration of either testosterone or oxandrolone nearly doubled 24-h growth hormone secretion (Ulloa-Aguirre et al., 1990); in a similar investigation, oxandrolone treatment increased serum concentrations of insulin-like growth factor I (Stanhope et al., 1988).

Anabolic steroids may also function as growth-promoting hormones through an anticatabolic regulation. This action would be expressed through the inhibition of glucocorticoid hormone mechanisms. This hypothesis has been considered attractive because of the elevated cortisol levels that accompany strenuous exercise in humans (Wheeler et al.,1984; Guglielmini et al., 1984; Villanueva et al., 1986; Urhausen & Kindermann, 1987; Mather et al., 1986). Glucocorticoid excess also causes total body and skeletal muscle catabolism through increased amino acid efflux, decreased rates of protein synthesis, and increased protein breakdown (Shoji & Pennington, 1977; Rannell & Jefferson, 1980; Odedra et al., 1983; Kayali et al., 1987). There are at least two ways that anabolic steroids may act to alter glucocorticoid action.

One method of anabolic steroid inhibition would be through binding to the glucocorticoid receptor. The number of glucocorticoid receptors is 20–50 fold higher than the number of androgen receptors, depending on muscle-fiber type (Hickson et al., 1983; Hickson et al., 1986). The availability of excess anabolic steroids, the limited androgen receptor capacity, and higher glucocorticoid receptor capacity within muscle cells would seem to present opportunistic conditions for "spillover" and occupancy of glucocorticoid binding sites by these compounds. However, the results of both in vitro and in vivo binding studies have been inconsistent. With in vitro binding experiments, Mayer and Rosen (1975), demonstrated androgen and anabolic steroid inhibition of dexamethasone binding to gastrocnemius muscle cytosols of adrenalectomized rats. Also, DuBois and Almon (1984) observed that low concentrations of dihydrotestosterone and testosterone inhibited 50% of dexamethasone binding.

On the contrary, other investigations have observed very low affinity of these androgens for the glucocorticoid receptor (Snochowski et al., 1980; Dahlberg et al., 1981; Sharpe et al., 1986; Capaccio et al., 1987). For instance, Capaccio et al. (1987) observed little or no competition by high concentrations of testosterone for triamcinolone acetonide binding in gastrocnemius muscle cytosols of either intact or adrenalectomized female rats.

There is no agreement regarding anabolic steroid binding to glucocorticoid receptors in muscle following in vivo hormone administration. In one study, fluoxymesterone reduced glucocorticoid binding by 77%, whereas testosterone had no effect following 4 d of treatment (Mayer & Rosen 1975). Other studies observed no inhibition of glucocorticoid binding by testosterone (Capaccio et al., 1987; Danhaive & Rousseau, 1988), whereas trenbolone administration resulted in an augmented glucocorticoid receptor binding (Danhaive & Rousseau, 1988). Sharpe et al. (1986) found that trenbolone acetate reduced glucocorticoid binding by 25–38% after 4–22 d of treatment, but concluded that the anabolic steroid was not occupying glucocorticoid receptor sites; rather, they suggested that the anabolic steroid was down-regulating glucocorticoid receptor content.

A second method whereby anabolic steroids may act as anti-catabolic hormones is at the gene level of glucocorticoid inducible proteins. Common DNA sequences in various genes, located prior to the transcription start site, are known to interact with the DNA binding site of the activated glucocorticoid receptor complex (Beato et al., 1987; Beato, 1989). A consensus hormone regulatory or response element (HRE) sequence, 15 nucleotides long, has been identified for the glucocorticoid receptor (glucocorticoid response element—GRE) from a variety of DNA binding sites (Beato et al., 1987; Beato, 1989). As yet, no clear consensus sequence for the androgen receptor has been shown to exist (Beato, 1989). Different steroid hormones are able to regulate the same set of genes, and the GRE does not have exclusive specificity for the glucocorticoid receptor. Recent evidence indicates that the GRE can mediate the induction of several genes by other steroid hormones, including androgens (Cato et al., 1987; Ham et al., 1988; Denison et al., 1989). Androgen induction of transcription at the GRE is inhibited by androgen receptor antagonists (Cato et al., 1987). The long-range physiological implications of several steroids operating through the same HRE are still unknown. But the potential of an anabolic steroid to act through its own receptor and alter the course of glucocorticoid action through the GRE of responsive genes could play a significant role in the regulation of muscle mass.

There is again an absence of consistency in the results of the limited number of studies that have examined the potential anti-catabolic functioning of androgens as glucocorticoid antagonists. Capaccio et al., (1987) observed that testosterone acetate administration was unable to prevent cortisol acetate-induced muscle wasting in slowly growing female rats. On the other hand, Danhaive and Rousseau (1988) reported that RU 486, i.e., RU 38486, testosterone, and trenbolone all attenuated corticosteroid-induced retardation of growth in several muscles examined in young, rapidly growing, adrenalectomized rats. Both studies observed enhanced total body and muscle growth due to androgenic/anabolic steroid treatment alone (Capaccio et al., 1987; Danhaive & Rousseau, 1988). Differences in steroids, dosages, hormonal state, age, and growth rates existed between these studies. It seems likely that there are multiple regulatory influences on the potential interference of androgens with glucocorticoid functioning.

In humans, Aakvaag et al. (1978) found a decrease in circulating testosterone and an increase in cortisol in military recruits undergoing severe physical and psychological stress. Other examples of training-induced increases in cortisol coupled to decreases in testosterone were shown by Wheeler et al. (1984), Guglielmini et al. (1984), Villanueva et al. (1986), Urhausen and Kindermann (1987), and Mather et al. (1986). In a recent study, Boone et al. (1990) did not observe an exercise-induced increase in plasma cortisol in anabolic/androgenic steroid users following 10 sets of squats. Plasma cortisol was increased in non-users performing the same exercise. Similarly, Doerr and Pirke (1976) showed that cortisol causes a decrease in the nocturnal rise in testosterone. Thus, one might speculate that one mechanism of action of exogenous anabolic/androgenic steroids is to counteract the catabolic effect of the increased cortisol found after high-intensity exercise by one or more of the mechanisms previously discussed.

The effect of anabolic/androgenic steroids on the biochemistry of the central nervous system is a third potential mechanism of anabolic/androgenic steroids ergogenicity. Androgen receptors have been found in both the brain and alpha-motor neurons (Sar & Stumpf, 1977; Stumpf & Sar, 1976). Vyskocil and Gutmann (1977) have implied that androgens can facilitate the release of acetylcholine at the neuromuscular junction as well as elevate monoamine levels in the central nervous system. Changes in electro-encephalograms reported by Itil (1976) and Itil et al. (1974) support the concept that androgens are active in the brain. Perhaps this activity is connected to the increase in aggressive behavior found in both animals (Simon et al., 1985) and humans (Persky et al., 1971; Kreuz & Rose, 1972;

Ehrenkranz et al., 1974; Scaramella & Brown, 1978). Aggressiveness in weight training rooms and at sports competitions can be a positive factor in the attainment of athletic goals.

Another suggestion has been made that the mechanism of action is solely a placebo effect. This is somewhat supported by the positive ergogenic effects of "steroid" placebos reported by Ariel and Saville (1972).

Most likely, there is not a single mechanism by which the anabolic/androgenic steroids provide any ergogenic effect. Some combination of the purported mechanisms discussed above or a heretofore unknown mechanism may be responsible.

Adverse Effects of Anabolic Steroids

Much has been written about the risks of androgen use in athletes. Suggestions that widespread steroid abuse would result in an epidemic of catastrophic, life-threatening adverse effects (Goldman, 1984; Ryan, 1981) have not been substantiated and have been a source of credibility loss by the medical community. There may be associations between androgen abuse and various adverse conditions, but the incidence of life-threatening adverse effects thus far has been extremely low in athletes. It also is important to realize that most, but not all, cases of the adverse effects of steroids are reversible when drug use ceases.

Unfortunately, there have been few studies of the short-term adverse effects of androgen use other than in the therapeutic literature. Most of the work in athletes is the result of case studies or retrospective studies on poorly selected samples. There have been no prospective or retrospective studies that have investigated the long-term adverse effects of androgen use in athletes.

The adverse effects commonly referred to in the literature as well as those that evoke the most concern will be discussed.

Liver Dysfunction and Tumors. Stang-Voss and Appel (1981) and Taylor et al. (1982) have demonstrated steroid-induced structural changes in the livers of rats and mice, respectively. Palva and Wasastjerna (1972) and Sacks et al. (1972), in therapeutic trials of anabolic/androgenic steroids in the treatment of refractory anemia in humans, reported cholestasis and jaundice. The remission of the jaundice after removal of the drug strengthened the connection between steroid use and liver dysfunction.

Farrell et al. (1975), Meadows et al. (1974), Mulvihill et al. (1975), and Zevin et al. (1981) reported benign hepatomas in patients using anabolic/androgenic steroids for various medical conditions. Falk et al. (1979), Johnson et al. (1972), and Stromeyer et al. (1979) reported malignant tumors of the liver with androgen therapy. The report by

Johnson et al. (1972) of tumor regression with removal of the drug strengthens the association between anabolic/androgenic steroids and the tumors. Overly et al. (1984) and Creagh et al. (1988) reported carcinoma of the liver in athletes who have used anabolic/androgenic steroids. The incidence of these life-threatening liver problems is not certain but seems low. However, for those few who are affected, liver pathology is obviously a cause for extreme concern.

Adverse Cardiovascular Effects. Adverse effects of anabolic/androgenic steroids on different aspects of the cardiovascular system have been reported. Appel et al. (1983), Behrendt (1977), Behrendt and Boffin (1977), and Weicker (1982) all reported disturbing morphological changes in the myocardium of animals treated with anabolic/androgenic steroids. These changes could have potential clinical significance in humans. More work is needed in this area, especially in view of the plight of a former steroid-abusing professional football player who has documented cardiomyopathy (Staff, 1989) and considering the cardiomyopathy reported in a dead high school athlete who used anabolic/androgenic steroids (Telander & Nodem, 1989). On the other hand, in a cross-sectional study comparing weightlifters who used or who did not use anabolic steroids, Salke et al. (1985) reported left ventricular hypertrophy in individuals who used anabolic steroids. There were no differences in size or function between those weightlifters who did or did not use anabolic/androgenic steroids. Hopefully, long-term follow up studies will be initiated to clarify the potential association between cardiomyopathy and anabolic/androgenic steroids abuse in athletes.

Adverse changes in serum lipids (i.e., a decrease in high density lipoprotein cholesterol and an increase in total cholesterol), which could potentially increase the risk of coronary artery disease, have been reported by Cohen et al. (1988), Hurley et al. (1984), Lenders et al. (1988), Olsson et al. (1974), and Webb et al. (1984), especially with orally administered steroids. The long-term effects of these commonly observed and potentially dangerous changes are not known.

Cerebrovascular accidents have been reported in two patients on androgen therapy (Shiozawa et al., 1982; Nagelberg et al., 1986) and two athletes using anabolic/androgenic steroids (Frankle et al., 1988; Mochizuki & Richter, 1988). A myocardial infarction was reported by McNutt et al. (1988) in a 22 year-old weightlifter who used anabolic/androgenic steroids.

The overall risks to the cardiovascular system seem potentially serious, but more work is needed to solidify the connection between anabolic/androgenic steroids and cardiovascular disease and also to identify the incidence of these problems.

Adverse Effects on the Male Reproductive System. Clerico et al. (1981), Hervey et al. (1976), Stromme et al. (1974), Kilshaw et al. (1975), and Remes et al. (1977) reported various effects on the male reproductive system, including oligospermia (small number of sperm in semen), azoospermia (lack of sperm in semen), decreased testicular tissue on biopsy, and reductions in circulating testosterone and gonadotropic hormones. Most of these effects are commonly observed in steroid users but seem to be reversible (Knuth et al., 1989). The time required for the hypothalamic-pituitary-testicular axis to return to normal after steroid withdrawal is not known, and even though there have been no reports of permanent changes, such changes are possible.

Adverse Effects on Psychological Status. Strauss et al. (1983) reported aggressive behavior, frequent mood swings, and libido changes in their survey of athletes using anabolic/androgenic steroids. Pope and Katz (1988) found psychotic symptoms and affective disorders in their retrospective study of athletes using anabolic/androgenic steroids. Furthermore, Tennant et al. (1988) and Brower et al. (1989) reported cases of dependency on anabolic/androgenic steroids similar to that for opiate dependency. These case reports raise questions concerning anabolic/androgenic steroids that need further study.

Other Adverse Effects. Other adverse effects of anabolic/androgenic steroids have been reported. These include premature closure of growth plates in bones of youths (Whitelaw et al., 1966); frequently observed masculinization in females, e.g., hirsutism, clitoromegaly, and irreversible deepening of the voice (Damste, 1967; Kruskemper, 1968; Wilson & Griffin, 1980); and weakening of connective tissue that would lead to increased incidence of musculoskeletal injury (Wood et al., 1988; Michna & Stang-Voss, 1983). This weakening of connective tissue could be significant to athletes because it potentially could predispose the user of anabolic steroids to musculoskeletal injuries. Calabrese et al. (1989) found a significant lowering of immunoglobulins (IgA, IgM) and enhanced natural killer activity in a small series of body builders who used anabolic/androgenic steroids. These effects were not seen in control groups of non-steroid-using bodybuilders and healthy non-weight-training subjects. The clinical significance of these changes is not known but could be a weakening of the body's defenses against infection as well as an increased susceptibility to harmful autoimmune responses.

GROWTH HORMONE

Growth hormone has been used by athletes in this decade both because of the perception that it might be more effective than anabolic steroids in maximizing size, strength, and performance, and because the improved techniques for detecting anabolic/androgenic steroids increase the risk of disqualification from athletic competition because of steroid use. Prior to the recent production of growth hormone through genetic engineering, the only source was human cadavers, and the hormone supply was very limited. Since the introduction of this genetically engineered drug, availability has increased, as has the reported use by athletes (Cowart, 1988; Taylor, 1985; Todd, 1983, 1984).

Biochemistry of Growth Hormone

Growth hormone is a polypeptide secreted by the anterior pituitary gland. Growth hormone concentration in the blood is increased by a number of factors including stress; physical exercise (Shephard & Sidney, 1975; Karagiorgos et al., 1979); hypoglycemia; L-DOPA; Clonidine, a central acting alpha-adrenergic anti-hypertensive drug; and arginine, an amino acid. In particular, Vanhelder et al. (1984) found that lifting heavy weights less frequently induced an increase in the concentration of circulating growth hormone that was not observed after lifting lighter weights more often.

The regulation of growth hormone secretion is a balance between the stimulatory action of the growth-hormone-releasing factor and the inhibitory somatostatin, both produced by the hypothalamus (Daughaday, 1989; Kostyo & Reagan, 1976). Control of growth hormone secretion is a complex and incompletely understood interaction of these substances.

Growth hormone has a direct growth-promoting action in striated muscle (Kostyo et al., 1959), cardiac muscle (Hjalmarson et al., 1969), and adipose tissue (Fain et al., 1965). This action is partly a function of increased amino acid transport into the growing cell. Also, increased lipolysis in muscle after growth hormone treatment has been found by Clemmons et al., (1981). However, the most substantial effect of growth hormone on skeletal muscle is indirect through the actions of the somatomedins (Salmon & DuVall, 1970).

Growth hormone has a short half-life. After intravenous injection of growth hormone, the concentration of circulating growth hormone peaks in 1 h and returns to baseline in 3 h (Hall, 1971). Hall also noted that somatomedin levels increased at approximately 3 h and remained elevated for 9–24 h. Thus, even though growth hormone itself has a relatively brief half-life that makes its detection prior to competition difficult, the prolonged increase in somatomedins can result in prolonged anabolic effects.

Incidence of Growth Hormone Use by Athletes

There is a paucity of data on the prevalence of growth hormone use by athletes. Salva and Bacon (1989) reported that 15 of 100 physicians surveyed reported a total of 52 inquiries about growth hormone. This simply verifies the interest in growth hormone but not the incidence of use. Other reports on this topic are anecdotal (Taylor, 1985; Todd, 1983, 1984; Cowart, 1988).

Actions of Growth Hormone

The three actions of growth hormone which the athlete perceives as beneficial or ergogenic are: 1) stimulation of protein and nucleic acid synthesis in skeletal muscle, 2) increase in lipolysis and overall decrease in body fat, and 3) enhancement of healing after musculoskeletal injuries (Taylor, 1985; MacIntyre, 1987; Rogol, 1989).

Anabolic Effects. The growth-hormone-induced stimulation of protein synthesis in skeletal muscle of hypophysectomized animals has been demonstrated by Kostyo and Nutting (1973). Goldberg (1967) found two types of skeletal muscle hypertrophy in rats. Growth-hormone-dependent hypertrophy occurred during developmental growth, whereas overload stress caused muscle hypertrophy even in the absence of growth hormone. Similarly, Goldberg and Goodman (1969) demonstrated that muscular hypertrophy can occur in hypophysectomized rats treated with growth hormone but without muscular overload.

In humans, Salomon et al. (1989) showed that growth hormone can affect body composition in growth-hormone-deficient adults. In a double-blind, placebo controlled study, they found significant increases in lean body mass and decreases in fat mass in the group treated with growth hormone. Basal metabolic rate also was significantly increased. Muscle performance was not measured.

Jorgensen et al. (1989) studied growth-hormone-deficient adults in a double-blind crossover study of the effects of growth hormone treatment on body composition and muscular performance. Muscle and adipose tissue volume (computerized tomography), percentage of body fat (subscapular skinfolds), isometric strength of quadriceps muscles (electronic dynamometer), and exercise capacity on a cycle ergometer were found to be affected by growth hormone. The authors observed an increase in muscle volume, a corresponding decrease in adipose tissue volume, and a decrease in subscapular skinfold thickness. Isometric quadriceps strength and exercise capacity were both increased in the treatment group. Thus, measures of muscular performance that could influence athletic prowess have been shown to be positively affected by growth hormone treatment in growth-hormone-deficient adults.

The anabolic effect of growth hormone in growth-hormone-deficient animals and humans is well-accepted. However, the question of the effects of exogenous growth hormone on anabolism in normal animals is another question. Bigland and Jehring (1952) studied the effect of growth hormone treatment on muscle size and tension in normal female rats. They reported increases in muscle fiber cross-sectional area in the hormone treated animals. However, the muscles of the treated animals produced less tension per gram of muscle than did the controls. These findings lead to questions about the quality and function of the growth-hormone-enhanced muscle mass.

Ullman et al. (1989) investigated in rats the effects of growth hormone on normal skeletal muscle and on muscle that had undergone ischemic necrosis or denervation. The weight of the muscles of rats treated with growth hormone was greater in all three groups, again demonstrating the anabolic effect of growth hormone on skeletal muscle. However, the functional ability of the muscle was not measured.

Crist et al. (1988) studied the effects of growth hormone on body composition (hydrodensitometry) in eight highly conditioned men who performed progressive resistance exercise. Using a double-blind technique, they found significant decreases in fat weight and increases in fat-free weight after growth hormone treatment when compared to a placebo. Unfortunately, the functional ability of the muscle was not reported.

The few studies reported are consistent with the hypothesis that growth hormone increases lean tissue mass and decreases fat mass. However, the quality and functional capabilities of any new muscle growth induced by growth hormone treatment remain unknown.

Lipolytic Effects. Federspil et al. (1975) reported increases in plasma free fatty acids after exercise in rats. This increase was abolished by hypophysectomy. Raben and Hallenberg (1959) found that in both dogs and humans, fat mobilization was increased by growth hormone administration. Hunter et al. (1965) reported elevations of circulating non-esterified fatty acids and a rising respiratory quotient after administration of growth hormone in humans. These changes also indicate increased fat mobilization.

The increased mobilization of fat is probably the mechanism responsible for the decrease in body fat seen after growth hormone treatment in the studies of Salomon et al. (1989), Jorgensen et al. (1989), and Crist et al. (1988). This could not only benefit the body composition of an athlete but may also be beneficial in the fuel selection process, if fatty acid utilization is increased, in an endurance event.

Effects On Healing of Injuries. The effects of growth hormone on healing have been studied in cases of bone fractures (Northmore-Ball et al., 1980), but there is controversy as to the efficacy of growth hormone. Koskinen (1959) found increased osteogenesis of the callus and more rapid callus formation in fractures in rats. This was contrary to the findings of Shepanek (1953), who reported no increase in rate of fracture healing with growth hormone treatment. Zadek and Robinson (1961) found healing of the radial defect of their dogs only in the group treated with growth hormone.

The effect of growth hormone administration on healing is not conclusively established. This is especially true in the area of soft tissue healing. There must be more evidence available prior to any conclusions concerning the effect of exogenous growth hormone on the healing process.

Potential Adverse Effects of Growth Hormone

Growth hormone excess causes gigantism in prepubertal individuals and acromegaly in adults. Randall (1989) reviewed these two syndromes and the adverse effects related to them. Common physical manifestations of acromegaly include thickening of the soft tissues, especially the face, hands, and feet. Excessive skeletal growth is found in the skull, mandible, hands, and feet. Pathological growth of the heart, liver, kidney, and colon may be found. Hypertension and cardiomyopathy may also be caused by excess growth hormone. Cardiomyopathy is the most common cause of death in acromegaly. Diabetes is also commonly seen in acromegalics.

There have been no reports or case studies of adverse effects associated with growth hormone in athletes. If the use of growth hormone escalates, as predicted by some, adverse effects may be reported in the future.

SUMMARY

Anabolic/androgenic steroid use by athletes has been documented in various athletes from sprinters to weightlifters. These athletes hope to enhance their fitness and their athletic performance. The evidence is contradictory and confusing, but a positive effect can often, but not always, be expected on lean mass and strength, but not on indirect measures of aerobic capacity. The scientific community has been limited in its attempts to replicate the actual pattern of use by athletes because of the ethical issues relating to subject selection, drug regimens, and reported adverse drug effects. Even though the anecdotal reports of athletes cannot be substantiated in research protocols because of these limitations, many scientists believe that there is substance in these anecdotal reports. The adverse effects of anabolic/androgenic steroids are real, but the incidence of serious health effects is believed to be low. To insure fair competition, organizations have banned the use of anabolic/androgenic steroids and use drug testing (urine tests) to enforce this ban.

Growth hormone is a polypeptide produced in the anterior pituitary. The anabolic and lipolytic actions of growth hormone make exogenous growth hormone attractive to the athlete. There is support for the contention that exogenous growth hormone can increase lean body mass in normal humans, but evidence is not available concerning the enhancement of athletic performance. The adverse effects of excess growth hormone are those seen in acromegaly and have not been reported in an athlete.

BIBLIOGRAPHY

Aakvaag, A., R. Bentdol, K. Quigstod, P. Walstod, H. Renningen, and F. Fonnum (1978). Testosterone and testosterone binding globulin (TeBg) in young men during prolonged stress. Int. J. Androl. 1:22–31.

Albrecht, H., and E. Albrecht (1969). Ergometric, rheographic, reflexographic and electrographic tests at altitude and effects of drugs on human physical performance. Fed. Proc. 28:1262–1267.

Alen, M., K. Hakkinen, and P.V. Komi (1984). Changes in neuromuscular performance and muscle fiber characteristics of elite power athletes self-administering androgenic and anabolic steroids. Acta. Physiol. Scand. 122:535–544.

American College of Sports Medicine (1987). Position stand on the use of anabolic-androgenic steroids in sports. Med. Sci. Sports Exerc. 19:534–539.

Anderson, W., and D. McKeag (1985). The substance use and abuse habits of college student-athletes. Technical Report. Mission, Kansas: National Collegiate Athletic Association.

Anderson, W., and D. McKeag (1989). Replication of the national study of substance use and abuse habits of college student athletes. Technical Report. Mission, Kansas: National Collegiate Athletic Association.

Appell, H., B. Heller-Umpfenback, M. Feraud, and H. Weicker (1983). Ultrastructural and morphometric investigations on the effects of training and administration of anabolic steroids on the myocardium of guinea pigs. Int. J. Sports Med. 4:268–274.

Ariel, G., and W. Saville (1972). Anabolic Steroids: The Physiological Effects of Placebos. Med. Sci. Sports. 4:123–126.

Beato, M. (1989). Gene regulation by steroid hormones. Cell. 56:335–344.

Beato, M., G. Arnemann, Chalepakis, E. Slater, and T. Williann (1987). Gene regulation by steroid hormones. J. Steroid Biochem. 27:9–14.

Behrendt, H. (1977). Effect of anabolic steroids on rat heart muscle cells, I. Intermediate Filaments. Cell Tissue Res. 180:303–315.

Behrendt, H., and H. Boffin (1977). Myocardial cell lesions caused by an anabolic hormone. Cell Tissue Res. 181: 337–338.

Bigland, B., and B. Jehring (1952). Muscle performance in rats, normal and treated with growth hormone. J. Physiol. 116:129–136.

Boje, O. (1939). Doping. Bull. Health Organization League of Nations. 8:439–469.

Boone, Jr., J.B., C.P. Lambert, M.G. Flynn, T.J. Michaud, J.A. Rodriguez-Zayas, and F.F. Andres (1990). Resistance exercise effects on plasma cortisol, testosterone and creatine kinase activity in anabolic-androgenic steroid users. Internat. J. Sports Med. 11:293–297.

Brower, K., F. Blow, T. Beresford, and C. Fuelling (1989). Anabolic-androgenic steroid dependence. J. Clin. Psychiatry. 50(1):31–33.

Buckley, W., C. Yesalis, K. Friedl, W. Anderson, A. Streit, and J. Wright (1988) Estimated prevalence of anabolic steroid use among male high school seniors. *JAMA* 260:3441–3445.

Calabrese, L., S. Kleiner, B. Barna, C. Skibinski, D. Kirkendall, R. Lahita, and J. Lombardo, (1989). The effects of anabolic steroids and strength training on the human immune response. *Med. Sci. Sports Exerc.* 21:386–392.

Capaccio, J.A., T.T Kurowski, S.M. Czerwinski, R.T. Chatterton, Jr., and R.C. Hickson (1987). Testosterone fails to prevent skeletal muscle atrophy from glucocorticoids. *J. Appl. Physiol.* 63:328–334.

Catlin, D., R. Kammerer, C. Hatton, M. Sekera, and J. Merdink (1987). Analytical chemistry at the games of the XXIIIrd Olympiad in Los Angeles. *Clin. Chem.* 33:319–327.

Cato, A.C.B., D. Henderson, and H. Ponta (1987). The hormone response element of the mouse mammary tumor virus DNA mediates the progestin and androgen induction of transcription in the proviral long terminal repeat region. *EMBO J.* 6:363–368.

Clemmons, D.R., L.E. Underwood, and J.J. Van Wyk (1981). Hormonal control of immuno-reactive somatomedin production by cultured human fibroblasts. *J. Clin. Invest.* 67:10–19.

Clerico, A., M. Ferdeghini, C. Palomba, et al. (1981). Effect of anabolic treatment on the serum levels of gonadotropins, testosterone, prolactin, thyroid hormones and myoglobin of male athletes under physical training. *J. Nuclear Med. Allied Sci.* 25: 79–88.

Cohen, J., T. Noakes, and A. Benade (1988). Hypercholesterolemia in male power lifters using anabolic-androgenic steroids. *Physician Sportsmed.* 16:49–56.

Cowart, V.S. (1988). Human growth hormone: the latest ergogenic aid? *Physician Sportsmed.* 16(3):175.

Creagh, T., A. Rubin, and D. Evans (1988). Hepatic tumors induced by anabolic steroids in an athlete. *J. Clin. Path.* 41: 441–443.

Crist, D.M., G.T. Peake, P.A. Egan, and D.L. Waters (1988). Body composition response to exogenous GH during training in highly conditioned adults. *J. Appl. Physiol.* 65(2):579–584.

Crist, D.M., P.J. Stackpole, and G.T. Peake (1983). Effects of androgenic-anabolic steroids on neuromuscular power and body composition. *J. Appl. Physiol.* 54:366–370.

Dahlberg, E., M. Snockowski, and J.A. Gustafsson (1981). Regulation of the androgen and glucocorticoid receptors in rat and mouse skeletal muscle cytosol. *Endocrinology* 108:1431–1439.

Damste, P.H. (1967). Voice change in adult women caused by virilizing agents. *J. Speech Hear. Disord.* 32:126–132.

Danhaive, P.A., and G.C. Rousseau (1988). Evidence for sex-dependent anabolic response to androgenic steroids mediated by muscle glucocorticoid receptors in the rat. *J. Steroid Biochem.* 29:575–581.

Daughaday, W.H. (1989). Growth hormone: Normal synthesis, secretion, control, and mechanisms of action. In: L.J. Degroot (ed.) *Endocrinology,* Philadelphia: W.B. Saunders, pp. 318–329.

Denison, S.H., A. Sands, and D.J. Tindall (1989). A tyrosine aminotransferase glucocorticoid response element also mediates androgen enhancement of gene expression. *Endocrinology* 124:1091–1093.

Dezelsky, T., J. Toohey, and R. Shaw (1985). Non-medical drug use behavior at five United States universities: a 15 year study. *Bull. Narcotics* 27:45–53.

Doerr, P., and K.M. Pirke (1976). Cortisol-induced suppression of plasma testosterone in normal adult males. *J. Clin. Endocrinol. Metab.* 43:622–629.

DuBois, D.C., and R.R. Almon (1984). Glucocorticoid sites in skeletal muscle: adrenalectomy, maturation, fiber type and sex. *Am. J. Physiol.* 247:E119–E125.

Ehrenkranz, J., E. Bliss, and M.H. Sheard (1974). Plasma testosterone; correlation with aggressive behavior and social dominance in man. *Psychosomatic Med.* 36(6):469–475.

Exner, G.U., H.W. Staudte, and D. Pette (1973). Isometric training of rats—effects upon fast and slow muscle and modification by an anabolic hormone (Nandrolone Decanoate) I. Female Rats. *Pflugers Arch.* 354:1–14.

Fahey, T.D., and C.H. Brown (1973). The effects of an anabolic steroid on strength, body composition and endurance of college males when accompanied by a weight training program. *Med. Sci. Sports* 5:272–276.

Fain, J.N., V.P. Kovacev, and R.O. Scow (1965). Effect of growth hormone and dexamethasone on lipolysis and metabolism in isolated fat cells of the rat. *J. Biol. Chem.* 240:3522–3529.

Falk, H., L. Thomas, H. Popper, and H.G. Ishak (1979). Hepatic angiosarcoma associated with androgenic-anabolic steroids. *Lancet* 2:1120–1123.

Farrell, G.C., D.E. Joshua, R.F. Uren, P.J. Baird, K.W. Perkins, and H. Kronenberg (1975). Androgen-induced hepatoma. *Lancet* 1:430.

Federspil, G., G. Udeschini, C. DePalo, and N. Sicalo (1975). Role of growth hormone in lipid mobilization stimulated by prolonged muscular exercise in the rat. *Horm. Metab. Res.* 7:484–488.

Forbes, T.R. (1947). Crowing hen; early observations on spontaneous sex reversals in birds. *Yale J. Biol. Med.* 19:955.

Fowler, W.M., Jr., G.W. Gardner, and G.H. Egstrom, (1965). Effect of an anabolic steroid on physical performance in young men. *J. Appl. Physiol.* 20:1038–1040.

Frankle, M., G. Cicero, and J. Payne (1984). Use of androgenic anabolic steroids by athletes, letter. *JAMA* 252:482.

Frankle, M., R. Eichberg, and S. Zachariah (1988). Anabolic-androgenic steroids and a stroke in an athlete: Case report. *Arch. Phys. Med. Rehab.* 69:632–633.

Goldberg, A.L. (1967). Work-induced growth of skeletal muscle in normal and hypophysectomized rats. *Am. J. Physiol.* 213:1193–1198.

Goldberg, A.L., and H.M. Goodman (1969). Relationship between growth hormone and muscle work in determining muscle size. *J. Physiol.* 200:655–666.

Golding, L.A., J.E. Freydinger, and S.S. Fishel (1974). The effect of an androgenic-anabolic steroid and a protein supplement on size, strength, weight and body composition in athletes. *Physician Sportsmed.* 2(6):39–45.

Goldman, B. (1984). *Death in the locker room.* South Bend, IN: Icarus Press, pp. 93–94.

Griggs, R.C., W. Kingston, R.F. Jozefowicz, B.E. Herr, G. Forbes, and D. Halliday (1989). Effect of testosterone on muscle mass and muscle protein synthesis. *J. Appl. Physiol.* 66:498–503.

Guglielmini, C., A.R. Paolini, and F. Conconi (1984). Variations of serum testosterone concentrations after physical exercises of different duration. *Int. J. Sports Med.* 5:246–249.

Hall, K. (1971). Effect of intravenous administration of human growth hormone on sulfation factor activity in serum of hypopituitary subjects. *Acta Endocrinol.* 66:491–497.

Ham, J., A. Thomson, M. Needham, P. Webb, and M. Parker (1988). Characterization of response elements for androgens, glucocorticoids and progestins in mouse mammary tumor virus. *Nucleic Acids Res.* 16:5256–5276.

Heitzman, R.J. (1976). The effectiveness of anabolic agents in increasing rate of growth in farm animals; report on experiments in cattle. In: F.C. Lu and J. Rendell (eds.) *Anabolic Agents in Animal Production.* Stuttgart: George Thieme, pp. 89–98.

Hervey, G.R., and I. Hutchinson (1973) The effects of testosterone on body weight and composition in the rat. *J. Endocrinol.* 57:xxiv–xxv.

Hervey, G.R., I. Hutchinson, A.V. Knibbs, L. Burkinshaw, P.R.M. Jones, N.G. Norgan, and M.J. Levell (1976). Anabolic effects of methandienone in men undergoing athletic training. *Lancet* 2:699–702.

Hervey, G.R., A.V. Knibbs, L. Burkinshaw, D.B. Morgan, P.R.M. Jones, D.R. Chettle, and D. Vartsky (1981). Effects of methandienone on the performance and body composition of men undergoing athletic training. *Clin. Sci.* 60:457–461.

Hickson, R.C., W.W. Heusner, W.D. VanHuss, D.E. Jackson, D.A. Anderson, D.A. Jones, and A.T. Psaledas (1976). Effects of Dianabol and high-intensity sprint training on body composition of rats. *Med. Sci. Sports* 8:191–196.

Hickson, R.C., T.M. Galassi, T.T. Kurowski, D.G. Daniels, and R.T. Chatterson Jr. (1983). Skeletal muscle cytosol [^{3}H] methyltrienolone receptor binding and serum androgens: effects of hypertrophy and hormonal state. *J. Steroid. Biochem.* 19:1705–1712.

Hickson, R.C., T.T. Kurowski, G.H. Andrews, J.A. Capaccio, and R.T. Chatterton Jr. (1986). Glucocorticoid cytosol binding in exercise-induced sparing of muscle atrophy. *J. Appl. Physiol.* 60:1413–1419.

Hjalmarson, A., O. Isaksson, and K. Ahren (1969). Effect of growth hormone and insulin on amino acid transport in perfused rat heart. *Am. J. Physiol.* 217:1795–1802.

Hunter, W.M., C.C. Fonseka, and R. Passmore (1965). The role of growth hormone in the mobilization of fuel for muscular exercise. *Quart. J. Exp. Physiol. Cogn. Med. Sci.* 50:406–416.

Hurley, B., D. Seals, J. Hagberg, A. Goldberg, S. Ostrove, J. Holloszy, W. Weist, and A. Goldberg (1984). High density lipoprotein cholesterol in bodybuilders and powerlifters (negative effects of androgens). *JAMA* 252:507–513.

Itil, T. (1976). Neurophysiological effects of hormones in humans; computer EEG profiles of sex and hypothalamic hormones. In: E.J. Sachar (ed.) *Hormones, Behavior and Psychotherapy.* New York: Raven Press, pp. 31–40.

Itil, T., C. Ackpinar, W. Harrman, and C. Patterson (1974). Psychotropic: action of sex hormones: computerized EEG in establishing the immediate CNS effects of steroid hormones. *Curr. Therapeutic Res.* 16:1147–1170.

Johnson, F.L., K.G. Lerner, M. Siegel, et al. (1972). Association of androgenic-anabolic steroid therapy with development of hepatocellular carcinoma. *Lancet* 2:1273.

Johnson, L.C., and J.P. O'Shea (1969). Anabolic steroid: effects on strength development. *Science* 164:957–959.

Johnson, L.C., G. Fisher, L.J. Silvester, and C.C. Hofheins (1972). Anabolic steroid: effects of strength, body weight, oxygen uptake and spermatogenesis upon mature males. *Med. Sci. Sports* 4:43–45.

Johnson, L.C., E.S. Roundy, P.E. Allsen, A.G. Fisher, and L.J. Silvester (1975). Effect of anabolic steroid treatment on endurance. *Med. Sci. Sports* 7:287–289.

Johnson, M., M.S. Jay, B. Shoup, and V. Rickert (1989). Anabolic steroid use by male adolescents. *Pediatrics* 83:921–924.

Jorgensen, J.O.L., L. Thuesen, T. Ingemann-Hansen, S.A. Pedersen, J. Jorgensen, N.E. Skakkebaek, and J.S. Christiansen (1989). Beneficial effects of growth hormone treatment in GH-deficient adults. *Lancet* 1221–1225, June 3.

Karagiorgos, A., J.F. Garcia, and G.W. Brooks (1979). Growth hormone response to continuous and intermittent exercise. *Med. Sci. Sports* 11:302–307.

Kayali, A.G., V.R. Young, and M.N. Goodman (1987). Sensitivity of myofibrillar proteins to glucocorticoid-induced muscle proteolysis. *Am. J. Physiol.* 252: E621–E626.

Kenyon, A.T., I. Sandiford, A.H. Bryan, K. Knowlton, and F.C. Koch (1938). The effect of testosterone propionate on nitrogen, electrolyte, water and energy metabolism in eunuchoidism. *Endocrinology* 23:135–153.

Keul, J., H. Deus, and W. Kindermann (1976). Anabole hormone; Schadigug, Leistungsfahigkeit und Stoffwechses. *Med. Klin.* 71:497–503.

Kilshaw, B.H., R.A. Harkness, B.M. Hobson, and A.W.M. Smith (1975). The effects of large doses of the anabolic steroid, methandrostenolone, on an athlete. *Clin. Endocrinol.* 4:537–541.

Knuth, U.A., H. Maniera, and E. Nieschlag (1989). Anabolic steroids and semen parameters in bodybuilders. *Fertil. Steril.* 52: 1041–1048.

Kochakian, C., and J. Murlin (1935). The effect of male hormone on the protein and energy metabolism of castrate dogs. *J. Nutr.* 10:437–459.

Kochakian, C.D. (1935). The effect of male hormone on protein metabolism of castrated dogs. *Proc. Soc. Exp. Biol. (NY)* 32: 1064–1065.

Kochakian, C.D. (1937). Testosterone and testosterone acetate and the protein and energy metabolism of castrate dogs. *Endocrinology* 21:750–755.

Kochakian, C.D., and B.R. Endahl (1959). Changes in body weight of normal and castrated rats by different doses of testosterone propionate. *Proc. Soc. Exper. Biol. Med.* 100:520–522.

Kochakian, C.D. (1976). *Anabolic-Androgenic Steroids*. Springer-Verlag, New York.

Konagaya, M., P.A. Bernard, and S.R. Max (1986). Blockage of glucocorticoid receptor binding and inhibition of dexamethasone-induced muscle atrophy in the rat by RU38486, a potent glucocorticoid antagonist. *Endocrinology* 119: 375–580.

Koskinen, E.V.S. (1959). The repair of experimental fractures under the action of growth hormone, thyrotropin and cortisone. A tissue analytic, roentgenologic and autoradiographic study. *Ann. Chir. Gynaecol. Fenn.* 48: Suppl 90.

Kostyo, J.L., J. Hotchkiss, and E. Knobil (1959). Stimulation of amino acid transport in isolated diaphragm by growth hormone added in vitro. *Science* 130:1653–1654.

Kostyo, J.L., and D.F. Nutting (1973). Acute in vivo actions of growth hormone on various tissue of hypophysectomized rats and their relationship to the levels of thymidine factor and insulin in the plasma. *Horm. Metab. Res.* 5:167–171.

Kostyo, J.L., and C.R. Reagan (1976). The biology of growth hormone. *Pharm. Ther.* 2:591–604.

Kruez, L.E. and R.M. Rose (1972). Assessment of Aggressive behavior and plasma testosterone in a young criminal population. *Psychosom. Med.* 34:321–332.

Kruskemper, H.L. (1968). *Anabolic Steroids*. New York: Academic Press, pp. 128–133, 162–164, 182.

Lamb, D.R. (1984). Anabolic steroids in athletics: How well do they work and how dangerous are they? *Am. J. Sports Med.* 12:31–38.

Lenders, J., P. Demacher, J. Vos, P. Jansen, A. Hoitsma, A. Van't Laar, and T. Thien (1988). Deleterious effects of anabolic steroids on serum lipoproteins, blood pressure and liver function in amateur body builders. *Int. J. Sports Med.* 9:19–23.

Liu, L., G.R. Merriam, and R.J. Sherins (1987). Chronic sex steroid exposure increases mean plasma growth hormone concentration and pulse amplitude in men with isolated hypogonadotropic hypogonadism. *J. Clin. Endocrinol. Metab.* 64:651–656.

Loughton, S. and R. Ruhling (1977). Human strength and endurance responses to anabolic steroid and training. *J. Sports Med.* 17:285–296.

Ljungqvist, A. (1975). The use of anabolic steroids in top Swedish athletes. *Br. J. Sports Med.* 9:82.

Lombardo, J. Ergogenic Effects of Anabolic-Androgenic Steroids. National Institute of Drug Abuse Monograph (in press).

MacIntyre, J.G. (1987). Growth hormone and athletes. *Sports Med.* 4:129–142.

Mather, D.N., A.L. Toriola, and O.A. Dada (1986). Serum cortisol and testosterone levels in conditioned male distance runners and nonathletes after maximal exercise. *J. Sports Med.* 26:245–250.

Mayer, M., and F. Rosen (1975). Interaction of anabolic steroids with glucocorticoid receptor sites in rat muscle cytosol. *Am. J. Physiol.* 229(5):1381–1386.

McClain, L. (1989). Anabolic steroids and high school students. Paper presented at the 29th Annual Meeting of the Ambulatory Pediatric Association. Washington, DC. May, 2–4.

McNutt, B., G. Ferenchick, P. Kirlin, and N. Hamlin (1988). Acute myocardial infarction in a 22 year old world class weightlifter using anabolic steroids. *Am. J. Cardiol.* 62:164.

Meadows, A.T., J.L. Naiman, and M. Valdes-Dapena (1974). Hepatoma associated with androgen therapy for aplastic anemia. *J. Pediatr.* 85:109–110.

Michna, H., and C. Stang-Voss (1983) [abstract]. The predisposition to tendon rupture after doping with anabolic steroids. *Int. J. Sports Med.* 4:59.

Mochizuki, R. and J. Richter (1988). Cardiomyopathy and cerebrovascular accident associated with anabolic steroid use. *Physician Sportsmed.* 16:109–115.

Mulvihill, J.J., R. L. Ridolfi, F.R. Schultz, M.S. Brozy, and P.B.T. Haughton (1975). Hepatic adenoma in Fanconi anemia treated with oxymetholone. *J. Pediatr.* 87:122–124.

Nagelberg, S., L. Laue, D. Loriaux, L. Liu, and R. Sherins (1986). Cerebrovascular accident associated with testosterone therapy in a 21 year old hypogonadal man. *New Engl. J. Med.* 314:649–650.

Nesheim, M.C. (1976). Some observations on the effectiveness of anabolic agents in increasing the growth rate in poultry. In: F.C. Lu and J. Rendell (eds.) *Anabolic Agents in Animal Production.* Stuttgart: Georg Thieme, pp. 110–114.

Newerla, G.H. (1943). The history of the discovery and isolation of the male hormone. *New Engl. J. Med.* 228:39–47.

Newman, M. (1986). Michigan Consortium of Schools Student Survey. Minneapolis, Minnesota: Hazelden Research Services.

Newman, M. (1987). Elite women athletes survey results. Minneapolis, Minnesota: Hazelden Research Services.

Northmore-Ball, M.D., M.R. Wood, and B.F. Meggitt (1980). A biomechanical study of the effects of growth hormone in experimental fracture healing. *J. Bone Joint Surg.* 62B:391–396.

Odedra, B.R., P.C. Bates, and D.J. Millward (1983). Time course of the effect of catabolic doses of corticosterone on protein turnover in rat skeletal muscle and liver. *Biochem. J.* 214: 617–627.

Olsson, A., L. Ono, and S. Rossner (1974). Effects of oxandrolone on plasma lipoproteins and the intravenous fat tolerance in man. *Atherosclerosis* 19:337–346.

O'Shea, J.P. (1971). The effects of an anabolic steroid on dynamic strength levels of weightlifters. *Nutr. Rep. Internat.* 4:363–370.

Overly, W.L., J.A. Dankoff, B.K. Wang, and U.D. Singh (1984). Androgens and hepatocellular carcinoma in an athlete. *Ann. Intern. Med.* 100:158–159.

Palva, I.P. and C. Wasastjerna (1972). Treatment of aplastic anaemia with methenolone. *Acta Haematol.* 47:13–20.

Persky, H., K.D. Smith, and G.K. Basu (1971). Relation of psychologic measures of aggression and hostility to testosterone production in man. *Psychosom. Med.* 33:265–277.

Pope, H., D. Katz, and R. Champoux (1988). Anabolic-androgenic steroid use among 1,010 college men. *Physician Sportsmed.* 16:75–81.

Pope, H.G., and D.L. Katz (1988). Affective and psychotic symptoms associated with anabolic steroid use. *Am. J. Psychiatry* 145: 487–490.

Raben, N.S., and C.H. Hallenberg (1959). Effect of growth hormone on plasma fatty acids. *J. Clin. Invest.* 38:484–488.

Randall, R.V. (1989). Acromegaly and Gigantism. In: L.J. Degroot (ed.) *Endocrinology.* Philadelphia: W. B. Saunders, pp. 330–350.

Rannell, S.R., and L.S. Jefferson (1980). Effects of glucocorticoids on muscle protein turnover in perfused rat hemicorpus. *Am. J. Physiol.* 238: E564–E572.

Remes, K., P. Vuopio, M. Jarvinen, H. Harkonen, and H. Adlercreutz (1977). Effect of short-term treatment with an anabolic steroid (methandienone) and dehydroepiandrosterone sulphate on plasma hormones, red cell column and 2,3-diphosphoglycerate in athletes. *Scand. J. Clin. Lab. Invest.* 7:577–586.

Richardson, J.A. (1977). A comparison of two drugs on strength increase in monkeys. *J. Sports Med. Phys. Fit.* 17:251–254.

Rogol, A. (1989). Growth Hormone: physiology, therapeutic use and potential for abuse. *Exer. Sports Sci. Rev.* 17:353–377.

Ryan, A. (1981). Anabolic steroids are fool's gold. *Fed. Proc.* 40:2682–2688.

Saartok, T., E. Dahlberg, and J-A. Gustafsson (1984). Relative binding affinity of anabolic/androgenic steroids: comparison of the binding to the androgen receptors in skeletal muscle and in prostate, as well as to sex hormone-binding globulin. *Endocrinology* 114:2100–2106.

Sacks, P., D. Gale, T.H. Bothwell, and K. Stevens (1972). Oxymetholone therapy in aplastic and other refractory anaemias. *S. Afr. Med J.* 46:1607–1615.

Salke, R.C., T.W. Rowland, and E.J. Burke (1985). Left ventricular size and function in bodybuilders using anabolic steroids. *Med. Sci. Sports Exerc.* 17(6):701–701.

Salmon, W.D., and M.R. DuVall (1970). In vitro stimulation of leucine incorporation into muscle and cartilage protein by a serum fraction with SF activity: Differentiation of effects from those of growth hormone and insulin. *Endocrinology* 87:1168–1180.

Salomon, F., R.C. Cuneo, R. Hesp, and P.H. Sonksen (1989). The effects of treatment with recombinant human growth hormone on body composition and metabolism in adults with growth hormone deficiency. *New Engl. J. Med.* 321:1797–1803.

Salva, P.S., and G.E. Bacon (1989). Anabolic steroids and growth hormone in the Texas Panhandle. *Texas Med.* 85:43–44.

Sar, M., and W. Stumpf (1977). Androgen concentration in motor neurons of cranial nerves and spinal cord. *Science* 197:77–79.

Scaramella, T.J., and W.R. Brown (1978). Serum testosterone and aggressiveness in hockey players. *Psychosom. Med.* 40:262–265.

Schmidt, T.J., and G. Litwack (1982). Activation of the glucocorticoid-receptor complex. *Physiol. Rev.* 62:1131–1192.

Sharpe, R.M., P.J. Buttery, and N.B. Haynes (1986). The effect of manipulating growth in sheep by diet or anabolic agents on plasma cortisol and muscle glucocorticoid receptors. *Br. J. Nutr.* 56:289–304.

Shepanek, L.A. (1953). The effect of endocrine substances (ACTH and growth hormone) on experimental fractures. *Surg. Gynecol. Obstet.* 96:200–204.

Shephard, R.J., and K.H. Sidney (1975). Effects of physical exercise on plasma growth hormone and cortisol levels in human subjects. *Exerc. Sport Sci. Rev.* 35:1–30.

Shiozawa, Z., H. Yamada, C. Mabuchi, T. Hotta, M. Saito, I. Sobue, and Y. Huang (1982). Superior sagittal sinus thrombosis associated with androgen therapy for hypoplastic anemia. *Ann. Neurol.* 12:578–580.

Shoji, S., and R.J.T. Pennington (1977). The effect of cortisone on protein breakdown and synthesis in rat skeletal muscle. *Mol. Cell. Endocrinol.* 6:240–245.

Simon, N.G., R.E. Whalen, and M.P. Tate (1985). Induction of male typical aggression by androgens but not by estrogens in adult female mice. *Horm. Behav.* 19:204–212.

Simonson, E., W. Kearns, and N. Enzer (1944). Effect of methyl testosterone treatment on muscular performance and the central nervous system of older men. *J. Clin. Endocrinol. Metab.* 4:528–534.

Snochowski, M., E. Dahlberg, and J.A. Gustafsson (1980). Characterization and quantification of the androgen and glucocorticoid receptors in cytosol from rat skeletal muscle. *Eur. J. Biochem.* 111:603–616.

Snochowski, M., E. Dahlberg, E. Ericksson, and J.A. Gustafsson (1981). Androgen and glucocorticoid receptors in human skeletal muscle cytosol. *J. Steroid Biochem.* 14:765–771.

Staff (1989). "Was the X factor a Factor?" *Sports Illus.* 70 (14):34.

Stamford, B.A., and R. Moffatt (1974). Anabolic steroid: effectiveness as an ergogenic aid to experienced weight trainers. *J. Sports Med. Phys. Fitness* 14:191–197.

Stang-Voss, C., and H-J. Appel (1981). Structural alterations of liver parenchyma induced by anabolic steroids. *Int. J. Sports Med.* 2:101–105.

Stanhope, R., C.R. Buchanan, G.C. Fenn, and M.A. Peece (1988). Double blind placebo controlled trial of low dose oxandrolone in the treatment of boys with constitutional delay of growth and puberty. *Arch. Dis. Child.* 63:501–505.

Starr, B. (1981). *Defying gravity: How to win at weightlifting.* Wichita Falls, TX: Five Starr Productions, pp. 84–94.

Strauss, R.H., H.E. Wright, G.A.M. Finerman, and D.H. Catlin (1983). Side effects of anabolic steroids in weight-trained men. *Physician Sportsmed.* 11:87–89.

Strauss, R.H., and T.J. Curry (1987). Magic, science and drugs. In: R.H. Strauss (ed.) *Drugs and Performance in Sports.* Philadelphia: W.B. Saunders, pp. 3–9.

Stromeyer, F.W., D.H. Smith, and K.G. Ishak (1979). Anabolic steroid therapy and intrahepatic cholangiocarcinoma. *Cancer* 43:440–443.

Stromme, S.B., H.D. Meen, and A. Aakvaag (1974). Effects of an androgenic-anabolic steroid on strength development and plasma testosterone levels in normal males. *Med. Sci. Sports* 6:203–208.

Stumpf, W., and W. Sar (1976). Steroid hormone target sites in the brain; The differential distribution of estrogen, progestin, androgen and glucocorticosteroid. *J. Steroid Biochem.* 7:1163–1170.

Taylor, W. (1985). *Hormonal Manipulation: A New Era of Monstrous Athletes.* Jefferson, NC: McFarland and Company.

Taylor, W.N. (1982). *Anabolic Steroids and the Athlete.* Jefferson, NC: McFarland and Company.

Taylor, W., S. Snowball, C.M. Dickson, and M. Lesna (1982). Alterations of liver architecture in mice treated with anabolic androgens and dimethylnitrosamine. NATO Adv. Study Inst. Series, Series A 52: 279–288.

Telander, R., and M. Nodem (1989). Death of an Athlete. *Sports Illus.* 70(8):68–78.

Tennant, F., D. Black, and R. Voy (1988). Anabolic steroid dependence with opioid-type features. *New Engl. J. Med.* 319:578.

Todd, T. (1983). The steroid dilemma. *Sports Illus.* 59:62–66.

Todd, T. (1984). The use of human growth hormone poses a grave dilemma for sport. *Sports Illus.* 60:8–12.

Todd, T. (1987). Anabolic steroids: the gremlins of sport. *J. Sport Hist.* 14:87–107.

Ullman, M., H. Alameddine, A. Skottner, and A. Oldfors (1989). Effects of growth hormone on skeletal muscle II. Studies on regeneration and denervation in adult rats. *Acta Physiol. Scand.* 135:537–543.

Ulloa-Aguirre, A., R.M. Blizzard, E. Garcia-Rubi, A.D. Rogol, K. Link, C.M. Christie, M.L. Johnson, and J.D. Veldhuis (1990). Testosterone and oxandrolone, a nonaromatizable androgen, specifically amplify the mass and rate of growth hormone (GH) secreted per burst without altering GH secretory burst duration or frequence or the GH half-life. *J. Clin. Endocrinol. Metab.* 71:846–854.

Urhausen A., and W. Kindermann (1987). Behavior of testosterone, sex hormone binding globulin (SHBG), and cortisol before and after a triathalon competition. *Int. J. Sports Med.* 8:305–308.

Vanhelder, W.P., M.W. Radomski, and R.C. Goode (1984). Growth hormone responses during intermittent weight lifting exercise in men. *Eur. J. Appl. Physiol.* 53:31–34.

Villaneuva, A.L., S. Schlosser, B. Hopper, J.H. Liu, D.I. Hoffman, and R.W. Rebar (1986). Increased cortisol production in women runners. *J. Clin. Endocrinol. Metab.* 63:133–136.

Vyskocil, E., and E. Gutmann (1977). Electrophysiological and contractile properties of the levator ani muscle after castration and testosterone administration. *Pflugers Arch.* 368:104–109.

Wade, N. (1972). Anabolic steroids: Doctors denounce them, but athletes aren't listening. *Science* 176:1399–1403.

Ward, P. (1973). The effect of an anabolic steroid on strength and lean body mass. *Med. Sci. Sports* 5:277–283.

Webb, O., P. Laskarzewski, and C. Glueck (1984). Severe depression of high-density lipoprotein cholesterol levels in weightlifters and bodybuilders by self-administered exogenous testosterone and anabolic-androgenic steroids. *Metabolism* 33:971–975.

Weicker, H., H. Hayle, B. Repp, and J. Kolb (1982). Influence of training and anabolic steroids on the LDH isozyme pattern of skeletal and heart muscle fibers of guinea pigs. *Int. J. Sports Med.* 3:90–96.

Wheeler, G.F., S.R. Wall, A.N. Belcasto, and D.C. Cumming (1984). Reduced serum testosterone and prolactin levels in male distance runners. *JAMA* 252:514–514.

Whitelaw, M.J., T.N. Foster, and W.H. Graham (1966). Methandrostenolone (Diabanol): a controlled study of its anabolic and androgenic effect in children. *Pediatric Pharm. Ther.* 68:291–296.

Wilson, J.D., and J.E. Griffin (1980). The use and misuse of androgens. *Metabolism* 29:1278–1295.

Wilson, J.D. (1988). Androgen abuse by athletes. *Endocrine Rev.* 9:181–199.

Windsor, R., and D. Dumitru (1989). Prevalence of anabolic steroid use by male and female adolescents: Survey. *Med. Sci. Sports Exerc.* 21:494–497.

Wood, T.O., P.H. Cooke, and A.E. Goodship (1988). The effect of exercise and anabolic steroids on the mechanical properties and crimp morphology of the rat tendon. *Am. J. Sports Med.* 16:153–158.

Wright, J. (1978). *Anabolic Steroids and Sports.* Natick, MA: Sports Science Consultants.

Yesalis, C.E., R.T. Herrick, W.E. Buckley, K.E. Friedl, D. Brannon, and J.E. Wright (1988). Self-reported use of anabolic-androgenic steroids by elite power lifters. *Physician Sportsmed.* 16:91–100.

Yesalis, C.E., J.E. Wright, and J.A. Lombardo (1989). Anabolic-androgenic steroids: a synthesis of existing data and recommendations for future research. *Clin. Sports Med.* 1:109–134.

Young, M., H.R. Crookshank, and L. Ponder (1977). Effects of an anabolic steroid on selected parameters in male albino rats. *Res. Quart. AAHPERD* 48:653–656.

Zadek, R.E., and R.A. Robinson (1961). The effect of growth hormone on healing of an experimental long-bone defect. *J. Bone Joint Surg.* 43-A:1261.

Zevin, D., H. Turani, A. Cohen, and J. Levi (1981). Androgen-associated hepatoma in a hemodialysis patient. *Nephron* 29:274–276.

DISCUSSION

HICKSON: With respect to a direct action of anabolic steroids on muscle, one of the classical approaches is to look at protein inducibility, that is, to see whether steroid hormones induce protein synthesis. No one has found a marker protein that androgens have induced in muscle as yet. This is very disappointing, and, in my opinion, it argues against a direct effect until such an inducible protein is found.

NADEL: Obviously, there is an increase in protein synthesis, and the fact that a marker protein hasn't been found suggests to me that this is a productive area of research. How fast do you think the proteins are increasing their synthetic rates?

HICKSON: I am not sure. The evidence for increased protein synthesis is that shown with whole body experiments. In one study, the investigators gave testosterone intramuscularly periodically for a few weeks and certainly increased muscle protein synthesis. The drawback with this is that they observed no change in muscle size, although the protein synthesis rate was increased. When they biopsied the muscle, they found no change in fiber size.

NADEL: Other proteins can be turned on rather rapidly when given the right stimulus, and the assumption is that this must be a similar type of response, but I am surprised that the protein markers have not been found.

HICKSON: I want to reaffirm that growth in normal male animals cannot be stimulated with huge doses of anabolic steroids alone.

NADEL: You need the exercise stimulus as well.

HEIGENHAUSER: Can you make some comments about discrepancies between athletes' use of steroids, e.g., with stacking of multiple drugs, and steroid research methods?

LOMBARDO: Most of the research studies have used rather moderate doses of a single drug. On the other hand, athletes use stacking the same way we treat people with multiple antihypertensive drugs. The idea is to use multiple drugs to get the maximal effect without going to a dangerous dose. Also, it is assumed that using multiple drugs working in different areas will give the best effect. What athletes are using now are two and three steroid drugs. They usually include a testosterone preparation. If they use an oral agent at all, it is usually either Oxandrolone or Stanazolol. They will probably use another injectable drug, generally of the equine variety, and it is either Boldenone (Equipoise) or Winstrol B (Stanazolol). They use those intermittently. The last thing they use in a drug cycle is human chorionic gonadotropin (HCG), which has the same structure as luteinizing hormone. The athletes use HCG to stimulate testicular function. The drug cycles typically last anywhere from 6–12 weeks. Then the athletes take a break for 6–12 weeks and subsequently start on the drugs again. We have had individuals using these drugs change their body composition in as little as 6 weeks by as much as 16 pounds of lean body mass with even greater changes in body weight.

HEIGENHAUSER: Chicken producers claim that beta agonists are the most potent anabolic agents for increasing muscle mass in chickens. The doses they use are very high. Is there is any indication that this treatment has any anabolic effect in man?

LOMBARDO: Not to my knowledge.

WILMORE: Are there any data on the use of steroids to speed recovery from training? This presumed effect is why middle distance runners and even long distance runners are now taking steroids.

LOMBARDO: There are no data. Research has basically stopped in this field, primarily because human subject review committees will not allow the use of anabolic steroids because of the potential adverse effects.

WILMORE: I am very confused about what I hear on drug testing. At one U.S. Olympic Committee meeting I learned that they can even tell what lipstick your girlfriend is wearing on the basis of a drug test done 6 months later. They say it is that accurate. Can you give us some information on the accuracy of drug testing and the effectiveness of the masking techniques that the athletes are using?

LOMBARDO: For the synthetic anabolic steroids, detection techniques are very good, especially with nandrolone, which stays in the system up to a year. The ratio of testosterone to epitestosterone (T:E) is another question. A study that was recently published showed that individuals can be given upwards of 100 mg/week of short-acting testosterone and not raise the T:E ratio to 6:1. An athlete on a maintenance dosage may need only 100–300 mg/week. The masking agents, including Probenecid and various diuretics, don't seem to be effective. If diuretics are used to produce dilute urine, we demand another specimen. I think that right now the testers are probably running even with the athletes, but they could quickly get behind unless they come up with some answers for testosterone.

ROBERTSON: Let me get at just a little bit of what is reality and what is myth regarding detection of steroid use. There is some thought that in the drug cycling, injectables and orals can be stacked in a way that can prevent detection. Is that true?

LOMBARDO: No, because the detection is based on the degradation of the drug itself. If you take two different drugs, the question is how fast your system can eliminate them. If they use the same degradation system, it may take longer.

ROBERTSON: But is there an advantage to certain regimens for sequencing injectables and orals?

LOMBARDO: From a scientific standpoint, we don't know.

COSTILL: One of the things that has intrigued me is the use of anabolic steroids by female body builders. Women who are not on steroids can usually develop their legs, but no matter how much weight lifting they do, their upper bodies do not seem to change much. When they go on anabolic steroids, it is very obvious that they suddenly gain an ability to hypertrophy muscles of the upper body. Is there any information available to tell us something about differential regional binding for androgens in muscle of various parts of the body?

HICKSON: The androgen receptor capacity in females is about twice as high as that in males, but that represents only two femtomoles versus one, and that is a questionable change. What probably is happening with anabolic steroid use in women is that they bring up the androgen concentration to the normal optimal level at which androgens function in men.

COSTILL: Why does this differentiate between the upper and lower body?

HICKSON: There are no known regional differences.

LAMB: In rodents there are sex-linked muscles that respond much more to androgens than do normal locomotor muscles. It seems that there is at least a precedence in the animal kingdom for differential responsiveness to androgens among different muscles.

EICHNER: One reason for women to take anabolic steroids is that it drives up their hemoglobin a little bit, and that probably somehow enhances erythropoietin. Also, while I do not have any direct evidence on gender effects on upper versus lower body muscle, there has been a burst of interest in medicine in the last five years on upper versus lower body fat. The investigator who first studied this 50 years ago described women who not only had their fat centrally located as in men, but who were also broader in the shoulders, as if some of their lean body mass was shifted centrally. You might think that those women had slightly higher androgen drive than their counterparts. This area may well be productive for research.

CLARKSON: I am interested in the mechanism of steroid action on muscle whereby androgens inhibit the glucocorticoid receptors. I have three points on that. First, that mechanism suggests a global effect of steroid use that would have nothing to do with the exercise of the muscle, yet exercise is required to get a positive effect of anabolic steroids. Secondly, this mechanism seems to be based on the idea that there is an exercise-induced increase in cortisol that causes catabolism, but is that ever shown after exercise? Does a rise in glucocorticoids during exercise actually cause catabolism after exercise? My third point is that to increase protein catabolism, the number of glucocorticoid receptors usually has to be increased. Are there enough of these receptors normally in steroid-using athletes? Is there enough cortisol to cause a catabolism effect?

LOMBARDO: You are not going to get an increase in muscle size simply by blocking glucocorticoids at rest without overload to the muscle. I don't know any literature that clearly demonstrates in humans that exercise causes an increased catabolism in muscle as a result of an increase in circulating cortisol.

HICKSON: With regard to muscle atrophy induced by denervation and/or immobilization, there is evidence that such atrophy is not glucocorticoid-mediated. The glucocorticoid may play a small role early on. Evidence for the absence of glucocorticoid-mediated atrophy under these circumstances is that glucocorticoids will down-regulate the glucocorticoid receptor, not up-regulate it. With regard to the cortisol point during exercise, both strength training and endurance training depress resting serum testosterone levels. I know there are some long-term studies showing that resting testosterone levels may increase in elite strength athletes after 2 years of training, but if you give these guys a high dose of lifting, the resting levels tend to decrease. This in conjunction with cortisol elevation may produce a synergistic effect to inhibit muscle growth.

EICHNER: I would like to express a note of concern about athletes who combine steroids with Lasix to lose water weight. In at least one reported case in a body builder, this led to a hematocrit of 71% at the time of competition. I am very worried about the likelihood of strokes and blood clots in such situations.

LOMBARDO: All of the adverse effects of various drug combinations are reported by case studies, but most physicians don't think to ask if a patient has used anabolic steroids. Unless we ask the question, we will never know. An oncologist once told me that he had three males with choreo carcinoma, and he did not understand how these healthy young males could have such a carcinoma. I asked him if they had taken steroids, and he said, "No, they were not on glucocorticoids." However, it turned out that all three were body builders on anabolic steroids. Those cases have never been reported. There are undoubtedly many cases like that sitting out there that have not been reported.

SAWKA: In at least two studies, steroids seem to be involved in weakening of connective tissue. My questions are: 1) What is actually known about the mechanism underlying this? 2) Have there been any reports by sports team physicians as to the incidence of these types of injuries?

LOMBARDO: Nobody has proved a mechanism as of yet, but there have been many reports by team doctors who feel that people on anabolic steroids get hurt more often and do not heal very well. My guess is that the stronger muscles generate more torque than ligaments can tolerate, either because the ligaments don't increase in density as fast as the muscle gets stronger or because the ligament is actually weakened by the steroids. Also, the athlete may be in an injury-susceptible state when he cycles off the drugs because it takes time for the natural production of testosterone to be re-established. We have only our clinical experience to guide us on this, but when we do surgery on steroid users, we supplement them with anabolic steroids when their testosterone levels go below 250–300, which is normal for our lab. Otherwise, I do not think that they are going to heal normally.

I think there are three reasons that we need to try to stop steroid use. One is that it is truly unfair because steroid use makes somebody else use steroids to remain competitive; it changes the normal behavior of those who don't want to use drugs. Second, I think the adverse effects are real and are going to be more and more commonly reported. For example, I have a 40 year old power lifter who has a cardiomyopathy and two-vessel heart disease with complete blockage of two coronary arteries. We are going to publish this case as soon as possible. The third reason is that athletes are role models, and drug use is not the type of behavior that should be modelled.

HEIGENHAUSER: How long does the steroid effect on body weight last, and can it be maintained by normal training?

LOMBARDO: Those are questions that have never been answered scientifically. Clinically, it appears that the power lifters and the body builders who get up for a major competition lose a lot of mass within a month or two if they do not train at the same intensity. They will maintain somewhere between 20% and 40% of their weight gains, but will lose the rest. This is clinical evidence based on athletes I have cared for. The ones who show the most dramatic weight loss are the ones that we operate on. We operate on a lot of steroid users who have torn their patellar tendons and their cruciate ligaments in lifting. They will lose anywhere from 20–60 pounds in 2 months.

HEIGENHAUSER: I am wondering how long the effects last. Do they get an adaptation with the drug such that they can later discontinue use of the drug, maintain a fairly high level of resistance training, and not lose the muscle mass they gained while using the drug?

LOMBARDO: Those who use steroids for the high-intensity part of their training cycle and then go into the taper claim that the strength and mass gains they have made are enough to get them through the rest of the training cycle. Swimmers and intermediate track runners would fall into this category. It is the big power people who need the weight and the strength who say that if they do not stay on the steroids until close to the time of competition they are going to lose enough muscle mass within 2–4 weeks to have a significant adverse effect on performance.

LAMB: Another reason for maintaining androgen use right up to competition is that some athletes want the aggression effect of the steroids.

LOMBARDO: Many of the relatively docile athletes take it for that reason. There are also some laid-back football players who claim that steroids give them the aggression they need to perform on the field at a high level.

KREIDER: I believe that drug testing has to be on a year-round, random basis to be effective. Also, the athletes see using steroids as no worse than tobacco smoking; they think that most of the adverse effects of steroids are overblown.

LOMBARDO: The testing program that we are putting on with the NFL is a random, year-round program so that every week somebody is going to get tested on each team. It is very costly. The NCAA is also going to an off-season testing program this year in Division I schools. If we reduce steroid abuse, it will be because of a greater risk of detection and not because athletes are afraid of the adverse effects. I think that the adverse effects area has been overblown. The serous adverse effect are real, but the incidence is extremely low. On the other hand, if you are the one in 100,000 who gets liver carcinoma, there is no cure, and you are going to die.

Chronic steroid users will almost always have some nuisance adverse effect, such as breast formation in males or hair loss, but most will not suffer life-threatening side effects.

KREIDER: There are a lot of state legislatures talking about giving steroid possession the same legal ramifications as marijuana or cocaine. We in Virginia Beach have had gyms raided and folks thrown in jail. I suspect this type of law enforcement will eventually have some impact.

8

Amphetamine, Caffeine, and Cocaine

Robert K. Conlee, Ph.D.

INTRODUCTION

Many of the chapters of this book deal with ethically acceptable methods for optimizing performance. These range from nutritional supplements and diet modification to improved equipment for bicycling. On the other hand, several of the chapters review practices that have received notoriety as ergogenic enhancers, but are nevertheless ethically unacceptable, e.g., anabolic steroids, blood doping, and beta blockers. The topics of this chapter fall into this latter category. Both cocaine and amphetamines are classified as controlled Class II drugs and are categorically banned by the International Olympic Committee (U.S. Olympic Committee, 1988) and by the U.S. National Collegiate Athletic Association (1988) under the classification of stimulants. Caffeine is also a banned stimulant, but because of its widespread availability in common foods and beverages (e.g. cola drinks, coffee, tea, chocolate, etc.), there is considerable tolerance by sport institutions for its presence in urine samples obtained for testing. Even though these three substances are deemed illegal drugs by various amateur and professional athletic associations, and in spite of the attendant risks associated with their use, each is used or has been used by athletes for the expressed purpose of improving performance (Wadler & Hainline, 1989). The purpose of this chapter is to establish why these drugs are potential ergogenic substances and then to review the literature which either verifies or refutes that notion. Finally, discussion will be presented regarding the health risks associated with use of these stimulants.

AMPHETAMINE

Source and Chemical Structure

The endogenous hormones and neurotransmitters of the sympathetic nervous system are known as catecholamines and include the substances epinephrine, norepinephrine, and dopamine. Upon release from nerve endings or the adrenal medulla, the catecholamines exert their effects on target tissues through interaction with specialized receptors known as α or β receptors. These receptors are further divided into α_1 or α_2, and β_1 or β_2. When catecholamines stimulate their respective receptors, they initiate the myriad of responses known collectively as the sympathetic response. These include increased respiratory and cardiac activity, fuel mobilization, redistribution of blood flow, and a heightened mental awareness. Exogenous substances that also cause these responses are referred to as sympathomimetics. Amphetamine and its derivatives (see Table 8-1) are classified specifically as sympathomimetic amines. Their chemical structures, shown in Figure 8-1, are somewhat similar to the catecholamines. All are derived from the parent compound, β-phenylethylamine, which consists of a benzene ring and the ethylamine side chain.

Catecholamines are characterized by the presence of hydroxyl groups (-0H) on the benzene ring. These hydroxyl groups are essential for interaction with the α and β receptors. Because the amphetamines do not contain these groups, they are not true catecholamines and do not exert direct sympathetic effects through α and β receptors.

For the sake of simplicity in the rest of this chapter, the terms amphetamine or amphetamines will refer to both benzedrine (a racemic mixture of the d and l isomers of amphetamine) and dexedrine (the d isomer only). Most of the findings discussed in this section are based on these two compounds. When appropriate, the specific form of the drug will be identified.

General Pharmacology

Central and Peripheral Effects. Outside the central nervous system, amphetamines act as indirect sympathomimetics by causing the release of norepinephrine from sympathetic nerve terminals (Weiner, 1985). They have no direct action on α or β receptors. The principal peripheral response to amphetamines is an increase in diastolic and systolic blood pressure due to norepinephrine-induced vasoconstriction. Heart rate may or may not be elevated (Fischman, 1987).

The primary effects of the drug take place in the central nervous system. Specifically, stimulants such as amphetamine and cocaine activate the pleasure or reward pathways of the brain. These are powerful reinforcement areas located in the mesolimbic or meso-

TABLE 8-1. *Common Amphetamines*

Generic Name	Trade Name	Street Name
Amphetamine	Benzedrine	Uppers, beanies
Dextroamphetamine	Dexedrine	Copilots, greenies
Methamphetamine	Methedrine	Speed, crystal, meth

Adapted from Wadler and Hainline (1989)

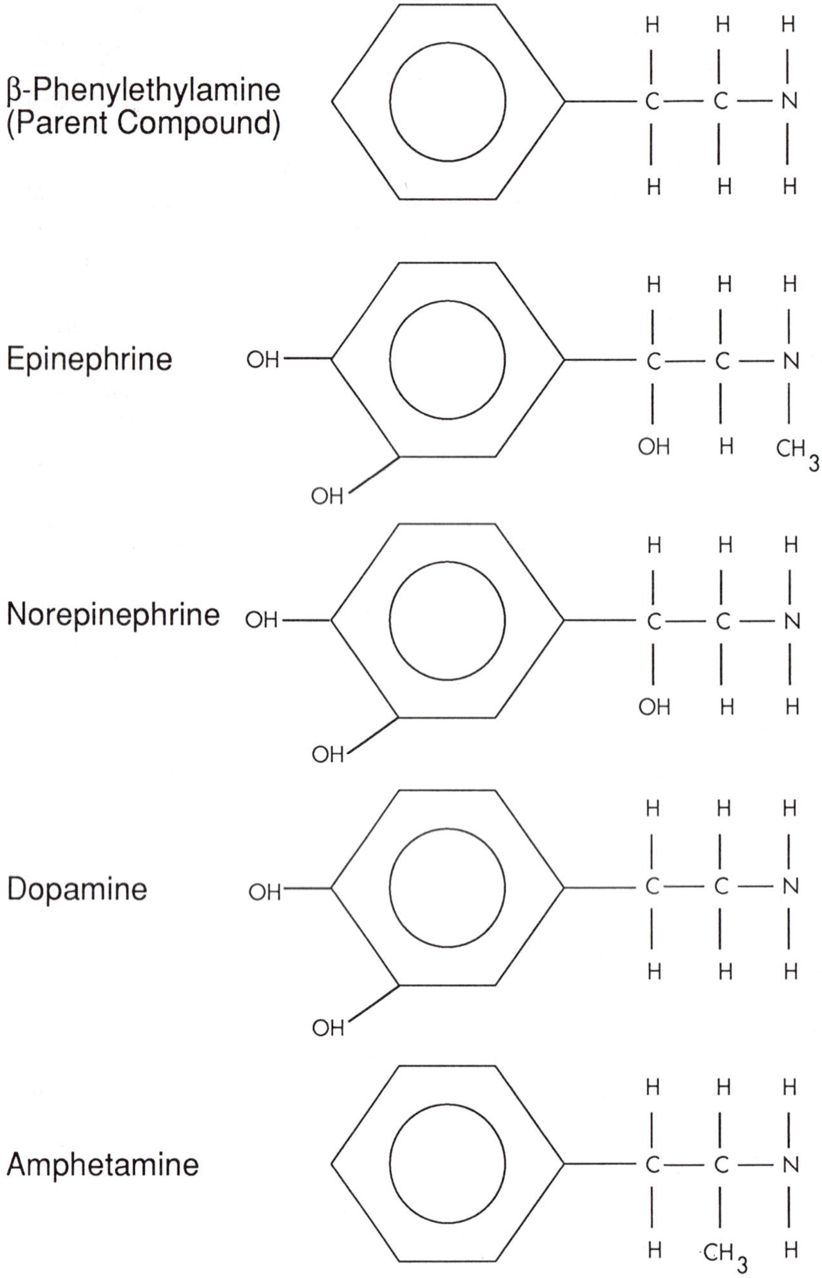

FIGURE 8-1. *Chemical structure of Amphetamine and the Catecholamines.*

cortical pathways (Gawin & Ellinwood, 1988). In addition, the drug has an effect on the reticular activating system and the hypothalamus. The result of a single dose of amphetamine, then, is a plethora of responses which include not only an elevation of mood and marked euphoria, but also a decreased sense of fatigue and an increased alertness in sleep-deprived individuals. Persons on amphetamine experience increased restlessness and tend to be more talkative; appetite is usually reduced (Weiner, 1985). Because some of these responses can have a positive effect on motor performance, the drug has been used extensively as an ergogenic aid.

Mechanism of Action. The mechanism by which amphetamines exert these responses is still not clear, but because most of these responses are mediated by the release of catecholamines in the brain, it is believed that the drug either enhances their release, interferes with their re-uptake, or inhibits their degradation (Fischman, 1987; Pitts & Marwah, 1988). In this regard, the catecholamine most responsible for the rewarding and reinforcing properties in the brain is dopamine (Gawin & Ellinwood, 1988). It is hypothesized that amphetamine treatment results in an increased release of dopamine because amphetamine responses can be blocked by the administration of selective dopamine receptor antagonists and mimicked by dopamine agonists (Carboni et al., 1989; Neilsen & Scheel-Krüger, 1988).

Absorption, Distribution, and Metabolism. Amphetamine is usually consumed as a 5 or 10 mg tablet. The drug is a white, water soluble powder; unlike epinephrine, amphetamine is easily absorbed from the gut and transported by the blood to the drug's site of action. Its effects are generally perceived within 30 min of ingestion, and the metabolic and physiological half life of the drug lasts from 3–6 h (Gawin & Ellinwood, 1988). The prolonged half life is probably due to the fact that the drug undergoes little or no metabolism to other intermediates before being excreted in the urine (Wadler & Hainline, 1989). Some amphetamine abusers dissolve the powder in water or saline and inject the drug intravenously. Such self-administration results in a rapid rush and extreme feeling of euphoria (Jaffe, 1985).

Side Effects. When taken acutely, amphetamines can induce restlessness, tremor, irritability, confusion, and psychotic behavior. The drug can induce vomiting, dry mouth, diarrhea, and abdominal cramps. Headache and various cardiovascular symptoms also may manifest themselves. Fatal poisoning may be due to cerebral hemorrhages. Chronic consumption leads to severe weight loss, hallucinations, and psychotic paranoia bordering on schizophrenia (Weiner, 1985). Some athletes have died as a direct result of amphetamine use (Wadler & Hainline, 1989). Such events should be strong warning to those who might consider using amphetamine for ergogenic purposes. A summary of adverse side effects is shown in Table 8-2.

Ergogenicity of Amphetamines

This topic has been the subject of numerous reviews since Heyrodt & Weissenstein (1940) revealed that amphetamines may enhance performance (Cooper, 1972; Hart & Wallace, 1975; Ivy, 1983; Ivy & Goetzl, 1943; Ivy & Krasno, 1941; Laties & Weiss, 1981; Lombardo, 1986; Lombardo, 1987; Lowenthal & Kendrick, 1985; Nuzzo & Waller, 1988; Wadler & Hainline, 1989; Weiss & Laties, 1962; Williams, 1974). Some of these reviews have been extensive and comprehensive, and the reader is referred to them for a more historical perspective (Weiss & Laties, 1962; Williams, 1974; Ivy, 1983). Of late, the topic has been quite adequately addressed by Wadler and Hainline (1989). It is apparent from the more recent reviews of the ergogenic effects of amphetamines that the topic has not been addressed as a research issue for the past 10 y. Since the well-conducted 1980 study by Chandler and Blair, not one original study using human subjects has been published that specifically addresses the ergogenicity of the amphetamines. This void is dramatic, but parallels the marked decline in the general abuse of the drug as determined by national survey (National Institute of Drug Abuse, 1989). This decline was inevitable when the drug was declared a controlled substance in 1970, thus precipitating a decrease in its availability (Wadler & Hainline, 1989). The decline in use also seems evident among

TABLE 8-2. *Adverse Effects of Amphetamine*

Acute, Mild	Acute, Severe	Chronic
Restlessness	Confusion	Addiction
Dizziness	Assaultiveness	Weight loss
Tremor	Delirium	Psychosis
Irritability	Paranoia	Paranoid delusions
Insomnia	Hallucinations	Dyskinesias
Euphoria	Convulsions	Compulsive/sterotypic/ repetitive behavior
Uncontrolled movements	Cerebral hemorrhage	Vasculitis
Headache	Angina/myocardial infarction	Neuropathy
Palpitations	Hypertension	
Anorexia	Circulatory collapse	
Nausea		
Vomiting		

Adapted from Wadler and Hainline (1989)

athletic populations. In his expose on the use of amphetamines in football, Mandell (1979) reported that approximately 66% of the National Football League players he interviewed during 1968–69 admitted to using amphetamines to improve performance. That contrasts to more recent surveys of collegiate athletes which detected only a 3–5% use rate (Anderson & McKeag, 1985; Newman, 1987).

Because the issue of ergogenicity has been addressed so thoroughly by Ivy (1983), and because there is no new research information, only the most pertinent findings will be summarized in this section. One can only conclude, in agreement with Laties and Weiss (1981), that the research generally supports an ergogenic benefit derived from amphetamine use. What is also apparent, however, in agreement with Chandler and Blair (1980), is that the beneficial effect of the drug is extremely variable and that the magnitude of performance enhancement depends on a number of factors including the responsiveness of the individual, the nature of the activity, the dose administered, and the timing of the administration.

Human Studies. A large number of studies was produced in the decade of the 1940s in response to the use of amphetamines by combat soldiers during World War II. These were designed to test the efficacy of the drug in reducing the effects of fatigue. Alles and Feigen (1942) showed quite nicely that work capacity was restored in fatigued muscle 30–120 min after administration of amphetamine in doses of 20, 30, or 40 mg. Knoefel (1943) observed a similar benefit. On the other hand, Foltz et al., in two separate studies (1943a, 1943b) observed no beneficial effect of amphetamine on recovery from previous fatiguing work. Probably the most notable of these early experiments was that of Cuthbertson and Knox (1947), who evaluated the effects of amphetamine on recovery from exhaustive exertion on either a leg or arm ergometer. Both 10 mg of methedrine and 15 mg of benzedrine, when administered during prolonged work at a point when fatigue was clearly evident, relieved fatigue and allowed the subject to work at a level similar to that prior to fatigue. In this same report, the authors also evaluated the effects of 15 mg of methedrine on the ability of military personnel to march 18 miles after not sleeping for 24 h. From subjective evaluations, the authors concluded that the drug significantly reduced the feelings of fatigue in the experimental group. They also reported that the treatment subjects were less likely to complain of severe blisters.

Finally, these same investigators reported from a third phase of their study that 15 mg of benzedrine kept subjects from sleeping between forced marches. Despite this, these men were still able to perform a subsequent 20-mile march. From these results, Cuthbertson and Knox (1947) concluded that amphetamines improved work output in previously fatigued soldiers and diminished the subjective feelings of fatigue due to sleeplessness. These findings were later corroborated when Tyler (1947) reported that benzedrine sulfate (either 10 or 15 mg doses) prevented the deterioration in certain motor skills and clearly improved the ability of the subjects to remain awake over the 72–112 h sleepless period. In contrast to these positive findings, Somerville (1946) was unable to detect an effect of amphetamine on improving performance of fatigued soldiers on an obstacle course or rifle range during 50 h of sleep deprivation.

These early studies were performed more as field studies with rather inadequate procedures for evaluation. In response to the need for better experimental controls, many studies assessed the effectiveness of amphetamines on laboratory tests of psychomotor skills such as tests of simple learning, reaction time, judgment, balance, and visual tracking. As a whole, they produced conflicting results. Some reported improved performance (Adler et al., 1950; Blum et al., 1964; Domino et al., 1972; Evans & Jewett, 1962; Kornetsky et al., 1959; Uyeda & Fuster, 1962), while others found no effect on performance (Evans et al., 1976; Goldstein et al., 1960; Hauty & Payne, 1957; Kornetsky, 1958; Wenzel & Rutledge, 1962). A common finding in the positive studies was that amphetamine was most effective under fatigued or sleep-deprived conditions (Adler et al., 1950; Blum et al., 1964; Domino et al., 1972; Kornetsky et al., 1959). It should also be pointed out that in the negative studies the drug was never reported to affect performance adversely, only that it gave no positive benefit.

In view of the conflicting results appearing in the literature regarding the ergogenic benefits of amphetamine and in response to the increasing use of amphetamine by athletes during the 1950s, the American Medical Association in 1957 commissioned Henry Beecher of Harvard University to undertake a study to test the effects of this stimulant on athletic performance (Ryan, 1959). The results of that study (Smith & Beecher, 1959) are the most supportive to date of the beneficial effects of amphetamine on performance. The authors reported that amphetamine (14 mg/70 kg body weight), administered 2–3 h prior to testing, improved swimming, running, and weight throwing performance in 75% of their collegiate athlete subjects. Throwers (shot put and hammer) exhibited the greatest improvement (3–4%), whereas runners (distances ranged from 600 m to 12.7 miles) improved by 1.5%, and swimmers (100–200 m distances) by 0.6–1.2%. It should be noted that the statistical analysis of this study has come under severe criticism (Pierson, 1961), which casts some doubt on the validity of the conclusions. The authors attempted to dispel that doubt by offering rebuttal to the criticism (Cochran et al., 1961) and by replicating certain aspects of the original study with similar positive results (Smith et al., 1963). Nevertheless, the findings of Beecher and his group must be accepted with caution. This is especially true in light of the results of Karpovich (1959), which were published at the same time as the original study of Smith and Beecher (1959). Karpovich (1959) also examined the effects of amphetamine on running and swimming performance using collegiate athletes. He administered 10 or 20 mg of amphetamine 30–60 min prior to testing and found no beneficial effects of the drug on performance. This is in marked contrast to the results of Smith and Beecher (1959), but illustrates the pattern of inconsistency observed in the literature. Subsequently, a variety of papers have been published which either support (Borg et al., 1972; Chandler & Blair, 1980; Lovingood et al., 1967; Smith & Beecher, 1961; Smith et al., 1963; Wyndham et al., 1971) or reject (Blyth et al., 1960; Borg et al., 1972; Chandler & Blair, 1980; Golding & Barnard, 1963; Hueting & Poulus, 1970; Williams & Thompson, 1973; Wyndham et al., 1971) the claim for ergogenicity of amphetamine. Many of these studies support both conclusions, depending on whether the tests of ergogenicity were administered before or after fatigue. The prevailing finding is that a beneficial effect of the drug is only observed under conditions of fatigue. The non-beneficial effects were almost always observed under non-fatigue conditions. When fatigue was incorporated as a variable, amphetamine usually improved performance compared to placebo. The notable exception was the study by Golding and Barnard (1963), who observed no effect of 15 mg of amphetamine on time to exhaustion either on the first run to exhaustion or on a second run in the exhausted state. It is possible that the workload, which resulted in exhaustion within 2–4 min, was too intense to observe an effect of the drug. Wyndham et al. (1971) used a less strenuous exercise test, which caused fatigue in 8–16 min, and found that amphetamine improved endurance in the fatigued condition.

The study of Chandler and Blair (1980) is representative of the contrasts in results obtained in previous investigations. The authors attempted to evaluate the effects of dexedrine (15 mg/70 kg) on strength, muscular power, running speed, acceleration, aerobic power, and anaerobic capacity. They reported that quadriceps extension was enhanced, but not elbow flexion. They also noted significant improvements due to amphetamine on measures of acceleration, anaerobic capacity, and time to exhaustion, but no improvement on VO_2max, muscular power, or speed. They pointed out in their discussion that the drug had no consistent effect for all people—a conclusion reached by most investigators—nor was the effect always predictable in the same individual.

Animal Studies. Almost all animal studies have shown that the drug improves endurance performance (Bättig, 1963; Bhagat & Wheeler, 1973; Estler & Gabrys, 1979; Gerald, 1978; Hanada et al., 1986; Kay & Birren, 1958; Latz et al., 1966; Molinengo & Orsetti, 1976), but some have reported that the positive effects are dose specific. For instance, endurance performance is increased at relatively low doses (Bättig, 1963; Gerald, 1978) and decreased at higher doses (Gerald, 1978; Latz et al., 1966). Unfortunately, as with the other studies reviewed in this section, this area is not without contradiction. Bhagat and Wheeler (1973) reported that low doses (1.25–5.0 mg/kg) were ineffective in influencing swim times to exhaustion in rats, but higher doses (10–20 mg/kg) proved beneficial. While there is no apparent explanation for these opposing results, it seems safe to conclude, based on the numerous reports supporting the view, that amphetamines at doses of 0.3–5.0 mg/kg are effective in improving endurance in animals (Gerald, 1978; Kay & Birren, 1958; Latz et al., 1966; Molinengo & Orsetti, 1976).

Hanada and coworkers (1986) reported the only important animal project since 1980. They showed that when mice were chronically treated with amphetamine (1–2 mg/kg) over a 7 d period, their ability to endure a prolonged swim (>120 min) increased with each daily administration of the drug. In addition, they found that 30 d after being drug free, the animals retained their previously enhanced swimming ability by swimming longer after an acute injection than they did after the first injection of their chronic treatment regimen. Interestingly, improvement in swimming only occurred when animals were allowed to swim after each daily injection. Animals restrained after each daily injection showed no improvement when finally given the opportunity to swim.

Summary and Future Research

In spite of much evidence to the contrary, it can be concluded with caution that amphetamine treatment can improve a number of indexes of physical performance. The results are most obvious and consistent when the subject is in the fatigued condition. Unfortunately, there are few, if any, studies which have attempted to deduce the mechanisms by which amphetamine may confer ergogenicity. Only one report attempted to correlate the exercise response to changes in the central nervous system. Stone (1970) reported that for 2 h following 20 min of swimming, control rats exhibited very little spontaneous motor activity and that this behavior was correlated to low endogenous levels of norepinephrine in the brain. When treated with amphetamine during recovery from swimming, spontaneous activity patterns reappeared rapidly coincident with increased levels of brain norepinephrine. The author postulated that the drug improved the synthesis of norepinephrine, thus relieving the depressant effects of the previous exercise stimulus.

In spite of the dearth of direct evidence, most explanations for the beneficial effect of amphetamine involve the central stimulatory effects of the drug and include the notion that amphetamine causes an euphoric effect and dulls the central perception of fatigue (Fischman, 1987). This may well be true, but fatigue is not just central in origin. The peripheral correlates of fatigue are numerous, and many of them involve the availability of energy substrates for maintenance of the excitation-contraction process (MacLaren et al., 1989).

The effects of amphetamine on the peripheral physiological and biochemical responses to exercise have not been well studied. Little insight has been gained from assessment of blood lactic acid responses (Chandler & Blair, 1980; Chatterjee et al., 1970; Wyndham et al., 1971). However, the work of Estler and Gabrys (1979) and Pinter and Pattee (1968) give some suggestion as to a potential mechanism by which amphetamine could prolong endurance. By raising free-fatty-acid levels in the blood prior to exercise, probably by the release of endogenous catecholamines, amphetamine could conceivably delay the breakdown of muscle glycogen stores and thus reduce fatigue (Conlee, 1987). However, this hypothesis was not supported by the data of Estler and Gabrys (1979), who found no evidence for glycogen sparing.

CAFFEINE

Source and Chemical Structure

Caffeine is one of the most widely consumed drugs in the world (Somani & Gupta, 1988). It is derived from a variety of plants and is consumed in coffee, tea, cocoa, soft drinks, and various foods. The amounts of caffeine in these various beverages and food sources are shown in Table 8-3.

Caffeine is an alkaloid and belongs to the group of drugs referred to as methylxanthines, which include caffeine, theophylline, and theobromine. The latter two substances are found abundantly in tea and cocoa, respectively. Xanthine is a dioxypurine, and the methylxanthines are derived from this basic compound. Their structures are shown in Figure 8-2. Their pharmacologic properties differ due to the methyl substitutions at position 1, 3, and 7 of the purine ring. Caffeine and theophylline are the most potent, whereas theobromine is considered to have little therapeutic value (Rall, 1985).

TABLE 8-3. *Caffeine Content in Popular Foods, Beverages and Drugs*

	Brewing Time	
TEA (mg/oz)	1 min	5 min
bagged*		
black	4.5 – 7.1 (5.8)	8.4 – 10.7 (9.9)
green	1.9 – 4.1 (3.0)	5.6 – 7.7 (6.6)
loose leaf*	3.2 – 6.4 (4.3)	4.3 – 8.6 (6.0)
instant*		2.5 – 7.3
iced**		1.8 – 3.0
COFFEE* (mg/oz)		
instant		13.1 – 15.0 (14.1)
percolated		20.8 – 26.8 (23.6)
dripolated		29.4 – 32.8 (31.3)
decaf		1.1 – 2.1 (1.5)
CARBONATED BEVERAGES** (mg/oz)		
w/caffeine		2.5 – 5.4 (3.9)
COCOA** (mg/oz)		1.0 – 1.5
CHOCOLATE		
Syrup (mg/2 Tbsp)		10.0 – 17.0
Milk Choco. (mg/oz)		6.0
Baking Choco. (mg/oz)		35.0
OVER THE COUNTER DRUGS (mg/tablet or capsule)		
Stimulants		100 – 200
Cold Remedies		0 – 30
Pain Relievers		30 – 65
Plain Aspirin		0

Values are ranges with the average value shown in parentheses.
* Usually served in 5 oz. cup
** Usually served in 12 oz. servings
Adapted from Bunker and McWilliams (1979) and Slavin and Joensen (1985)

General Pharmacology

Central and Peripheral Effects. Caffeine appears to have an effect on almost every system of the body. The most obvious effects occur in the central nervous system (CNS). The drug is considered a stimulant and affects the cortex, medulla, and spinal cord. General responses to caffeine at low doses (2–10 mg/kg) include increased alertness or less drowsiness, relief from fatigue, and decreased reaction time, but also decreased performance of some motor tasks (Curatolo & Robertson, 1983), and increased respiration (Powers et al., 1986). Because of the effects of the drug on breathing behavior, it has been used successfully as a treatment for apnea in the premature infant (Neims & von Borstel, 1983). At higher doses (over 15 mg/kg), the drug produces nervousness, restlessness, insomnia, and tremors. Caffeine also stimulates the cardiovascular system, but its effects are not always consistent. It can both raise heart rate by

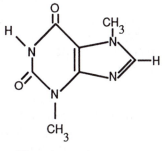

Purine

Xanthine

Caffeine

Theophylline

Theobromine

FIGURE 8-2. *Chemical structure of Caffeine, Theophylline, Theobromine, and their pre-cursors.*

direct effect on the myocardium, or lower heart rate by medullary vagal stimulation (Arnaud, 1987). Likewise, caffeine can cause both dilation and constriction of blood vessels. In noncaffeine users, caffeine causes an increase in both systolic and diastolic blood pressures. However, these effects are not observed in the chronic user (Robertson et al., 1981). In the kidney, caffeine causes a mild diuresis. In the lung, it causes bronchial dilation and has been used as an anti-asthmatic (Arnaud, 1987). Caffeine also stimulates the release of gastric secretions and may therefore exacerbate peptic ulcer conditions (Rall, 1985).

More relevant to the topic of this chapter is the direct effect of caffeine on muscle. It has been established that caffeine potentiates twitch tension in directly stimulated muscles *in vitro* and in indirectly stimulated muscle-nerve preparations (Connett et al., 1983; MacIntosh et al., 1981; Varagic & Zugic, 1971; Yamaguchi, 1975). Caffeine increases the metabolic rate of muscle, either directly or indirectly, through release of catecholamines (Rall, 1985). Catecholamines can activate the enzyme system responsible for glycogenolysis in muscle and liver as well as the enzymes responsible for lipolysis in muscle and adipose tissue (Van Handel, 1983). These effects result in an elevation in plasma free fatty acid (FFA) concentrations (Bellet et al., 1968), increased fatty acid oxidation in muscle, and eventual glycogen sparing (cf. Conlee, 1987).

Mechanism of Action. It is clear from this brief presentation of the pharmacologic actions of caffeine that the drug has the potential for ergogenicity in a variety of activities. This accounts for its reputation as the most used and abused drug in sports. As reviewed in a number of sources (Arnaud, 1987; Fredholm, 1985; Neims & von Borstel, 1983; Rall, 1985; Somani & Gupta, 1988), three major mechanisms have been proposed to explain the pharmacological responses to the drug. The first mechanism, and one relevant to the observations that caffeine augments the twitch response in skeletal muscle, is that caffeine increases the mobilization of calcium from the sarcoplasmic reticulum (S.R.) and thereby affects contraction (Blinks et al., 1972). This is thought to be due to an increased sensitization of the mechanism of Ca^{++} release or to an increased permeability of the S.R. This mechanism also has relevance to other processes controlled by Ca^{++} concentration, such as catecholamine release from the adrenal medulla (Rall, 1985).

The second mechanism proposes that caffeine inhibits the enzyme cAMP phosphodiesterase which is responsible for the breakdown of cAMP (Butcher & Sutherland, 1962). Cyclic AMP is the second messenger in target tissues of the catecholamines and is responsible for initiating the cascading activation of phosphorylated enzymes such as lipase in fat cells and glycogen phosphorylase in liver and muscle. By inhibiting cAMP phosphodiesterase, caffeine causes cAMP to accumulate in cells so that the hormonal responses are exaggerated. Such a mechanism could explain the caffeine-induced increase in plasma free-fatty-acids commonly observed in a number of studies (Beavo et al., 1970; Bellet et al., 1965; Bellet et al., 1968; Patwardhan et al., 1980). Both of these first two mechanisms have been criticized of late because they require doses of caffeine significantly higher than those attainable *in vivo* (Rall, 1985; Arnaud, 1987).

Presently, the mechanism most favored to explain the actions of caffeine and theophylline involves competitive antagonism at extracellular adenosine receptors (Sattin & Rall, 1970). Adenosine is present in all mammalian tissues and tends to exert its inhibitory effects through A_1 receptors. Those effects often include inhibition of adenylate cyclase, the enzyme responsible for the rapid formation of cAMP in response to catecholamine stimulation. Caffeine is an antagonist to A_1 receptors, thus negating the inhibitory effect of adenosine and propagating a variety of responses such as increased blood pressure, catecholamine release, CNS activity, lipolysis, and renin release (Somani & Gupta, 1988). Future research will likely confirm the importance of this mechanism and identify others not yet postulated so that the myriad effects of caffeine can be explained.

Absorption, Distribution, and Metabolism. Regardless of the form in which it is consumed (e.g., coffee, tea, chocolate, etc.), caffeine is rapidly absorbed from the gut and reaches peak plasma concentrations within 15–120 min, depending on the rate of gastric emptying (Arnaud, 1987). It is rapidly distributed to all tissues of the body, easily passes the blood-brain barrier, and exhibits a plasma half-life of 2.5–4.5 h. Only a small percentage (0.5–4%) is cleared in the urine as caffeine; most is degraded enzymatically in the liver (Arnaud, 1987; Rall, 1985).

Side Effects. It has been estimated that in the United States of America alone the average intake of caffeine is 206 mg per person per day (Somani & Gupta, 1988). As much as 10% of the population consumes greater than 1000 mg/d (Greyden, 1974). The therapeutic dose is supposedly 100–200 mg (1–3 mg/kg). Doses greater than 15 mg/kg may produce one or more of the adverse effects shown in Table 8-4. It is clear that tolerance to caffeine occurs rapidly, because many of the pharmacologic effects observed in the caffeine-naive are not seen in chronic users (Robertson et al., 1981). Nevertheless, high doses (>200 mg/kg) have reportedly resulted in seizures, coma, and death (Wadler & Hainline, 1989). Chronic use has also been implicated as a contributing factor in heart disease, cancer, and birth defects, although those claims are not universally supported (Somani & Gupta, 1988).

TABLE 8-4. *Adverse Effects of Caffeine*

Acute, Mild	Acute, Severe	Chronic
Nervousness	Peptic ulcer	Increased serum cholesterol
Irritability	Delirium	? Increased ischemic heart disease
Insomnia	Seizures	? Increased teratogenicity
Sinus tachycardia	Coma	? Increased carcinogenesis
Hypertension	Arrhythmia	? Increased fibrocystic breast disease
Gastrointestinal distress	Supraventricular Ventricular Death	

Modified from Wadler and Hainline (1989)

Ergogenicity of Caffeine

The possible role of caffeine as an ergogenic aid has been supported by a considerable body of literature. Excellent reviews are available (Eichner, 1986; Jacobson & Kulling, 1989; Lombardo, 1986, 1987; Powers & Dodd, 1985; Van Handel, 1983; Wadler & Hainline, 1989; Weiss & Laties, 1962; Wenger, 1988; Williams, 1974). In particular, the review by Van Handel (1983) is most noteworthy.

Psychomotor Responses. There is a considerable body of literature devoted to the effect of caffeine on psychomotor responses. However, it is not possible in the space available to provide a thorough review of this literature. The reader is referred to the excellent reviews of Weiss and Laties (1962) and Williams (1974) for an historical perspective as well as that of Jacobson and Kulling (1989) for a more up-to-date analysis. In summary, caffeine has been shown to improve reaction and movement time at lower doses (200–300 mg) (Jacobson & Kulling, 1989), but this effect is less evident with more complex movement patterns. In fact, the drug has been shown to impair task performance when the cognitive processing demands were high (Foreman et al., 1989). Coordination is also disrupted as the dose of caffeine increases. Caffeine appears to provide a beneficial effect on mental alertness. It delays the onset of sleep, but higher doses cause nervousness that could be detrimental to performance of fine motor tasks (Jacobson & Kulling, 1989). From these observations it may be safely concluded that the effects of caffeine on psychomotor tasks are contradictory and equivocal.

Muscle Strength. As discussed earlier, caffeine has been shown to potentiate twitch tension in *in vitro* and *in situ* muscle preparations (Connett et al., 1983; MacIntosh, 1981; Varagic & Zugic, 1971; Yamaguchi, 1975). These findings have led to the question of whether caffeine has a direct stimulatory effect on human muscle *in vivo*. The most often cited study in this regard is that of Lopes et al. (1983), who examined the effects of 500 mg of caffeine on voluntary and electrically stimulated contractions of the adductor pollicis. They found that caffeine treatment significantly increased force output at low frequencies of electrical stimulation (10–50 Hz) but did not alter maximum voluntary contractions (MVC) or force output at the highest stimulation frequency (100 Hz). There was no significant effect on muscle endurance at 50% MVC, although the authors argued that a real effect may have been masked by experimental insensitivity because a trend for improvement was apparent. This expectation is supported by the report of Supinski et al. (1986), who found that submaximal breathing endurance at various respiratory levels was significantly improved by caffeine. They reasoned that this improvement could have resulted directly from an effect of caffeine on the respiratory muscles or indirectly from an effect on the medullary respiratory centers. Evidence for a central effect was provided by lower ratings of perceived exertion in the caffeine trials compared to the placebo trial at the same workload. However, the authors found no beneficial effect on maximum inspiratory strength, even though the subjects consumed 600 mg of caffeine 60 min prior to the experimental task.

Williams and co-workers (1987) studied the effects of caffeine (7 mg/kg, 50 min prior to testing) on handgrip strength and found no enhancing effect of the drug on maximum strength. There was no effect on maximum motor unit recruitment as determined from integrated EMG. The authors also observed no changes in the ability to sustain a 50% MVC or the corresponding EMG pattern. They concluded that caffeine had no ergogenic benefit for activities requiring strength and/or short-term endurance. That conclusion substantiated the earlier findings of Perkins and Williams (1975), who reported no effect of caffeine at various doses ranging from 4–10 mg/kg on time to exhaustion (approximately 5 min) during high-intensity work performed on a bicycle ergometer. Similarly, in a followup project, Williams and co-workers (1988) found no beneficial effects of 7 mg/kg of caffeine (ingested 50 min prior to exercise) on peak power output, total work, and fatigue as assessed by a 15 s maximal exercise bout on a cycle ergometer.

In spite of earlier reports to the contrary (cf. Weiss & Laties, 1962; Williams, 1974), based on evidence from the above-mentioned studies and from other work (Bond et al., 1986; Bugyi, 1980), it appears that caffeine does not increase one's maximal force output. Therefore, little benefit to power activities would be expected. This contrasts with the perception that athletes have of its ergogenicity. It has been reported that weight lifters and throwers (discus, shotput, hammer) use the drug prior to competition to maximize performance (Brooks & Fahey, 1984). Any benefit derived under those circumstances may be due more to a placebo effect than to a physiological response. The explanation put forth by Van Handel (1983) for the lack of effect of caffeine in high power efforts still seems applicable: "Under these conditions, it is possible that 1) the sympathetic response to work stress is of such a magnitude that it masks the caffeine-induced alterations seen in *in vitro, in situ,* or resting *in vivo* studies, 2) the homeostatic adjustments *in vivo* preclude effects on contractibility seen *in vitro* or *in situ,* or 3) the dose relative to the muscle mass involved is too small."

Endurance Performance. There is considerable evidence in the early literature to infer that caffeine can improve physical endurance (Asmussen & Boje, 1948; Foltz et al., 1942; Rivers & Weber, 1907; Seashore & Ivy, 1953). Though these studies may be criticized for inadequate controls, subjective evaluations, or small numbers of observation, they have nevertheless provided the impetus for much of the research into the ergogenicity of caffeine.

Human Studies. That caffeine exerts an ergogenic benefit to endurance activities derives from a series of papers by Costill and coworkers (Costill et al., 1978; Essig et al., 1980; Ivy et al., 1979). In the first study (Costill et al., 1978), subjects who consumed 330 mg of caffeine 60 min before pedaling to exhaustion at a workload of 80% $\dot{V}O_2$max exhibited a 19.5% increase in endurance time (90.2 min vs. 75.5 min, caffeine vs. placebo, respectively). The authors speculated that caffeine caused an increased availability of free-fatty-acids to the muscle, resulting in an increased rate of fat oxidation for energy. Using more fat for energy production could reduce muscle glycogen utilization and thereby retard the onset of fatigue. This position was supported by a decrease in respiratory exchange ratios (R values) and an increase in plasma glycerol levels. Both conditions are indicative of greater fat mobilization and utilization. Unfortunately, plasma free-fatty-acid values were not significantly different between placebo and drug treatments. In addition, the investigators did not measure muscle glycogen concentrations to verify glycogen sparing.

In the second study (Ivy et al., 1979), subjects ingested 250 mg of caffeine 60 min before beginning a 2 h ride on an isokinetic cycling device. They were given an additional 250 mg in divided doses during the ride. The caffeine allowed the subjects to work at a higher $\dot{V}O_2$ during the ride and to produce more work (7% greater than control) over the 2 h. The authors postulated that the increased work capacity may have been due to central stimulatory effects of the drug in addition to increased oxidation of fat and reduced carbohydrate utilization. Again, muscle glycogen was not measured; plasma fatty acids were elevated at the end of exercise, but not at the beginning, as would be expected.

In the final study of the series (Essig et al., 1980), subjects received caffeine (5 mg/kg) 60 min prior to exercising for 30 min at 65–75% $\dot{V}O_2$max on a bicycle ergometer. (One improvement in the methodology in this study was that the dose of caffeine was administered relative to body weight.) This time muscle glycogen changes were measured, and the investigators observed a 42% sparing of glycogen due to the caffeine treatment. In addition, they showed that muscle triglyceride use was increased by 150%. This utilization of muscle triglyceride could have contributed to the reduced R values observed in the caffeine-treated group in the initial study of the series (Costill et al., 1978). They also were able to show an elevated plasma free-fatty-acid concentration prior to exercise, a result that was not observed in their prior studies. The authors postulated that the glycogen sparing effect of caffeine may have occurred as a result of a combination of factors. First, the elevation of free-fatty-acids and their subsequent oxidation exerts an inhibitory feedback on glycogen degradation (Neely et al., 1968). Second, caffeine may have exerted a direct inhibitory effect on glycogen degradation. Third, caffeine may have stimulated enough muscle triglyceride breakdown to provide the necessary energy, thus sparing glycogen. The authors then proposed a number of variables that must be controlled in order to discover the definitive effects of caffeine during exercise. Among those were body composition, muscle mass, caffeine dosage, hormonal responses, substrate turnover, and drug tolerance of the subjects. As we shall see, the failure to control these variables has resulted in the prevailing lack of consensus regarding the ergogenicity of caffeine.

Since 1980, only three reports have supported the idea that caffeine ingestion prior to exercise can improve endurance performance. One of those was a field study. Caffeine ingestion (6 mg/kg) 60 min prior to racing was shown to improve cross country ski times by 59 to 152 s compared to placebo times (Berglund & Hemmingsson, 1982). These results seem to establish the practical relevance for use of the drug to enhance performance. Unfortunately, the study is open to criticism because the authors did not analyze the ski times directly, but developed a normalization procedure to take into consideration differences in race conditions on different days. Further, the study provided no supporting metabolic data to help elucidate the mechanism by which caffeine may have enhanced performance. The authors did state, however, that ratings of perceived exertion were not different between placebo and caffeine runs.

If the exercise intensity on the caffeine trial was higher, as it surely must have been to have produced faster times, then the same perceived exertion suggests that a central effect on the perception of fatigue may have been operative and could explain the improvement in performance.

The other two studies that show a direct effect of caffeine on endurance were laboratory studies. Sasaki et al. (1987a) gave caffeine to their trained subjects 60 min before (300 mg), immediately before (60 mg), and during (60 mg), an exhaustive treadmill run at 80% max $\dot{V}O_2$. Caffeine increased the run time significantly from 40 min (control) to 52 min. Likewise, McNaughton (1987) showed an improved performance on an incremental bicycle ergometer test in subjects who consumed caffeine in doses of 10 or 15 mg/kg 1 h before the test. Average endurance times ranged from 7 min and 10 s in the control trial to 7 min and 40 s in the treatment groups. The mechanism by which performance was improved in these two studies appeared to be consistent with that proposed by the Costill group. In both studies, free-fatty-acid levels were elevated prior to and during the work tests in the caffeine treated group. Based on R values, this resulted in an increased fat utilization. These findings are quite surprising, especially in the case of McNaughton, when we consider the high intensity of the work and the brevity of the effort. It should be noted that there was no direct evidence of carbohydrate sparing in either of these latter two studies.

Erickson and his colleagues (1987) evaluated the effects of caffeine (5 mg/kg) during a 90-min cycling exercise at 65–70% $\dot{V}O_2$max. In contrast to previous studies in this section, these investigators did not examine endurance. This study is noteworthy, however, because muscle biopsies revealed a significant glycogen sparing effect due to the caffeine treatment. Even though glycogen sparing is the principal explanation for the ergogenic effects of caffeine, this study is the only one other than that of Essig et al. (1980) that attempted to directly measure muscle glycogen concentrations. The Erickson study also illustrates the ambiguity in this field. Even though they observed a glycogen sparing effect, the authors could not attribute it to an increased fat oxidation, because R values were not different and plasma free-fatty-acid levels were not altered by caffeine.

In contrast to these positive results, five other reports since 1980 concluded that caffeine did not improve endurance. Four of these involved cycling exercise. Powers and coworkers (1983) observed no effect of the drug (5 mg/kg) on an exhaustive cycle ergometer ride (20–22 min endurance time), in spite of increases in plasma free-fatty-acids. Similar results were observed by Bond et al. (1987), who reported no influence of the drug (5 mg/kg) on a test to exhaustion that lasted approximately 27 min for both placebo and experimental groups. In this latter study, the drug had no effect on any variables related to substrate utilization. Butts and Crowell (1985) also employed cycling as the performance test, but they had their subjects exercise at 75% $\dot{V}O_2$max. Times to exhaustion were 60–70 min, and no effect of caffeine was observed.

In the final two studies to be described in this section, the investigators tested the effects of caffeine on near-maximal endurance capacity after previous prolonged exercise. For instance, Sasaki et al. (1987b) ran their subjects for 2 h at 60% max $\dot{V}O_2$, during which time they ingested 800 mg of caffeine over four 30-min intervals, followed by a run to exhaustion at greater than 90% $\dot{V}O_2$max. Run times lasted from 15 to 17.5 min; no beneficial effect of caffeine was observed, in spite of the caffeine-induced higher plasma free-fatty-acid levels. Finally, Falk and associates (1989) tested their subjects after a 40-km march. Caffeine (5 mg/kg) ingestion did not improve endurance time on a maximal intensity ride on a cycle ergometer, in spite of a decreased perceived exertion. These studies raise questions as to whether caffeine is truly an ergogenic substance. The discrepancies cannot be attributed to mode of exercise (e.g., running or cycle ergometer), nor to intensity of exercise because positive and negative results were obtained in both modes at modest to high intensities.

Other investigative teams that have attempted to predict improvement of performance from metabolic measurements have not clarified whether caffeine is an ergogenic aid. For instance, Knapik and coworkers (1983) used trained and untrained runners to test the effects of 5 and 9 mg/kg caffeine on R values and plasma free-fatty-acids levels obtained during an hour run on the treadmill at 60% $\dot{V}O_2$max. They noted a trend for a caffeine-stimulatory effect on plasma glycerol, but no effect on free-fatty-acids or on the R values.

In another study (Casal & Leon, 1985), caffeine treatment (6 mg/kg) failed to alter substrate utilization in trained marathon runners during 45 min of treadmill exercise, despite a caffeine-induced elevation in pre-exercise values for plasma free-fatty-acids. Neither the study by Casel and Leon nor the study by Knapik et al. measured muscle glycogen directly or attempted to assess endurance.

Casel and Leon attempted to explain why caffeine was ineffective by reasoning that because exercise is a powerful sympathetic enhancer that mobilizes free-fatty-acids, exercise probably overrides and masks the caffeine-induced elevation of free-fatty-acids. This might negate any ergogenic benefit of the drug. In addition, because training optimizes lipid oxidation during exercise, there is probably little caffeine-induced potentiation of lipid oxidation in the trained subject. The literature makes it clear that it is tenuous to try to predict the effects of caffeine on endurance from indirect measures because endurance and these measures are not always correlated. For instance, Costill and co-workers (Costill et al., 1978; Ivy et al., 1979) observed an increased work output without corresponding evidence of increased plasma free-fatty-acids. Similarly, Erickson's team (Erickson et al., 1987) observed a glycogen sparing effect without supporting evidence of altered substrate utilization (e.g., R values or fatty acid availability). Further, in other studies that detected no positive effects on performance, supporting metabolic data would have suggested otherwise (Powers et al., 1983; Butts & Crowell, 1985; Sasaki et al., 1987b).

While most authors recognize these inconsistencies, only a few have designed studies to try to control the variables that might account for them. McNaughton's (1987) use of relatively naive caffeine users for subjects is one such study. Most other studies reviewed thus far paid no attention to this variable in spite of the 1981 study by Robertson et al. (1981) that showed caffeine tolerance in chronic caffeine users. After 4 d on caffeine, the characteristic increases in blood pressure and plasma catecholamines in response to a caffeine treatment are completely attenuated. Fisher and colleagues (1986) were aware of this finding and designed their study to test the effects of caffeine on the exercise response in habitual users following 4 d of withdrawal. When caffeine (5 mg/kg) was administered to the habitual users prior to withdrawal, it had a modest stimulatory effect on pre-exercise plasma fatty acid levels, but no effect relative to placebo treatment on norepinephrine levels during exercise. However, after 4 d of withdrawal, caffeine nearly doubled the pre-exercise plasma fatty acid values and significantly elevated exercise norepinephrine values. These results show that the response to caffeine during exercise may be blunted in subjects who are chronic caffeine users, at least at the doses tested. It is possible that caffeine users may require higher doses to produce clear physiological effects. That question needs to be answered by further research.

As was pointed out at the beginning of this section, the average intake of caffeine in the U.S.A. is 200 mg/d, and a majority of the population consumes caffeine as part of the normal diet. This includes the athletic population. Knowing this, Tarnopolsky et al. (1989) designed a study to specifically assess the effects of caffeine in habitual users in a manner similar to that in the study by Fisher and coworkers (1986) just described. Trained male runners who were also chronic caffeine users (200 mg/d) were given caffeine (6 mg/kg) 60 min prior to running on the treadmill for 90 min at 70% $\dot{V}O_2max$. Prior to exercise, caffeine induced a small but significant increase in plasma free-fatty-acids which persisted for 60 min into the exercise. This did not, however, produce a change in substrate metabolism because R values were similar between the caffeine and placebo treats. Caffeine treatment also did not alter plasma catecholamine concentrations before or during exercise relative to those of the placebo trial. These findings in combination with those of Fisher et al. (1986) argue strongly against an ergogenic effect of caffeine in habitual users of the drug.

Tarnopolsky et al. (1989) stated that one other variable in their study may have also been a factor in the results. They fed their subjects a high carbohydrate meal 2 h prior to the ingestion of caffeine and 3 h prior to exercise in an attempt to simulate the pattern normally followed by endurance athletes prior to competition. However, Weir and her colleagues (1987) had shown earlier that such a procedure may attenuate the stimulatory effects of caffeine. They had one group of subjects consume a high carbohydrate diet for 3 d and a high carbohydrate meal 3 h prior to running on the treadmill for 120 min at 75% $\dot{V}O_2$max. When caffeine was given under these circumstances 3 h prior to exercise, there was no appreciable effect on free-fatty-acid levels either before or during the exercise. Likewise, respiratory exchange ratios during exercise were not different from the placebo condition. When the caffeine was given to these same subjects in the non-carbohydrate loaded condition, it stimulated a 50–100% increase in resting free-fatty-acid levels, which peaked 3 h after caffeine ingestion. These results point to the fact that the simultaneous use of caffeine and carbohydrate loading prior to exercise may be of no more benefit than carbohydrate loading alone and that carbohydrate loading may ameliorate the potential effects of caffeine.

One final point deserves mention. Almost without exception, the administration of caffeine in these studies occurred 60 min prior to exercise testing, probably because this time represents the peak availability of the drug in the blood (Robertson et al., 1981). However, Bellet et al. (1968) and Weir and colleagues (1987) noted that the peak free-fatty-acid level occurred 3 h after ingestion. This may prove to be another important variable that deserves attention in future studies.

It should be clear from this review of all the human studies performed since 1980 that the ergogenicity of caffeine is controversial. Such controversy reflects the diverse and non-uniform approach research teams have taken to address the issue. It may also reflect the diverse and subtle effects of the drug that are only discernable under the most favorable of research conditions. It certainly is not clear why some designs result in positive findings while similar designs show no effects. The question is, what are the optimal conditions under which caffeine would exert an ergogenic benefit? The literature suggests that those conditions may include use of untrained subjects who have a history of abstinence or infrequent use of caffeine, caffeine doses of 6–10 mg/kg, abstinence from high carbohydrate diets, and caffeine use in prolonged activities at intensities of 70–85% $\dot{V}O_2$max. Clearly, we still do not have the definitive answer.

Animal Studies. This review would not be complete without reference to those recent studies which have used animals to study the ergogenicity of caffeine. Of initial interest is the 1978 study of Estler et al., who examined the effects of both acute and chronic consumption of caffeine on swim times to exhaustion in mice. Six weeks of chronic ingestion (150 mg $\cdot$ kg$^{-1}\cdot$d^{-1}) resulted in severely depressed endurance, whereas a single subcutaneous injection (50 mg/kg) given 90 min prior to swimming either had no effect or had a negative effect. This study is remarkable in that the doses used are extremely high. In spite of that, the drug had no effect on muscle or liver glycogen concentrations at rest. Resting free-fatty-acid levels were elevated prior to exercise, and there was evidence for glycogen sparing in the chronically-treated, but not the acutely-treated mice.

The most extensive investigations into the ergogenic effects of caffeine using animals are those of Winder and co-workers. In the first of a series of three experiments Winder (1986) found that caffeine in acute doses of 5–50 mg/kg had no effect on the rate of muscle or liver glycogenolysis during 60 min of treadmill running in rats. The drug also had no effect on plasma free-fatty-acid levels, although pre-exercise values were elevated 60 min after the 25 mg/kg dose. In fasted rats caffeine treatment (25 mg/kg, 60 min prior to exercise) raised pre-exercise plasma free-fatty-acid levels but also failed to spare muscle glycogen during a subsequent 60 min treadmill run at 21 m/min up a 15% grade (Arogyasami et al., 1989b). This was important to evaluate because pre-exercise diet may influence the caffeine response (Weir et al., 1987). In fact, the authors noted that the rate of glycogen degradation after the first 15 min of exercise had been accelerated in the caffeine treated animals, resulting in a simultaneous concomitant elevation in blood lactate concentrations. Others have noted an elevation in lactate production in response to caffeine and attributed it to a direct glycogenolytic effect of the drug (Casal & Leon, 1985; Gaesser & Rich, 1985).

Finally, Winder's group examined the effects of caffeine on exercise endurance and glycogenolysis in trained rats (Arogyasami et al., 1989a). Using doses of 5 or 25 mg/kg they found that caffeine had no beneficial effect on running time to exhaustion (average run times ranged between 149 and 176 min). Caffeine treatment did not alter plasma free-fatty-acid concentrations during exercise; effects at baseline before exercise were not reported. Similarly, neither dose exerted any effect on the rate of muscle nor liver glycogenolysis during the exercise period. From these studies (Winder, 1986; Arogyasami et al., 1989a; Arogyasami et al., 1989b), the authors concluded that caffeine does not reduce the rate of glycogenolysis in muscle during exercise in spite of elevated plasma free-fatty-acid levels and has no beneficial effect on prolonged exercise. One might question the applicability of these animal studies to the human experience, especially in light of the differences in muscle glycogen storage capacity between the two species (cf. Conlee, 1987). It should be pointed out, however, that both man and rat experience similar increases in endurance and similar glycogen-sparing effects when presented with marked elevations in plasma free-fatty-acids, e.g., after heparin-induced lipolysis (cf. Conlee, 1987). That caffeine has no effect in the rat should not be surprising considering the lack of consistent effect seen in most of the human studies reviewed in this section.

Summary and Future Research

Since the series of studies from Costill's lab was published in 1978–1980 laying claim to an ergogenic benefit to caffeine, subsequent research has been less than supportive of that notion (see Table 8-5 for summary). Studies reviewed here have demonstrated that the results can be influenced by a number of experimental factors, including: 1) dose, 2) type of exercise, 3) intensity of exercise, 4) pre-exercise feedings, 5) previous caffeine use, 6) training status of the subjects, and 7) individual variation.

The possible mechanisms by which caffeine may exert a beneficial effect are quite varied, but include: 1) a stimulatory effect on the central nervous system, 2) enhanced release of catecholamines, 3) free-fatty-acid mobilization from adipose tissue and subsequent oxidation by muscle, thus sparing muscle glycogen, 4) increased use of muscle triglycerides, thus sparing muscle glycogen, and 5) indirect inhibition of muscle glycogenolysis, thus sparing muscle glycogen. The primary mechanism originally proposed by the Costill group, i.e., glycogen sparing due to enhanced lipid oxidation, is still attractive and plausible, but it has not been consistently supported. That hypothetical lipid-oxidation effect was based on earlier observations that an elevation in plasma fatty acids after treatment with heparin injection and fat consumption was shown to provide a significant glycogen sparing effect during prolonged exercise with a concomitant delay in fatigue (see Conlee, 1987, for review). But, the heparin-fat treatment promoted a 200–300% increase in plasma free-fatty-acid levels; the free-fatty-acid response to caffeine is substantially less. That caffeine treatment does not conclusively enhance performance or spare glycogen is probably due to the fact that the natural catecholamine response to exercise may obscure the effects of caffeine during prolonged exercise. This may be especially true in the trained individual. Future designs, then, should focus on controlling the confounding variables listed previously, while at the same time incorporating conditions that most likely represent those in competition. It may be that those who most desire the benefit of the drug (e.g., trained athletes in the carbohydrate loaded state) would be the least sensitive to its effects. This implies that any perceived benefit by those who feel a compulsion to use the drug may simply be due to its placebo effect.

COCAINE

Source and Chemical Structure

Cocaine is an alkaloid derived from the leaves of the plant genus *Erythroxylum*, of which the most notable species is *Erythroxylum coca*. These plants grow extensively throughout the countries of northern South America, and this region is the primary source of the world's cocaine supply. The drug is extracted from the leaves by soaking them in an organic solvent, which leaves an impure coca paste. The so-called "free-base" is purified from this paste as a white crystalline solid. To make it more soluble, the free-base is converted to cocaine hydrochloride. Both forms are depicted in Figure 8-3. Cocaine is actually benzoylmethylecgonine and belongs to the tropane family of alkaloids which also includes the compound, atropine. Although their chemical structures are similar, their pharmacological properties are quite different.

General Pharmacology

Central and Peripheral Effects. Cocaine's main therapeutic use is as a local anesthetic. It was extensively used in ophthalmology, but has since fallen out of favor because of its side effects and potential for abuse. Now it is restricted to topical use, usually in the respiratory tract (Ritchie & Greene, 1985). As an anesthetic, it blocks nerve conductance by altering the membrane permeability of the nerve axon to sodium ions (Ritchie & Greene, 1985). It also exerts a local vasoconstriction which inhibits its own absorption, thus prolonging and potentiating its anesthetic properties.

By far the most striking effect of cocaine is its ability to stimulate the central nervous system. This effect is manifested by a feeling of

TABLE 8–5. *Summary of Human Studies on the Ergogenic Effects of Caffeine on Endurance*

Reference	Dose	Exercise Mode	Exercise Intensity	Performance Measure	Plasma FFA	RER	Glycogen Sparing	Fat Oxidat.	Perceived Exertion
POSITIVE ERGOGENIC EFFECTS									
Costill et al. (1978)	330 mg	Cycling	80% $\dot{V}O_2$max	↑ end time (75 → 90 min)	—	→	N.M.	↑	→
Ivy et al. (1979)	500 mg	Cycling	70–75% $\dot{V}O_2$max	↑ work in 2 h	↑	↓	N.M.	↑	—
Berglund & Hemmingson (1982)	6 mg/kg	X-C Skiing	Variable	↓ race times	N.M.	N.M.	N.M.	N.M.	—
McNaughton (1987)	10–15 mg/kg	Cycling	Incremental	↑ end time (7'11" → 7'48")	N.M.	→	N.M.	N.M.	N.M.
Sasaki et al. (1987a)	420 mg	Running	80% $\dot{V}O_2$max	↑ end time (40 min → 52 min)	N.M	→	N.M.	↑	N.M.
NO ERGOGENIC EFFECTS									
Powers et al. (1983)	5 mg/kg	Cycling	Incremental	Time to Exhaustion (20–22 min)	↑	—	N.M.	N.M.	N.M.
Butts & Crowell (1985)	300 mg	Cycling	75% $\dot{V}O_2$max	Time to Exhaustion (60–70 min)	N.M.	—	N.M.	N.M.	—
Bond et al. (1987)	5 mg/kg	Cycling	Incremental	Time to Exhaustion (27 min)	N.M.	—	N.M.	N.M.	N.M.
Sasaki et al. (1987b)	800 mg	Running	90% $\dot{V}O_2$max	Time to Exhaustion (15–17 min)	↑	—	N.M.	N.M.	N.M.
Falk et al. (1989)	5 mg/kg	Cycling	90% $\dot{V}O_2$max	Time to Exhaustion (4–6)	—	N.M.	N.M.	N.M.	→

↑ = increase, ↓ = decrease, — = no effect, N.M. = not measured

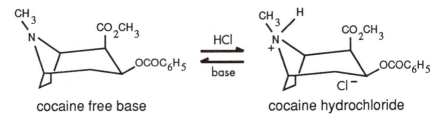

cocaine free base   cocaine hydrochloride

FIGURE 8-3. *Chemical structure of two forms of Cocaine.*

euphoria and a positive alteration in mood state. There is a decreased sense of fatigue, greater wakefulness, and increased motor activity; however, learning acquisition is diminished. The drug is also a powerful anorectic. It can be characterized as a sympathomimetic drug and produces pharmacological responses similar to those of amphetamine. Experienced users cannot always discriminate between the two (Fischman et al., 1976). Cocaine is a potent reinforcer with major effects occurring in the mesocorticolimbic dopamine system of the brain (Koob & Hubner, 1988). These reinforcing properties are so strong that in studies with monkeys, it has been observed that when given a choice between food and cocaine, or between cocaine and social interaction with other monkeys, the animals will always choose cocaine (Aigner & Balster, 1978). In the periphery, cocaine potentiates the sympathetic responses. It increases the heart rate and blood pressure either by direct action on the heart and vascular system or by indirect effects operating through the release of catecholamines. It does not, however, affect respiration at low doses. At higher doses, it is markedly pyrogenic because it enhances heat production through increased motor activity and decreases heat dissipation by constricting cutaneous blood vessels (Ritchie & Greene, 1985).

    Mechanism of Action. The sympathomimetic responses to cocaine in the periphery can be explained by three possible mechanisms. The one most often cited is the ability of cocaine to block the re-uptake of norepinephrine at the pre-synaptic terminals of the sympathetic nerves (Trendelenburg, 1959). This would potentiate the effects of catecholamines. The second mechanism suggests that cocaine directly stimulates the release of catecholamines from peripheral nerve endings (Langer & Enero, 1974); this hypothesis has been questioned by Levy and Blattberg (1978). Finally, the peripheral effects of the drug could be due to cocaine-induced effects on the central nervous system that result in the release of adrenal catecholamines (Chiueh & Kopin, 1978). This latter possibility is highly plausible because of the varied effects the drug exerts centrally.

The mechanisms responsible for the central effects are complex and not well understood. They seem to involve interference with the re-uptake of numerous neurotransmitters of the brain such as norepinephrine, serotonin, and acetyl choline (Jones, 1984), but especially dopamine (Carboni et al., 1989). Considerable research effort has focused on trying to explain the reinforcing effects of cocaine. The prevailing opinion is that cocaine effects are mediated through the dopamine-specific D_2 receptor. The drug blocks the re-uptake of dopamine, resulting in increased concentrations of this neurotransmitter at the receptor site (Woolverton & Kleven, 1988; Ritz et al., 1988). Unlike amphetamine, cocaine does not appear to stimulate dopamine release (Carboni et al., 1989).

Absorption, Distribution, and Metabolism. Cocaine is self-administered orally, intravenously, intranasally, or by smoking. The least effective of these is oral. The other routes allow a rapid assimilation of the drug with euphoric effects apparent within 1–2 min after intravenous injection or smoking and 5–10 min after intranasal administration. The half-life of the drug is short (30–40 min) compared to that for amphetamine (3–6 h) (Johanson & Fischman, 1989). The drug is rapidly metabolized by esterases in the blood and liver. Some of the metabolic by-products (e.g., norcocaine nitroxide) are extremely hepatotoxic. Seventy percent of a dose of cocaine can be accounted for by the elimination of benzoylecgonine in the urine within 3 h of administration. This substance is detectable for up to 2 d after an acute treatment and is the substance usually measured during drug testing procedures (Turner et al., 1988).

Side Effects. Of the three drugs discussed in this chapter, cocaine warrants the greatest concern with respect to its adverse side effects. This is emphasized by the publicized deaths of well-known sports figures after cocaine use (Wadler & Hainline, 1989). Cocaine reportedly causes cardiac seizures in individuals with or without coronary vascular problems (Cregler & Mark, 1986). It was recently shown that even a therapeutic dose of cocaine (2 mg/kg) similar to that used in topical anesthesia caused vasoconstriction of the left coronary artery and decreased myocardial blood flow (Lange et al., 1989). The drug is highly addictive, and under its influence the user often acts irrationally, becomes psychotic, and can experience deep depression. During chronic use, symptoms of paranoia, delirium, and confusion persist. Seizures are common. Numerous other medical complications have been correlated to cocaine abuse, among which is the increased risk of Acquired Immune Deficiency Syndrome (AIDS) due to intravenous administration of the drug (Table 8-6) (Wadler & Hainline, 1989).

Ergogenicity of Cocaine

Unlike the extensive body of literature for amphetamine and caffeine, the literature for cocaine is scant and obscure (Wadler & Hainline, 1989; Lombardo, 1987; Wenger, 1988). However, the recent concern about the rampant use of cocaine by professional athletes has stimulated an increased interest in its potential ergogenic effects, and several studies have been published more recently addressing the issue. A few poorly controlled studies published prior to 1988 concluded that cocaine did exert an ergogenic benefit. The more recent literature, however, argues against that notion.

The Literature Prior to 1983. It had been known for centuries that the natives of South America chewed the coca leaves to promote vigor and increase efficiency (Williams, 1974). But the first published experiments with the drug came from the lab of Sigmund Freud in 1884. Using himself as the primary subject, Freud tested the effects of 0.1 g of cocaine hydrochloride on hand grip strength and reaction time. He concluded that strength was increased within minutes of taking the drug intranasally. The effects were more profound if he was already in a fatigued state or after prolonged sleeplessness. Similar results were obtained from the reaction time experiments (Freud, 1885).

TABLE 8-6. *Complications of Cocaine Use*

Cardiac	Central	Peripheral
Ventricular arrhythmia	Cerebrovascular	Spontaneous abortion
Sudden death	Cerebral hemorrhage	Congenital malformations of fetus
Angina pectoris	Subarachnoid hemorrhage	Breast milk transfer to infant and secondary acute toxicity
Myocardial infarction	Transient ischemic attacks	Sexual dysfunction
Myocarditis	Addiction	Liver toxicity
	Seizures	Osteolytic sinusitis
	Headache	Gastrointestinal ischemia
	Visual scotoma/ blindness	Necrosis/perforation of nasal septum
	Insomnia	Loss of smell
	Euphoria/dysphoria	Hyperthermia/tachycardia
	Confusion	
	Delirium	
	Paranoia	
	Psychosis	
	Repetitive behavior	
	Anorexia	

Modified from Wadler and Hainline (1989)

For years after Freud's experiments, there were only suggestions in the literature that cocaine had ergogenic effects (cf. Williams, 1974). However, in the early 1930s two German papers were published which again tended to extol the virtues of cocaine. Theil and Essing (1930) gave 0.1 g of cocaine to subjects prior to exercising on a cycle ergometer to exhaustion and reported that work efficiency was improved based on $\dot{V}O_2$ measurements per unit work. They also noted longer work times and attributed the improved performance to a reduced central nervous system perception of fatigue. This agreed with the opinion of Freud (1885). One year later, a similar study was performed using trained subjects (Herbst & Schellenberg, 1931). The cocaine treatment (0.1 g) had no effect on endurance or work efficiency on a cycle ergometer, but recovery after the exercise was more rapid under the influence of cocaine.

The next study involving the ergogenicity of cocaine was published in 1948. Using a standardized ergometer test, Asmussen and Boje (1948) found no improvement in the rate at which their subjects could complete either 35 or 450 revolutions on a bicycle ergometer after 120 mg of cocaine was administered in capsule form 15 min prior to exercise. This result would be expected, given the now recognized slow absorption rate of cocaine after oral ingestion (Johansen & Fischman, 1989).

Jacob and Michaud (1961), in the first study to test the effects of cocaine using animals, swam mice to exhaustion in a bath with artificial waves at a water temp of 20° C. Mean exhaustion time of controls was a brief 5.6 min. The authors evaluated the effects of cocaine chlorohydrate at doses ranging from 3–200 mg/kg at either 30 or 120 min after intraperitoneal (IP) injection. Cocaine appeared to give marginal improvement at the lowest dose 30 min after injection (swim time ranged 5.9–7.0 min). Detrimental effects were observed at doses greater than 50 mg/kg. Surprisingly, the authors concluded that cocaine does not influence performance.

In the early 1970s Hanna performed two studies designed to test the effects of coca leaf chewing on work performance on Andean natives. First, Hanna (1970) compared the exercise response to 'box stepping' between chewers and non-chewers. The amount of leaves chewed was not controlled during the hour prior to the test. Chewers had higher exercise blood pressure, but lower exercise and recovery heart rates. The author postulated that if work intensity was extrapolated to maximum heart rate, then the chewers would perform at a lower $\dot{V}O_2$. Because of the poor controls imposed during this study, Hanna (1971) performed a second one designed to again examine the effects of coca chewing on cardiovascular and respiratory responses during work. In this study, habitual chewers and non-chewers performed all tests before and after chewing. Coca chewing caused an elevation in heart rate—not a decrease as observed in the first study—and no effect on blood pressure. There was no evidence of improved work capacity during submaximal cycle exercise, and there was no consistent improvement in performance during a maximal test. Hanna (1971) concluded that cocaine does not improve performance and that any purported beneficial effect from cocaine would be due to its central stimulatory effects, which act to reduce the perception of fatigue.

These few studies are the extent of the literature prior to 1983. Most reviews on the pharmacological effects of cocaine universally mention the results of Freud's experiments as the proof for potential ergogenicity (Johansen & Fischman, 1989; Ritchie & Greene, 1985). Surely, a field in which the premier paper is one in which the lone subject is the author deserves much more scientific attention. Such attention appears to have increased since 1983.

The Literature Since 1983. This period began with the appearance of two abstracts. Kershner et al. (1983) reported that rats receiving intraperitoneal (IP) injections of either 10 or 25 mg/kg cocaine-HCl were able to run longer at high-intensity exercise (run times averaged 14–16 min), and achieved higher max $\dot{V}O_2$ levels. The authors concluded their brief report by stating that the potential for ergogenicity deserves serious study. The second abstract by Avakian (1986) reported the effects of 26 d of chronic cocaine administration (10 mg $\cdot$ kg^{-1} $\cdot$ d^{-1}, IP) on exercise endurance time and on various substrate and hormonal variables. The addicted animals had reduced resting muscle and liver glycogen concentrations and elevated plasma catecholamine levels. This could have contributed to the severely depressed exercise time to exhaustion. Because this latter study has not appeared as a complete report, it is not possible to assess the experimental details. For example, the time after the last injection of cocaine was not stated. Nonetheless, these brief reports were the impetus for the subsequent studies of Conlee and co-workers, which provide a clearer picture of the effects of cocaine on the physiology of exercise.

The first study in that series tested the effects of an acute injection (IP) of cocaine-HCl (20 mg/kg) on exercise endurance of rats running on the treadmill (Bracken et al., 1988). Control animals ran for 75 min, whereas the cocaine-injected group averaged only 29 min. In this latter group, blood lactate concentration was nearly 12 mM at exhaustion, compared to only 5 mM in the control exercisers. The rate of glycogen degradation in muscle was accelerated in the drug-treated animals. Bracken and co-workers (1989) subsequently evaluated the dose-response (0.1–20.0 mg/kg body weight) for a run to exhaustion on the treadmill. Cocaine had no beneficial effect on running times at any dose and was clearly detrimental at doses of 12.5 and 20.0 mg/kg. Again, the rate of glycogen degradation in red and white vastus lateralis muscles appeared to be increased in the cocainized animals, with a concomitant elevation in blood lactate levels. However, the pattern of response of the plasma catecholamines was quite variable and not instructive with respect to formulating a mechanism by which cocaine reduced endurance.

Because these first two studies suggested that cocaine altered skeletal muscle glycogen metabolism during exercise, a third study evaluated whether cocaine altered myocardial glycogen stores during exercise (Conlee et al., 1989). It was postulated that if cocaine did have an inhibitory effect on myocardial blood flow, as suggested by recent reports (Lange et al., 1989; Wilkerson, 1988), then the rate of myocardial glycogen degradation could be enhanced. Conlee and coworkers (1989) found that such was not the case, at least during 20 min of exercise at intravenous (IV) doses ranging from 1.25 to 10 mg/kg. They noted that this area still deserved further research.

The most recent paper from this group (Conlee et al., 1990) was an effort to address design problems associated with the first two studies and to gain insight into potential mechanisms of action of cocaine. Their prior studies were confounded by the use of electric shock employed to force animals to run to exhaustion; this might have affected glycogen and hormonal responses. In this latest study, animals ran voluntarily for only 30 min at a steady rate. The results were enlightening. Cocaine (12.5 mg/kg, IV or IP) caused an additive effect on circulatory levels of epinephrine and norepinephrine during exercise beyond that attributed to exercise or cocaine alone. In addition, there was a clear increase in glycogen degradation in the fast twitch muscles of the hindlimb during exercise in the cocaine animals compared to saline-treated rats. This probably contributed to the significant elevation in blood lactate concentration. These results verified that cocaine alters muscle glycogen metabolism during exercise and also exaggerates the normal exercise-induced sympathetic response. The authors proposed several possible mechanisms by which cocaine exerts its detrimental effects on endurance performance. First, a drug-stimulated catecholamine release could increase the rate of glycogenolysis and lactate production and lead to early fatigue. Second, cocaine may cause vasoconstriction of the vasculature serving skeletal muscle during exercise; this could lead to a diminished oxygen delivery, an increased rate of glycogenolysis and lactate production, and early fatigue. Finally, cocaine itself may have a direct effect on stimulating muscle glycogenolysis. Confirmation of these mechanisms awaits further research.

Summary and Future Research

There is evidence, albeit questionable, that cocaine may elicit an ergogenic effect on activities that are of high intensity and short duration. This effect may not be due to a direct peripheral effect of the drug, but more likely to its central stimulatory effects that result in euphoria and a masking of the subjective effects of fatigue. On the other hand, the literature is very persuasive, based primarily on animal studies, that cocaine has no beneficial effect on prolonged exercise and can be quite detrimental.

Future work should re-examine the findings of Avakian (1986) on chronic cocaine exposure. For instance, does chronic cocaine treatment affect the ability to adapt to training? Other avenues of interest would be to 1) attempt to determine any cause and effect relationship between cocaine use, recreational exercise, and cardiac seizures, 2) continue to explore the dose-response and dose-time studies initiated by Bracken et al. (1989) and Conlee and associates (1990), and 3) attempt to elucidate the mechanisms by which cocaine exerts its peripheral effects. Such studies will be of significant importance if the use and abuse of cocaine continues as at the present.

ETHICAL CONSIDERATIONS

All of the drugs reviewed in this chapter have been banned by various athletic governing boards. The rationale underlying this action includes the conclusions that 1) use of the drugs could provide an artificial enhancement of performance above that due to natural endowment and dedicated preparation, and 2) use of the drugs has great potential for self-destructive effects that not only jeopardize the health of the athlete but have ramifications that extend to family, friends, and society. This rationale provides a valid basis for legislative sanctions against the use of these agents. In addition, one cannot overestimate the potential adverse effects of highly visible elite athletes fostering drug abuse among the impressionable youth in society. This obligates responsible behaviors on the part of all those associated with sports. Similarly, scientists have a responsibility to identify and report any adverse effects of drug treatments that are observed. Such is my purpose in this section of the chapter. The trivial, i.e., non-medical, use of amphetamine, caffeine, and cocaine can impose serious health-threatening and even fatal side effects. These drugs should never be used for the purpose of enhancing sport performance. Those who do so risk the inherent consequences to self and society and demonstrate a lack of respect for the moral principles that should prevail.

SUMMARY

This chapter has reviewed the literature pertaining to the ergogenicity of amphetamine, caffeine, and cocaine. Amphetamine has been shown to improve prolonged submaximal endurance, especially in exhausted or sleep-deprived individuals. Amphetamine also improves psychomotor responses under similar fatigued conditions. The ergogenic effect of amphetamine on muscular power is equivocal.

The literature relating to the ergogenicity of caffeine tends to show that caffeine has little or no effect on muscle contraction *in vivo*, in spite of its potentiating effects on contraction *in vitro* and *in situ*. Maximal voluntary contraction is not enhanced by caffeine. On the other hand, there is considerably more evidence for a positive effect of caffeine on endurance. This effect has not been shown conclusively, and there is considerable question concerning its validity. Previous caffeine use, training status, and prior diet are among many confounding variables that cause confusion on this issue. If caffeine does exert a beneficial effect on endurance performance, the mechanism underlying that effect is also obscure. Any beneficial effect may be centrally mediated or may be caused by alteration of substrate metabolism. Both potential mechanisms have been supported in the literature.

Cocaine appears to be less ergogenic than either amphetamines or caffeine. It is not well studied, but recent literature suggests that the drug has no beneficial effect on endurance across a wide range of doses and may be severely detrimental. Because of its additive effect on the sympathetic response to exercise, its use prior to exercise by individuals with pre-existing heart conditions may be hazardous.

ACKNOWLEDGEMENTS

This work was partially funded by the National Institute on Drug Abuse Grant No. DA04382. I wish to express appreciation to my graduate students—K. Patrick Kelly and Dong Ho Han— for their valuable assistance in the preparation of this manuscript and to my secretary Deanna Ostergaard for her spirit of cooperation in this effort. Finally, I thank my colleagues Ronald Terjung, Ph.D., and Scott Powers, Ph.D., for their editorial suggestions which improved the chapter significantly.

BIBLIOGRAPHY

Adler, H.F., W.L. Burkhardt, A.C. Ivy, and A.J. Atkinson (1950). Effect of various drugs on psychomotor performance at ground level and at simulated altitudes of 18,000 feet in a low pressure chamber. *J. Aviat. Med.* 21:221–236.

Aigner, T.G., and R.L. Balster (1978). Choice behavior in rhesus monkeys: cocaine versus food. *Science* 201:534–535.

Alles, G.A., and G.A. Feigen (1942). The influence of benzedrine on work-decrement and patellar reflex. *Am. J. Physiol.* 136:392–400.

Anderson, W.A., and D.B. McKeag (1985). The substance use and abuse habits of college student athletes. *Research paper no. 2: General findings* . Mission, Kansas: National Collegiate Athletic Association.

Arnaud, M.J. (1987). The pharmacology of caffeine. In: E. Jucker (ed.) *Progress in Drug Research.* Boston: Birkhäuser Verlag, pp. 273–313.

Arogyasami, J., H.T. Yang, and W.W. Winder (1989a). Effect of caffeine on glycogenolysis during exercise in endurance trained rats. *Med. Sci. Sports Exerc.* 21:173–177.

Arogyasami, J., H.T. Yang, and W.W. Winder (1989b). Effect of intravenous caffeine on muscle glycogenolysis in fasted exercising rats. *Med. Sci. Sports Exerc.* 21:167–172.

Asmussen, E., and O. Bøje (1948). The effect of alcohol and some drugs on the capacity for work. *Acta Phys. Scand.* 15:109–118.

Avakian, E.V. (1986). Effect of chronic cocaine administration on adrenergic and metabolic responses to exercise. *Fed. Proc.* 45:1060.

Bättig, K. (1963). Die Wirkung und training und amphetamin auf ausdauer und geschwindigkeit der schwimmleistund der ratte. *Psychopharmacologia* 4:15–27.

Beavo, J.A., N.L. Rogers, O.B. Crofford, J.G. Hardman, E.W. Sutherland, and E.V. Newman (1970). Effects of xanthine derivatives on lipolysis and an adenosine 3′,5′-monophosphate phosphodiesterase activity. *Mol. Pharmacol.* 6:597–603.

Bellet, S., A. Kershbaum, and E.M. Finck (1968). Response of free fatty acids to coffee and caffeine. *Metabolism* 17:702–707.

Bellet, S., A. Kershbaum, and J. Aspe (1965). The effect of caffeine on free fatty acids. *Arch. Intern. Med.* 116:750–752.

Berglund, B., and P. Hemmingsson (1982). Effects of caffeine ingestion on exercise performance at low and high altitudes in cross-country skiers. *Int. J. Sports Med.* 3:234–236.

Bhagat, B., and N. Wheeler (1973). Effect of amphetamine on the swimming endurance of rats. *Neuropharmacology* 12:711–713.

Blinks, J.R., C.B. Olson, B.R. Jewell, and P. Braveny (1972). Influence of caffeine and other methylxanthines on mechanical properties of isolated mammalian heart muscle. *Circ. Res.* 30:367–92.

Blum, B., M.H. Stern, and K.I. Melville (1964). A comparative evaluation of the action of depressant and stimulant drugs on human performance. *Psychopharmacologia* 6:173–177.

Blyth, C.S., E.M. Allen, and B.W. Lovingood (1960). Effects of amphetamine (dexedrine) and caffeine on subjects exposed to heat and exercise stress. *Res. Quart.* 31:553–559.

Bond, V., K. Gresham, J. McRae, and R.J. Tearney (1986). Caffeine ingestion and isokinetic strength. *Brit. J. Sports Med.* 20:135–137.

Bond, V., R. Adams, B. Balkissoon, J. McRae, E. Knight, S. Robbins, and M. Banks (1987). Effects of caffeine on cardiorespiratory function and glucose metabolism during rest and graded exercise. *J. Sports Med. Phys. Fit.* 27:47–52.

Borg, G., C-G Edström, H. Linderholm, and G. Marklund (1972). Changes in physical performance induced by amphetamine and amobarbital. *Psychopharmacologia* 26:10–18.

Bracken, M.E., D.R. Bracken, A.G. Nelson, and R.K. Conlee (1988). Effect of cocaine on exercise endurance and glycogen use in rats. *J. Appl. Physiol.* 64:884–887.

Bracken, M.E., D.R. Bracken, W.W. Winder, and R.K. Conlee (1989). Effect of various doses of cocaine on endurance capacity in rats. *J. Appl. Physiol.* 66:377–383.

Brooks, G.A., and T.D. Fahey (1984). *Exercise Physiology: Human Bioenergetics and Its Applications* New York: John Wiley & Sons, pp. 626–627.

Bugyi, G.J. (1980). The effects of moderate doses of caffeine on fatigue parameters of the forearm flexor muscles. *Amer. Corr. Ther. J.* 34:49–53.

Bunker, M.L., and M. McWilliams (1979). Caffeine content of common beverages. *J. Amer. Dietetic Assoc.* 74:28–32.

Butcher, R.W., and E.W. Sutherland (1962). Adenosine 3′,5′-phosphate in biological materials. *J. Biol. Chem.* 237:1244–1250.

Butts, N.K., and D. Crowell (1985). Effect of caffeine ingestion on cardiorespiratory endurance in men and women. *Res. Quart.* 56:301–305.

Carboni, E., A. Imperato, L. Perezzani, and G. Di Chiara (1989). Amphetamine, cocaine, phencyclidine and nomifensine increase extracellular dopamine concentrations preferentially in the nucleus accumbens of freely moving rats. *Neuroscience* 28:653–661.

Casal, D.C., and A.S. Leon (1985). Failure of caffeine to affect substrate utilization during prolonged running. *Med. Sci. Sports Exerc.* 17:174–179.

Chandler, J.V., and S.N. Blair (1980). The effect of amphetamines on selected physiological components related to athletic success. *Med. Sci. Sports Exerc.* 12:65–69.

Chatterjee, A.K., S.A. Jacob, R.K. Srivastava, P.R. Pabrai, and A. Ghose (1970). Influence of methylamphetamine on blood lactic acid following exercise. *Jap. J. Pharmac.* 20:170–172.

Chiueh, C.C., and E.J. Kopin (1978). Centrally mediated release by cocaine of endogenous epinephrine and norepinephrine from the sympathoadrenal medullary system of unanesthetized rats. *J. Pharmacol. Exp. Ther.* 205:148–154.

Cochran, W.G., G.M. Smith, and H.K. Beecher (1961). A reply. *J. Amer. Med. Assoc.* 177:347–349.

Conlee, R.K. (1987). Muscle glycogen and exercise endurance: A twenty-year perspective. *Exerc. Sport Sci. Rev.* 15:1–28.

Conlee, R.K., D.W. Barnett, K.P. Kelly, and D.H. Han (1991). Effects of cocaine on plasma catecholamine and muscle glycogen concentrations during exercise in the rat. *J. Appl. Physiol.* 70:1323–1327.

Conlee, R.K., T.L. Berg, D.H. Han, K.P. Kelly, and D.W. Barnett (1989). Cocaine does not alter cardiac glycogen content at rest or during exercise. *Metabolism* 38:1039–1041.

Connett, R.J., L.M. Ugol, M.J. Hammack, and E.T. Hays (1983). Twitch potentiation and caffeine contractures in isolated rat soleus muscle. *Comp. Biochem. Physiol.* 74C:349–354.

Cooper, D.L. (1972). Drugs and the athlete. *J. Amer. Med. Assoc.* 221:1007–1011.

Costill, D.L., G.P. Dalsky, and W.J. Fink (1978). Effects of caffeine ingestion on metabolism and exercise performance. *Med. Sci. Sports* 10:155–158.

Cregler, L.L. and H. Mark (1986). Medical complications of cocaine abuse. *N. Engl. J. Med.* 315:1495–1500.

Curatolo, P.W., and D. Robertson (1983). The health consequences of caffeine. *Ann. Intern. Med.* 98:641–653.

Cuthbertson, D.P., and J.A.C. Knox (1947). The effects of analeptics on the fatigued subject. *J. Physiol.* 106:42–58.

Domino, E.F., J.W. Albers, A.R. Potvin, B.S. Repa, and W.W. Tourtellotte (1972). Effects of d-amphetamine on quantitative measures of motor performance. *Clin. Pharmacol. Therap.* 13:251–257.

Eichner, E.R. (1986). The caffeine controversy: Effects on endurance and cholesterol. *Phys. Sportsmed.* 14:124–132.

Erickson, M.A., R.J. Schwarzkopf, and R.D. McKenzie (1987). Effects of caffeine, fructose, and glucose ingestion on muscle glycogen utilization during exercise. *Med. Sci. Sports Exerc.* 19:579–583.

Essig, D., D.L. Costill, and P.J. Van Handel (1980). Effects of caffeine ingestion on utilization of muscle glycogen and lipid during leg ergometer cycling. *Int. J. Sports Med.* 1:86–90.

Estler, C.J., H.P.T. Ammon, and C. Herzog (1978). Swimming capacity of mice after prolonged treatment with psychostimulants. *Psychopharmacology* 58:161–166.

Estler, C.J., and M.C. Gabrys (1979). Swimming capacity of mice after prolonged treatment with psychostimulants. II. Effect of Methamphetamine on swimming performance and availability of metabolic substrates. *Psychopharmacology* 60:173–176.

Evans, M.A., R. Martz, L. Lemberger, B.E. Rodda, and R.B. Forney (1976). Effects of dextroamphetamine on psychomotor skills. *Clin. Pharmacol. Therap.* 19:777–781.

Evans, W.O., and A. Jewett (1962). The effect of some centrally acting drugs on disjunctive reaction time. *Psychopharmacologia* 3:124–127.

Falk, B., R. Burstein, I. Ashkenazi, O. Spilberg, J. Alter, E. Zylber-Katz, A. Rubinstein, N. Bashan, and Y. Shapiro (1989). The effect of caffeine ingestion on physical performance after prolonged exercise. *Eur. J. Appl. Physiol.* 59:168–173.

Fischman, M.W. (1987). Cocaine and the amphetamines. In: H.Y. Meltzer (ed.) *Psychopharmacology: The Third Generation of Progress.* New York: Raven Press, pp. 1543–1553.

Fischman, M.W., C.R. Schuster, L. Resnekov, J.F.E. Schick, N.A. Krasnegor, W. Fennell, and D.X. Freedman (1976). Cardiovascular and subjective effects of intravenous cocaine administration in humans. *Arch. Gen. Psych.* 33:983–989.

Fisher, S.M., R.G. McMurray, M. Berry, M.H. Mar, and W.A. Forsythe (1986). Influence of caffeine on exercise performance in habitual caffeine users. *Int. J. Sports Med.* 7:276–280.

Foltz, E.E., A.C. Ivy, and C.J. Barborka (1943a). The influence of amphetamine (benzedrine) sulfate, d-desoxyephedrine hydrochloride (pervitin), and caffeine upon work output and recovery when rapidly exhausting work is done by trained subjects. *J. Lab. Clin. Med.* 28:603–606.

Foltz, E.E., M.J. Schiffrin, and A.C. Ivy (1943b). The influence of amphetamine (benzedrine) sulfate and caffeine on the performance of rapidly exhausting work by untrained subjects. *J. Lab. Clin. Med.* 28:601–603.

Foltz, E., A. Ivy, and C. Barborka (1942). The use of double work periods in the study of fatigue and the influence of caffeine. *Am. J. Physiol.* 136:79–86.

Foreman, N., S. Barraclough, C. Moore, A. Mehta, and M. Madon (1989). High doses of caffeine impair performance of a numerical version of the stroop task in men. *Pharm. Biochem. Behav.* 32:399–403.

Fredholm, B.B. (1985). On the mechanism of action of theophylline and caffeine. *Acta. Med. Scand.* 217:149–53.

Freud, S. (1885). On the general effects of cocaine. *Medicinisch-Chirurgisches Central-Blatt* 20:374–375.

Gaesser, G.A., and R.G. Rich (1985). Influence of caffeine on blood lactate response during incremental exercise. *Int. J. Sports Med.* 6:207–211.

Gawin, F.H., and E.H. Ellinwood (1988). Cocaine and other stimulants. *New Engl. J. Med.* 318:1173–1182.

Gerald, M.C. (1978). Effects of (+)-amphetamine on the treadmill endurance performance of rats. *Neuropharmacology* 17:703–704.

Golding, L.A., and J.R. Barnard (1963). The effect of d-amphetamine sulfate on physical performance. *J. Sports Med. Phys. Fit.* 3:221–224.

Goldstein, A., B.W. Searle, and R.T. Schimke (1960). Effects of secobarbital and of d-amphetamine on psychomotor performance of normal subjects. *J. Pharmacol. Exp. Therap.* 130:55–58.

Greyden, J.F. (1974). Anxiety or Caffeinism: A diagnostic dilemma. *Am. J. Psych.* 131:1089–1092.

Hanada, S., K. Hijikuruo, and H. Kaneto (1986). Reverse tolerance to the swimming time prolonging effect of d-amphetamine in mice. *Jap. J. Pharmacol.* 41:81–86.

Hanna, J.M. (1970). The effects of coca chewing on exercise in the Quechua of Peru. *Human Biol.* 42:1–11.

Hanna, J.M. (1971). Further studies on the effects of coca chewing on exercise. *Human Biol.* 43:200–209.

Hart, J.B., and J. Wallace (1975). The adverse effects of amphetamines. *Clin. Toxicol.* 8:179–790.

Hauty, G.T., and R.B. Payne (1957). Effects of dextro-amphetamine upon judgment. *J. Pharmacol. Exp. Therap.* 120:33–37.

Herbst, R., and P. Schellenberg (1931). Cocain und muskelarbeit. *Arbeitsphysiologie* 4:203–216.

Heyrodt, H., and H. Weissenstein (1940). Uber Steigerung korperlicher Leistungfahigkeit durch Pervitin. *Arch. Exp. Pathol. Pharmokol.* 195:273–275.

Hueting, J.E., and A.J. Poulus (1970). Amphetamine, performance, effort, and fatigue. *Pfluger's Arch.* 318:260.

Ivy, A.C., and F.R. Goetzl (1943). D-desoxyephedrine: A review. *War Med.* 3:60–77.

Ivy, A.C., and L.R. Krasno (1941). Amphetamine (benzedrine) sulfate: a review of its pharmacology. *War Med.* 1:15–42.

Ivy, J.L. (1983). Amphetamines. In: M.H. Williams (ed.) *Ergogenic Aids in Sport.* Illinois: Human Kinetics, pp. 101–127.

Ivy, J.L., D.L. Costill, W.J. Fink, and R.W. Lower (1979). Influence of caffeine and carbohydrate feedings on endurance performance. *Med. Sci. Sports* 11:6–11.

Jacob, J., and G. Michaud (1961). Actions de divers agents pharmacologiques sur les temps d'épuisement et le comportement de souris nageant a 20° C. *Arch. Int. Pharmacodyn.* 133:101–115.

Jacobson, B.H., and F.A. Kulling (1989). Health and ergogenic effects of caffeine. *Br. J. Sports Med.* 23:34–40.

Jaffe, J.H. (1985). Drug addiction and drug abuse. In: A.G. Gilman, L.S. Goodman, and A. Gilman (eds.) *The Pharmacological Basis of Therapeutics.* (7th ed.) New York: Macmillan, pp. 532–581.

Johanson, C-E., and M.W. Fischman (1989). The pharmacology of cocaine related to its abuse. *Pharm. Rev.* 41:3–52.

Jones, R.T. (1984). The pharmacology of cocaine. In: J. Grabowski (ed.) *Cocaine: Pharmacology, Effects, and Treatment of Abuse.* Washington, D.C.: Natl. Inst. Drug Abuse Res. Monograph 50, pp.34–53.

Karpovich, P.V. (1959). Effect of amphetamine sulfate on athletic performance. *J. Amer. Med. Assoc.* 170:558–561.

Kay, H., and J.E. Birren (1958). Swimming speed of the albino rat: II. Fatigue, practice and drug effects on age and sex differences. *J. Gerontol.* 13:378–385.

Kershner, P.L., J.G. Edwards, and C.M. Tipton (1983). Effect of cocaine on the running performance of rats. *Med. Sci. Sports Exerc.* 15:12.

Knapik, J.J., B.H. Jones, M.M. Toner, W.L. Daniels, and W.J. Evans (1983). Influence of caffeine on serum substrate changes during running in trained and untrained individuals. In: H.G. Knuttgen, J.A. Vogel, and J. Poortmans (eds.) *Biochemistry of Exercise.* Illinois: Human Kinetics, pp. 514–519.

Knoefel, K. (1943). The influence of phenisopropylamine and phenisopropyl methylamine on work output. *Fed. Proc.* 2:83.

Koob, G.F., and C.B. Hubner (1988). Reinforcement pathways for cocaine. In: D. Clouet, K. Asghar, and R. Brown (eds.) *Mechanisms of Cocaine Abuse and Toxicity.* Washington, D.C.: U.S. Dept. of Health and Human Serv., pp. 137–159.

Kornetsky, C. (1958). Effects of meprobamate, phenobarbital and dextro-amphetamine on reaction time and learning in man. *J. Pharmacol. Exp. Therap.* 123:216–219.

Kornetsky, C., A.F. Mirsky, E.K. Kessler, and J.E. Dorff (1959). The effects of dextro-amphetamine on behavioral deficits produced by sleep loss in humans. *J. Pharmacol. Exp. Therap.* 127:46–50.

Lange, R.A., R.G. Cigarroa, C.W. Yancy, J.E. Willard, J.J. Popma, M.N. Sills, W. McBride, A.S. Kim, and L.D. Hillis (1989). Cocaine-induced coronary-artery vasoconstriction. *New Engl. J. Med.* 321:1557–1562.

Langer, S.Z., and M.A. Enero (1974). The potentiation of responses to adrenergic nerve stimulation in the presence of cocaine: its relationship to the metabolic fate of released norepinephrine. *J. Pharmacol. Exp. Ther.* 191:431–443.

Laties, V.G., and B. Weiss (1981). The amphetamine margin in sports. *Fed. Proc.* 40:2689–2692.

Latz, A., C. Kornetsky, G. Bain, and M. Goldman (1966). Swimming performance of mice as affected by antidepressant drugs and baseline levels. *Psychopharmacologia* 10:67–88.

Levy, M.N., and B. Blattberg (1978). The influence of cocaine and desipramine on the cardiac responses to exogenous and endogenous norepinephrine. *Eur. J. Pharmacol.* 48:37–49.

Lombardo, J.A. (1986). Stimulants and athletic performance (part 1 of 2): Amphetamines and caffeine. *Phys. Sportsmed.* 14:128–140.

Lombardo, J.A. (1987). Stimulants. In: R.H. Strauss (ed.) *Drugs & Performance in Sports.* Philadelphia: W.B. Saunders, pp. 69–85.

Lopes, J.M., M. Aubier, J. Jardim, J.V. Aranda, and P.T. Macklem (1983). Effect of caffeine on skeletal muscle function before and after fatigue. *J. Appl. Physiol.* 54:1303–1305.

Lovingood, B.W., C.S. Blyth, W.H. Peacock, and R.B. Lindsay (1967). Effects of d-amphetamine sulfate, caffeine, and high temperature on human performance. *Res. Quart.* 38:64–71.

Lowenthal, D.T., and Z.V. Kendrick (1985). Drug-exercise interactions. *Ann. Rev. Pharmacol. Toxicol.* 25:275–305.

MacIntosh, B.R., R.W. Barbee, and W.N.Stainsby (1981). Contractile response to caffeine of rested and fatigued skeletal muscle. *Med. Sci. Sports* 13:95.

MacLaren, D.P., H. Gibson, M. Parry-Billings, and R.H.T. Edwards (1989). A review of metabolic and physiological factors in fatigue. *Exerc. Sport Sci. Rev.* 17:29–66.

Mandell, A.J. (1979). The Sunday syndrome: A unique pattern of amphetamine abuse indigenous to American professional football. *Clin. Toxicol.* 15:225–232.

McNaughton, L. (1987). Two levels of caffeine ingestion on blood lactate and free fatty acid responses during incremental exercise. *Res. Quart.* 58:255–259.

Molinengo, L., and M. Orsetti (1976). Drug action on the "grasping" reflex and on swimming endurance: An attempt to characterize experimentally antidepressant drugs. *Neuropharmacology* 15:257–260.

National Collegiate Athletic Association (1988). The 1988–89 NCAA drug testing program. Mission, Kansas.

National Institute of Drug Abuse (1989). Americans' Current Illicit Drug Use Drops 37 Percent. *NIDA Notes* 4:42–43.

Neely, J.R., R.H. Bowman, and H.E. Morgan (1968). Conservation of glycogen in the perfused rat heart developing intraventricular pressure. In: Whelan W.J. (ed.) *Control of Glycogen Metabolism.* New York: Academic Press, pp. 49–64.

Neims, A.H., and R.W. von Borstel (1983). Caffeine: Metabolism and biochemical mechanisms of action. In: R.J. Wurtman and J.J. Wurtman (eds.) *Nutrition and the Brain.* Vol. 6, New York: Raven Press, pp. 1–30.

Newman, M. (1987). Elite Women Athletes Survey Results. Minneapolis: Hazelden Health Promotion Services.

Nielsen, E.B., and J. Scheel-Krüger (1988). Central nervous system stimulants: neuropharmacological mechanisms. In: F.C. Colpaert and R.L. Balster (eds.) *Psychopharmacology Series 4 Transduction Mechanisms of Drug Stimuli.* Berlin: Springer-Verlag, pp. 57–72.

Nuzzo, N.A., and D.P. Waller (1988). Drug Abuse in Athletes. In: J.A. Thomas (ed.) *Drugs, Athletes, and Physical Performance.* New York: Plenum Medical Book, pp. 141–167.

Patwardhan, R.V., P.V. Desmond, R.F. Johnson, G.D. Dunn, D.H. Robertson, A.M. Hoyumpa, and S. Schenker (1980). Effects of caffeine on plasma free fatty acids, urinary catecholamines, and drug binding. *Clin. Pharmacol. Ther.* 28:398–403.

Perkins, R., and M.H. Williams (1975). Effect of caffeine upon maximal muscular endurance of females. *Med. Sci. Sports* 7:221–224.

Pierson, W.R. (1961). Amphetamine sulfate and performance. *J. Amer. Med. Assoc.* 177:345–347.

Pinter, E.J., and C.J. Pattee (1968). Fat-mobilizing action of amphetamine. *J. Clin. Invest.* 47:394–402.

Pitts, D.K., and J. Marwah (1988). Cocaine and central monoaminergic neurotransmission: A review of electrophysiological studies and comparison to amphetamine and antidepressants. *Life Sci.* 42:949–968.

Powers, S.K., R.J. Byrd, R. Tulley, and T. Callender (1983). Effects of caffeine ingestion on metabolism and performance during graded exercise. *Eur. J. Appl. Physiol.* 50:301–307.

AMPHETAMINE, CAFFEINE, AND COCAINE   **323**

Powers, S.K., and S. Dodd (1985). Caffeine and endurance performance. *Sports Med.* 2:165–174.

Powers, S.K., S. Dodd, J. Woodyard, and M. Mangum (1986). Caffeine alters ventilatory and gas exchange kinetics during exercise. *Med. Sci. Sports Exerc.* 18:101–106.

Rall, T. (1985). The methylxanthines. In: A.G. Gilman, L.S. Goodman, and A. Gilman (eds.) *Pharmacological Basis of Therapeutics.* (7th ed.) New York: Macmillan, pp. 589–603.

Ritchie, J.M., and N.M. Greene (1985). Local anesthetics. In: A.G. Gilman, L.S. Goodman, and A. Gilman (eds.) *The Pharmacological Basis of Therapeutics.* (7th ed.) New York: MacMillan, pp. 302–321.

Ritz, M.C., R.J. Lamb, S.R. Goldberg, and M.J. Kuhar (1988). Cocaine self-administration appears to be mediated by dopamine uptake inhibition. *Prog. Neuro-Psychopharmacol. & Biol. Psychiat.* 12:233–239.

Rivers, W., and H. Webber (1907). The action of caffeine on the capacity for muscular work. *J. Physiol.* 36:33–47.

Robertson, D., D. Wade, R. Workman, R.L. Woosley, and J.A. Oates (1981). Tolerance to the humoral and hemodynamic effects of caffeine in man. *J. Clin. Invest.* 67:1111–1117.

Ryan, A.J. Use of amphetamines in athletics (1959). *J. Amer. Med. Assoc.* 170:562.

Sasaki, H., J. Maeda, S. Usui, and T. Ishiko (1987a). Effect of sucrose and caffeine ingestion on performance of prolonged strenuous running. *Int. J. Sports Med.* 8:261–265.

Sasaki, H., I. Takaoka, and T. Ishiko (1987b). Effects of sucrose or caffeine ingestion on running performance and biochemical responses to endurance running. *Int. J. Sports Med.* 8:203–207.

Sattin, A., and T.W. Rall (1970). The effect of adenosine and adenine nucleotides on the adenosine 3′,5′-phosphate content of Guinea-pig cerebral cortex slices. *Mol. Pharmacol.* 6:13–23.

Seashore, R.H., and A.C. Ivy (1953). Effects of analeptic drugs in relieving fatigue. *Psychol. Monogr.* 67:1–16.

Slavin, J.L., and D.J. Joensen (1985). Caffeine and sports performance. *Phys. Sportsmed.* 13:191–193.

Smith, G.M., and H.K. Beecher (1959). Amphetamine sulfate and athletic performance. I. Objective effects. *J. Amer. Med. Assoc.* 170:542–557.

Smith, G.M., and H.K. Beecher (1961). Amphetamine, secobarbital, and athletic performance. *J. Amer. Med. Assoc.* 172:1502–1514.

Smith, G.M., M. Weitzner, and H.K. Beecher (1963). Increased sensitivity of measurement of drug effects in expert swimmers. *J. Pharmacol. Exp. Therap.* 139:114–119.

Somani, S.M., and P. Gupta (1988). Caffeine: A new look at an age-old drug. *Int. J. Clin. Pharm. Ther. Toxicol.* 26:521–533.

Somerville, W. (1946). The effect of benzedrine on mental or physical fatigue in soldiers. *Canadian Med. Assoc. J.* 55:470–476.

Stone, E.A. (1970). Swim-stress-induced inactivity: Relation to body temperature and brain norepinephrine, and effects of d-amphetamine. *Psychosomatic Med.* 32:51–59.

Supinski, G.S., S. Levin, and S.G. Kelsen (1986). Caffeine effect on respiratory muscle endurance and sense of effort during loaded breathing. *J. Appl. Physiol.* 60:2040–2047.

Tarnopolsky, M.A., S.A. Atkinson, J.D. MacDougall, D.G. Sale, and J.R. Sutton (1989). Physiological responses to caffeine during endurance running in habitual caffeine users. *Med. Sci. Sports Exerc.* 21:418–424.

Theil, D., and B. Essing (1930). Cocain und muskelarbeit. I. Der einfluss auf leistung und gasstoffwechsel. *Arbeitsphysiologie* 3:287–297.

Trendelenburg, V. (1959). The supersensitivity caused by cocaine. *J. Pharmacol. Exp. Ther.* 125:55–65.

Turner, C.E., B.S. Urbanek, G.M. Wall, and C.W. Waller (1988). *Cocaine. An Annotated Bibliography* Vol. I. Jackson, Mississippi: University Press of Mississippi, p xiii.

Tyler, D.B. (1947). The effect of amphetamine sulfate and some barbiturates on the fatigue produced by prolonged wakefulness. *Amer. J. Physiol.* 150:253–262.

U.S. Olympic Committee, Division of Sports Medicine and Science: Drug Education & Control Policy (1988). Colorado Springs.

Uyeda, A.A., and J.M. Fuster (1962). The effects of amphetamine on tachistoscopic performance in the monkey. *Psychopharmacologia* 3:463–467.

Van Handel, P. (1983). Caffeine. In: M.H. Williams (ed.) *Ergogenic Aids in Sport.* Illinois: Human Kinetics, pp. 128–163.

Varagic, V.M., and M. Zugic (1971). Interactions of xanthine derivatives, catecholamines and glucose-6-phosphate on the isolated phrenic nerve diaphragm preparation of the rat. *Pharmacology* 5:275–286.

Wadler, G.I., and B. Hainline (1989). *Drugs and the Athlete.* Philadelphia: F.A. Davis Company.

Weiner, N. (1985). Norepinephrine, epinephrine, and the sympathomimetic amines. In: A.G. Gilman, L.S. Goodman, and A. Gilman (eds.) *Pharmacological Basis of Therapeutics.* (7th ed.) New York: Macmillan, pp. 145–180.

Weir, J., T.D. Noakes, K. Myburgh, and B. Adams (1987). A high carbohydrate diet negates the metabolic effects of caffeine during exercise. *Med. Sci. Sports Exerc.* 19:100–105.

Weiss, B., and V.G. Laties (1962). Enhancement of human performance by caffeine and the amphetamines. *Pharm. Rev.* 14:1–36.

Wenger, Galen R. (1988). CNS stimulants and athletic performance. In: J.A. Thomas (ed.) *Drugs, Athletes, and Physical Performance.* New York: Plenum Medical Book, pp. 217–234.

Wenzel, D.G., and C.O. Rutledge (1962). Effects of centrally-acting drugs on human motor and psychomotor performance. *J. Pharmaceut. Sci.* 51:631–644.

Wilkerson, R.D. (1988). Cardiovascular toxicity of cocaine. In: D. Clouet, K. Asghar, and R. Brown (eds.) *Mechanisms of Cocaine Abuse and Toxicity, National Institute for Drug Abuse Research Monograph 88.* Washington, D.C.: U.S. Government Printing Office, pp. 304–324.

Williams, J.H., J.F. Signorile, W.S. Barnes, and T.W. Henrich (1988). Caffeine, maximal power output and fatigue. *Brit. J. Sports Med.* 22:132–134.

Williams, J.H., W.S. Barnes, and W.L. Gadberry (1987). Influence of caffeine on force and EMG in rested and fatigued muscle. *Amer. J. Phys. Med.* 66:169–182.

Williams, M.H. (1974). *Drugs and Athletic Performance.* Springfield: Charles C. Thomas, pp. 20–55.

Williams, M.H., and J. Thompson (1973). Effect of variant dosages of amphetamine upon endurance. *Res. Quart.* 44:417–422.

Winder, W.W. (1986). Effect of intravenous caffeine on liver glycogenolysis during prolonged exercise. *Med. Sci. Sports Exerc.* 18:192–196.

Woolverton, W.L., and M.S. Kleven (1988). Multiple dopamine receptors and the behavioral effects of cocaine. In: D. Clouet, K. Asghar, and R. Brown (eds.) *Mechanisms of Cocaine Abuse and Toxicity, National Institute for Drug Abuse Research Monograph 88.* Washington, D.C.: U.S. Government Printing Office, pp. 160–184.

Wyndham, C.H., G.G. Rogers, A.J.S. Beade, and N.B. Strydom (1971). Physiological effects of the amphetamines during exercise. *S. Afr. Med. J.* 45:247–252.

Yamaguchi, T. (1975). Caffeine-induced potentiation of twitches in frog single muscle fiber. *Jap. J. Physiol.* 25:693–704.

DISCUSSION

POWERS: When discussing the ergogenicity of caffeine, we must classify exercise regimens according to intensity and duration. It isn't fair to compare the effect of caffeine on the duration of high-intensity exercise that lasted 7–9 min to exercise lasting 3 h or more, in which glycogen depletion might have been a limiting factor. Such comparisons lead to confusion. I also wonder if the "lack of response" seen in regular caffeine users is related to inadequate doses of the drug being administered. Would we see a physiological response in these people if we increased the dosage to something higher than 10 mg/kg?

CONLEE: That's a valid question. The highest dose given was in a study where subjects increased their endurance from 440 s to 460 s on a caffeine dose of 15 mg/kg. The pharmacological literature suggests that with a dose above 15 mg/kg one could begin to experience some adverse acute effects of the caffeine. It may be difficult to get approval for higher doses from human subject committees.

With regard to your point about the variability in intensities of exercise, there was a wide range of intensities of exercise used in these experiments. The problem is that there were benefits to both high-intensity and more moderate-intensity exercise. Therefore, a positive effect of caffeine is possible even with very high-intensity exercise. If glycogen depletion is the fatigue mechanism being affected, glycogen depletion must occur in those motor units being called on during high-intensity exercise. If the ergogenic effect of caffeine operates by way of the substrate metabolism mechanism as proposed initially by Dave Costill and his group, then caffeine could have an effect at both high and moderate intensity, even though we don't normally associate a positive effect with high-intensity exercise.

SHERMAN: To minimize the variability in performance data among studies that use apparently similar designs, we need to pay a lot more attention to the protocols employed to detect changes in performance. For example, we should use subjects who are very familiar with the protocols; we should use repeated-measures designs with subjects serving as their own controls; we should counterbalance the design; we should establish well-defined criteria of fatigue; and we should carefully train the people who will monitor the performance aspect of these trials.

WILMORE: It's also very important to try to get performance data in conditions as similar to a competitive situation as possible. It would be fascinating to test some of these "erogenic" aids in a series of 10 km races under controlled competitive conditions, including, perhaps, some prizes for race winners.

SPRIET: I would like to mention a study that we have recently completed. We used well-trained, high quality runners (30 min/10 km) and gave them a caffeine dose that produced urinary caffeine measurements that were right on the borderline of the International Olympic Committee's legal limit. Our rationale was that if we could show that there was no effect at that level, then we might convince athletes that caffeine would not be an ergogenic aid and that there would be no sense in taking it. We also had these athletes eat their normal pre-race high carbohydrate diet. They were asked to run to exhaustion at a race pace intensity of 80–85% $\dot{V}O_2$max. They exercised in both placebo and caffeine conditions both during running and during cycling to get at the modality question. To our surprise, we saw very large increases in performance, both on the treadmill and on the bike, in every one of the seven subjects. With caffeine, they increased their endurance by 25–40% over the 45–60 min control times. We saw a very large increase in plasma epinephrine throughout the exercise in the caffeine condition. Based on epinephrine changes, there is apparently something going on metabolically.

WILMORE: When did you give the caffeine dose?

SPRIET: About 70–75 min before exercise.

CONLEE: How about their previous caffeine use?

SPRIET: We didn't control for that because our hypothesis was that we would see no difference. We had three definite non-users and four who were moderate users, but there responses to caffeine were similar. They were asked to abstain from caffeine use 24 h before exercise. The point I would like to make is that a lot of the studies have used low doses and have fasted their people ahead of time; that is not what an athlete would do coming into a competition. These points should be taken into account whenever we do these studies.

CONLEE: Your results are contrary to those found in studies where a high carbohydrate diet prior to the caffeine use negated the effects of caffeine.

COSTILL: I have been puzzled by the fact that there is such a wide diversity of findings with caffeine because in the first couple of studies we did, the effect was very clear—like night and day— in the performance changes. Looking at it over the years, I have often wondered if it didn't have a great deal to do with the selection of our subjects. In both studies we used some of the same subjects, and we found that there were some people who always responded with the greatest improvements. I have come to a subjective conclusion that subject selection may be the most important factor in explaining the variability in results for caffeine. If you study people who respond positively to caffeine, I'll bet you will always find that they will respond well, but by throwing in a mixed bag of subjects or random sampling, you will find no statistical difference because the variance is so great.

COYLE: How much of the beneficial effect seen with caffeine is due to increased fatty acid metabolism as opposed to a central nervous system effect? Subjects who benefit from caffeine note that early in exercise they feel more coordinated and more powerful. I wonder if caffeine might not cause a better coordination of muscle groups.

CONLEE: One of Ivy's hypotheses was that caffeine caused central nervous system effects such as euphoria because they did not see the elevation of fatty acids or other metabolic changes. Cocaine and amphetamines, as well as caffeine, produce euphoria, increased alertness, and increased attentiveness to the task. These effects certainly are consistent with a propensity for ergogenicity.

COGGAN: I also think we have greatly overemphasized the potential ergogenic effects of changes in fatty acids of the magnitude observed after ingesting caffeine. In five human subjects, we used heparin and lipid infusion to double plasma free-fatty acid levels from 1 mM to 2 mM, and under those conditions during 90 min of exercise, we reduced R values only by 0.01 or 0.02. We could not show any difference in glucose turnover or oxidation, but the biopsy measurements have not been completed. If you can't show an effect with that large of a difference in circulating fatty acids, I think it is unlikely that there will be much of an effect when fatty acids go up only 0.1–0.2 mM with caffeine.

HEIGENHAUSER: In studies of free-fatty acid turnover rates during high intensity exercise that we did in the late 1970s, R values did not give us a satisfactory indication of what free-fatty acid utilization was. Turnover studies must be done to gain any insight on fatty acid utilization, and even then one can't be sure of what is happening in the muscles.

CONLEE: Basically, I have similar concerns with using R values as representing what is happening metabolically. There are studies where all the so-called indicators were in line with improving performance, and yet performance was not improved. On the other hand, when performance was improved, there were often no metabolic indicators, such as increased fatty acids or lowered R values, that would have suggested it.

HEIGENHAUSER: In the animal studies that have been done in England, there seems to be a selective response of different fiber types to caffeine. Caffeine has a greater effect on the slow-twitch oxidative fibers than on the fast-twitch fibers. Therefore, subjects with a high proportion of slow-twitch fibers may be good responders to caffeine.

CONLEE: In all three of the studies from Winder's group, they found no effect of caffeine with respect to fiber type on glycogen sparing or alterations in glycogen. In fact, in one of their studies they found increased use of glycogen in the caffeine-treated animals.

HEIGENHAUSER: On another point, I think the detrimental effect of caffeine has probably been exagerrated. That area right now is just one big can of worms. One week a paper claims that use of caffeine is associated with heart disease, but the next week another paper says it's not. This topic could be the subject of an entire epidemiology paper itself.

ROBERTSON: There seems to be a thread of similarity with respect to the perception of exertion that runs through the literature with all three of these drugs. You suggest that if the effect of attenuating the perception of exertion is present, it's a central phenomenon. I wonder where the site of the action is. There seems to be some agreement that signals of exertion are primarily a function of a feed-forward mechanism with some corollary discharge being copied in the sensory cortex. Is it your speculation that the site of the action is at those corollary discharges? In other words, is there a blockade of some sort that occurs independent of any kind of peripheral metabolic function?

CONLEE: Those who have studied the central nervous system effects of these drugs, especially of cocaine and amphetamines, conclude that the attenuation of perceived exertion is a central receptor effect, regardless of the exercise response. It is not a metabolic factor or the effect of negating any metabolic feedback. It is more of a euphoric response, perhaps due to the release of dopamine in the meso-cortical limbic system, which is the system responsible for arousal and pleasure. The drugs cause neurotransmitter release, or they block the uptake of the neurotransmitter to cause the euphoria.

MURRAY: I am struck by the 1947 paper of Cuthbertson and Knox who fatigued subjects with arm and leg ergometry. Their subjects went along quite nicely and then began to fatigue as would be predicted, presumably because of depletion of substrate such as glucose or blood glucose. Yet, when they were administered amphetamine, the work output shot right back up. Obviously, the muscles were oxidizing something, and substrate wasn't limiting. This perhaps indicates a very strong peripheral effect. When one deals with amphetamines and caffeine, it is easy to get locked into a metabolic rationale for fatigue.

HEIGENHAUSER: Some rat studies at McMaster found that dopamine was depleted in certain areas of the brain with fatigue. If they injected amino acid precursors of dopamine, they could significantly increase endurance time. This suggests that some of the central neuron transmitters might be responsible for the fatigue. Similarly, the data from Everest II indicate that neurotransmitter could have been the limiting factor for performance rather than any change in the muscles.

CONLEE: In support of that idea are results of experiments on brain concentrations of norepinephrine. When the animal was exhausted and displayed very little enthusiasm for any activity, the brain concentration of norepinephrine was very low. When they gave those animals amphetamines, the concentration of norepinephrine in brain tissue was elevated. The amphetamine-treated animals responded by being much more active. The investigators proposed that the amphetamines somehow stimulated a repletion of norepinephrine in the brain tissue, which allowed the animals to feel more energetic.

LOMBARDO: Amphetamines are indirect acting sympathomimetics that seem to work through the catecholamine system. Do you think that one of the reasons there is such diversity in the amphetamine studies is that there are so many other factors that also influence catecholamines?

CONLEE: Yes, that could easily be the source of some of the variability in results.

LAMB: What is the level of amphetamine abuse among athletes these days? My impression is that 10–15 years ago it was being used much more widely than it is now.

CONLEE: I don't know.

LOMBARDO: The use of amphetamines is believed to be down among athletes, and I think that is directly related to the deaths attributed to amphetamines. Athletes can feel the heart palpitations when they take amphetamines, and that seems to be a real concern to them. Also, athletes sense a loss of control if they are on amphetamines during a competition.

9

Alcohol, Marijuana and Beta Blockers

MELVIN H. WILLIAMS, PH.D.

331

INTRODUCTION

Doping, as the term is applied to sport, is generally interpreted today as the illegal use of ergogenic drugs, or similar ergogenic aids, as a means to enhance performance. In the distant past, however, doping was seen in a different light, for drugs were often given surreptitiously to one's opponents in an attempt to impair their performance. Although this practice seems to have disappeared, a number of drugs that athletes consume today for medicinal or social purposes may actually impair their own performance. Moreover, athletes taking certain drugs for an ergogenic effect may actually experience the opposite, a deterioration in performance. As contrasted to ergogenic drugs, Eichner (1989) has coined the term "ergolytic drugs" for those drugs that may impair performance.

This chapter will center on three dissimilar, and yet in several ways similar, drugs which may commonly be used by athletes— alcohol, marijuana, and beta blockers. Alcohol and marijuana are primarily used as social drugs, but may also be used medicinally, whereas beta blockers are primarily used as medications. All three drugs may possess ergogenic potential for certain sports, but may be ergolytic for others. Although medical and social implications for the athlete will be incorporated into the discussion where appropriate, the primary focus of this chapter will be upon the ergogenic and ergolytic properties of each drug. It is important to note, however, that in relation to physiological and psychological effects, all three drugs may elicit highly variable interindividual responses. Furthermore, particularly in the case of alcohol and marijuana, highly variable intraindividual responses are affected by factors such as tolerance to the drug, preexisting mood, expectancy, and environment (Lowenthal et al., 1987; Mathew et al., 1989; Mitchell, 1985).

ALCOHOL

Alcohol (ethyl alcohol, ethanol) is a simple two-carbon molecule with the chemical formula, C_2H_5OH. Although alcohol is a drug, technically it may also be classified as a nutrient because it provides energy, one of the major functions of nutrients. One gram of alcohol contains 7 kcal of energy. On the other hand, alcohol may also be classified as an antinutrient because it may interfere with the proper metabolism of other nutrients (Lieber, 1983).

Alcohol is found in a wide variety of beverages, the most common being beer, wine and liquor, which may contain additional nutrients. Table 9–1 provides a summary of the alcohol, carbohydrate, and caloric content of some common beverages, along with amounts

TABLE 9-1. *Approximate Nutrient Content of Selected Alcoholic Beverages*

	Regular Beer (12 oz.)	Light Beer (12 oz.)	Red Wine (4 oz.)	White Wine (4 oz.)	Liquors (80 Proof) (1.25 oz.)
Energy (kcal)	150	100	100	90	100
Alcohol (g)	13	11	12	12	14
Carbohydrate (g)	13	7	4	3	0
Protein (g)	1	1	.2	.2	0
Thiamin (mg)	.02	.03	.006	.005	0
Riboflavin (mg)	.09	.10	.033	.006	0
Niacin (mg)	1.6	1.4	.100	.080	0
Calcium (mg)	18	18	9	10	0
Iron (mg)	.1	.14	.5	.35	0
Potassium (mg)	89	64	131	94	0

of several selected vitamins and minerals. Approximately the same amount of alcohol (14 g of 100% ethanol) is found in 12 ounces of beer, 4 ounces of wine, and 1.25 ounces of 80-proof liquor, each being designated as one drink.

Following ingestion, alcohol is absorbed rapidly from the stomach and the small intestine, although the rate of absorption may be retarded by the presense of other food and fluids in the gastrointestinal tract (Pikaar et al., 1988). The distribution of alcohol in the body is governed by the water content. Since ethanol is completely water soluble, organs with a high water content and rich blood supply, such as the brain, receive the highest initial concentration (Dubowski, 1985). Although alcohol may affect almost all tissues in the body, its most prevalent effects are upon the central nervous system (CNS). Wadler and Hainline (1989) noted that no known receptor exists for alcohol and that its molecular mechanisms of action are not understood; nevertheless, alcohol appears to influence synaptic funtion, possibly by modifying resting membrane permeability, neurotransmitter release, or postsynaptic excitation.

The psychological and physiological effects of alcohol are dependent primarily upon the blood alcohol concentration (BAC), which is usually expressed as mg% or mmol/L. The molecular weight of alcohol is 46.07, so 1 mmol/L = 46 mg/L or 4.6 mg/dL. A BAC of 21.7 mmol/L is the equivalent of 100 mg/dL, which is 100 mg%, (0.10 g/dL), the legal definition for intoxication. One drink in the average-size male will lead to a BAC of approximately 0.025 g/dL, so four drinks, containing approximately 56 g of alcohol, will result in a BAC of approximately 0.10 g/dL. Approximately 90% of the ingested alcohol is eliminated by the liver at a rate of 8 g/h. An additional 10% is excreted in the urine, breath, and perspiration. In total, the equivalent of a BAC of 0.015 g/dL is excreted in 1 h.

Theoretical Ergogenic or Ergolytic Considerations

Alcohol consumption prior to and during performance has a long history of use by athletes for ergogenic purposes. Jokl (1968) reported evidence that alcohol was in wide use on the European sport scene at the turn of the century; he cited cases of endurance athletes imbibing rum, champagne, cognac, or beer during competition. Boje (1939) and Wolf (1963) indicated that in cases of extreme athletic exertion or in events of brief maximal effort, alcohol has been given to athletes to serve as a stimulant by releasing inhibitions and lessening the sense of fatigue.

A biphasic hypothesis regarding the effects of alcohol has been advanced, i.e., it may produce a transitory sensation of excitement followed by depressive effects. Gould (1970) indicated that stimulation may be caused by the depresssive action of ethanol on the reticular activating system, releasing inhibitory control. However, Doctor and Perkins (1961) and Perman (1958) attributed the excitatory effect of alcohol to increased sympathetic nervous system activity and increased secretions of epinephrine from the adrenal medulla. More recently, increases of 30–40% in plasma norepinephrine concentrations have been reported following alcohol intake, but no increase was noted in plasma epinephrine (Kelbaek et al., 1987, 1988). Although the rise in norepinephrine following alcohol ingestion is not consistent across all studies, Kelbaek and others (1987, 1988) have provided support for the concept that an increased sympathetic nervous activity is induced by alcohol intoxication. However with increasing time and dosage, alcohol exerts its depressive effects. Relative to the biphasic hypothesis alcohol has been ascribed ergogenic qualities for both its potential stimulating and depressive actions, but, as described later, some of its effects may also be ergolytic.

Potential Ergogenic Effects. Alcohol has been used by athletes primarily for its psychological effects, but it may also affect physiological responses important to exercise. Psychologically, alcohol may theoretically benefit performance by improving self-confidence through a central nervous system disinhibition effect or an enhanced sympathetic effect. Alcohol may also decrease sensitivity to pain and may remove psychological barriers to performance by a central nervous system depression effect. However, its most prevalent use in athletic competition appears to be its effect to reduce anxiety and tremor, one of its beneficial medical applications for patients with essential tremor (Koller & Biary, 1984). In this regard, Shephard (1972) noted that two pistol shooters were disqualified during the 1968 Olympics, allegedly because they used alcohol in an attempt to improve their competitive ability. Alcohol may also have been used for its potential stimulant effect upon the cardiovascular system. In an earlier review of the literature, Williams (1974) indicated that the effects of alcohol ingestion upon the resting heart rate were variable; five studies showed an increase and five a decrease. Similarly findings of an increased heart rate (Kelbaek et al., 1988; Kelbaek et al., 1987) and no effect in response to alcohol (Stromberg et al., 1988) have been reported more recently. The increased heart rate has been attributed to the sympathetic effect noted previously (Kelbaek et al., 1988). This sympathetic activation also affects energy substrate for exercise because increased splanchnic release of glucose (Juhlin-Dannfelt et al., 1977a) and free fatty acids (FFA) (Markiewicz & Cholewa, 1978) have been reported following alcohol ingestion. Moreover, alcohol has been evaluated as a potential energy source during exercise (Schurch et al., 1982).

Prior to the 1968 Olympics, alcohol was listed as a doping agent by the International Olympic Committee (IOC). However, because wine and beer may be part of the athlete's normal diet, Fischbach (1972) reported that alcohol was deleted and not listed as a specific doping agent for most athletes in the 1972 Olympics. Fischbach also noted that alcohol is called "goldwater" by athletes involved in shooting competition and the use of alcohol is now banned in shooting sports.

Potential Ergolytic Effects. Alcohol may also elicit negative psychological and physiological events that could impair physical performance. These effects may range on a continuum from euphoria and reduced tension to coma and even death (Sollman, 1956). Table 9–2 indicates the typical BAC in relation to number of drinks and the typical effects. Obviously, many of the adverse psychomotor effects could significantly worsen athletic performance.

A number of the physiological effects of alcohol could also impair performance. Gould (Gould, 1970; Gould et al., 1971) reported nearly 20 y ago that alcohol may be a myocardial depressant, decreasing the cardiac output without a change in heart rate. Stratton and others (1981) also reported a decreased contractile strength of the heart following alcohol ingestion. A series of recent experiments has shown that a BAC in the range of 21–45 mmol/L could depress left ventricular function in healthy subjects by approximately 5–10 percent (Lang et al., 1985; Kelbaek et al., 1987; Kelbaek et al., 1985), the higher dosage being associated with the largest impairment (Kelbaek et al., 1985). However, in another study by Kelbaek's research group (Kelbaek et al., 1988) the left ventricular ejection frac-

TABLE 9-2. *Typical Effects of Increasing Blood Alcohol Content*

Number of drinks in two hours	Blood alcohol level (g/dL)	Typical effects
2–3	.02–.04	Reduced tension, relaxed feelings, relief from daily stress
4–5	.06–.09	Impaired judgement, euphoria, impaired fine motor ability and coordination
6–8	.11–.16	Legally drunk, slurred speech, impaired gross motor coordination, staggering gait
9–12	.18–.25	Loss of control of voluntary activity, erratic behavior, impaired vision
13–18	.27–.39	Stuporous, total loss of coordination
>19	>.40	Coma, depression of respiratory centers, death

Based upon body weight of 72.6 KG (160 pounds)
One drink = 12 ounces regular beer; four ounces wine; 1.25 ounces liquor.
Adapted from Williams, M.H., *Lifetime fitness and wellness.* Dubuque: Wm. C. Brown Publishers, 1990.

tion (LVEF) decreased 3% at a BAC of 35 mmol/L during early intoxication, but increased during late intoxication (21 mmol/L) by 6%.

Other physiological effects of alcohol at rest, if they persisted during exercise, would also impair aerobic endurance. These effects include agglutination of red blood cells, which could decrease oxygen transport (Pennington & Knisely, 1973); vasoconstriction in resting musculature (Fewings et al., 1966; Graf & Strom, 1960), which could lead to an increased lactic acid production in muscle (Chui et al., 1978); cutaneous vasodilation and a decreased release of antidiuretic hormone from the pituitary gland, which could lead to problems with temperature regulation; and an impaired gluconeogenesis with resultant hypoglycemia (Jorfeldt & Juhlin-Dannfelt, 1978). Relative to this latter point, Mezey (1985) noted that ethanol may cause hyperglycemia or hypoglycemia, depending on whether hepatic glycogen stores are adequate. When liver glycogen is low, ethanol inhibits hepatic gluconeogenesis, which could be detrimental to athletes in prolonged endurance events.

A potential problem for an athlete who may substitute alcohol energy for carbohydrate energy is a loss of weight, possibly as lean muscle mass. Reinus and others (1989) noted that weight loss during short-term (7 d) ethanol infusion is unrelated to overall negative energy balance, stems primarily from decrements in protein, minerals, and fluid, and may in part be mediated by the reduction in insulin secretion that accompainies switching from dietary glucose to ethanol. They observed weight loss on a zero energy balance, noting losses of nitrogen, potassium, phosphorus, magnesium, and sodium.

Effects on Sports-related Performance

Psychomotor Performance. For the purpose of this chapter, psychomotor performance will include tests of strength, power, speed, local muscular endurance, and perceptual-motor skills. Perceptual-motor skills may be tested in the laboratory in a variety of ways. Perceptual ability is usually tested by simple reaction time. Attention is evaluated by a test of choice reaction time, in which two or more stimuli are presented requiring distinct responses, or by a test of reaction time measured under conditions of divided attention. Sensorimotor coordination is measured by tests such as pursuit rotor tracking, body sway, or the finger to finger apposition test. Rate of information processing is tested by the interaction between speed and accuracy in choice reaction tests (Mitchell, 1985).

Although athletes may consume alcohol to improve psychological function, research suggests that most types of psychomotor functions associated with performance in sport are impaired. A decreased ability to process information, i.e., to interpret stimuli and produce an appropriate response, is a consistent research finding. In a critical review of earlier literature from 1940–1960, Carpenter (1962) has noted that most psychomotor processes associated with driving skills, including reaction time, are typically impaired at low and moderate blood alcohol levels. In a more recent review, Mitchell (1985) supported the earlier conclusions of Carpenter, noting that the degree of impairment is dose related. Representative studies have shown that small to moderate doses of alcohol may impair choice reaction time (Franks et al., 1976; Huntley, 1974, Huntley, 1972; Moskowitz & Burns, 1971; Moskowitz & Roth, 1971; Moskowitz et al., 1985; Nelson, 1959, Stromberg et al., 1988; Tharp et al., 1974), hand-eye coordination (Collins et al., 1971; Forney et al., 1964; Sidell & Pless, 1971), accuracy (Nelson, 1959; Rundell & Williams, 1979), balance (Begbie, 1966; Stromberg et al., 1988), complex coordination or gross motor skills (Belgrave et al., 1979; Hebbelinck, 1961; Nelson, 1959; Tang & Rosenstein, 1967), and even the operation of a bicycle (Schewe et al., 1984).

However, Mitchell (1985) noted that the psychomotor effects of alcohol are not identical or strictly linear for all behaviors. He concluded that there is no consistent evidence that BACs below 0.05 g/dL impair any psychomotor behavior in most individuals, although there is considerable interindividual variability. Simple reaction time is least susceptible to the adverse effects of alcohol and may not be affected at levels up to 0.08 g/dL. Other studies have reported no significant influence of alcohol on various psychomotor tasks, particularly simple reaction time, even at BACs approximating 0.10 g/dL (Baylor et al., 1989; Fagan et al., 1987; Rohrbaugh et al., 1988). On the other hand, Mitchell (1985) also noted that above a BAC of 0.10 g/dL, almost all behavioral skills are impaired by alcohol. Mitchell further observed that deterioration is greatest in tasks such as complex reaction time that require cognitive funtioning, the effect being noted in BACs above 0.05 g/dL and markedly affected above 0.10 g/dL. Complex skills may be impaired at even lower BACs. For example, Moskowitz and others (1985) reported that a variety of psychomotor skills, including tracking, a visual search-and-recognition task, and a divided attention display were impaired with a BAC as low as 0.015 g/dL. In addition, Collins and associates (1971) noted that alcohol was more likely to adversely affect tracking performance under dynamic as opposed to static conditions. Several studies have also suggested that the deteriorative effect of alcohol upon psychomotor performance becomes greater with time on task during vigilance tasks including tests of auditory reaction time (Gustafson, 1986a), visual reaction time (Gustafson, 1986b), and visual detection of degraded target stimuli (Rohrbaugh et al., 1988). Rohrbaugh and his associates (1988) also noted that the deteriorative effects were dose related.

The effects of alcohol appear to be mediated by a deleterious effect upon central processing capacity (Rohrbaugh et al., 1988). In support of this claim, Baylor and others (1989), using both simple and choice reaction time tasks, fractionated reaction time into premotor (central) and motor (peripheral, contractile) components and found that a BAC of 0.17 g/dL impaired all components involving central processing (response time, reaction time, and premotor time), but peripheral components (contractile time and movement time) were little affected.

Strength, power, speed and local muscular endurance. Alcohol was one of the first drugs to be tested for its ergogenic effect relative to strength and local muscular endurance, but the results of this early research, ranging from tremendous increases to modest decreases in performance, were confounded by improper experimental methodology. The interested reader may consult Rivers (1908) and Williams (1974) for extensive reviews.

In more contemporary laboratory and field experiments with strength, speed, power, and local muscular endurance, alcohol appears to exert no ergogenic effect; rather, it may be ergolytic. The ingestion of alcohol in small to moderate doses, i.e., the equivalent of BACs approximating 0.05–0.10 g/dL, exerted no significant acute effects upon static strength of various muscle groups (Giles et al., 1982; Hebbelinck, 1959; Hebbelinck, 1963; Ikai & Steinhaus, 1961; Williams, 1969), upon intermittent isometric muscular endurance (Williams, 1969), upon maximal muscular work on a bicycle ergometer designed to simulate a 100 m dash (Asmussen & Boje, 1948), or upon speed in a 100 m dash (McNaughton & Preece, 1986). In several studies, a detrimental effect has been noted upon dynamic strength (Hebbelinck, 1963), isometric grip strength (Nelson, 1959), power (Hebbelinck, 1959), and speed in an 80 m dash (Hebbelinck, 1963) and 200 m and 400 m dashes (McNaughton & Preece, 1986); however, because the details of the methodology were not specified in these latter two studies, the effect could be on the reaction time component.

Precision Shooting Sports. Theoretically, the best application of alcohol to sports as an ergogenic aid is to use alcohol in tension reduction, because alcohol has been shown to reduce stress-related emotional arousal (Vogel & Netter, 1989). Unfortunately, this area has received little research attention.

S'Jongers and others (1978) found that acute effects of one ounce of 40% alcohol significantly improved the shooting precision of pistol shooters, but so, too, did a placebo, suggesting that the placebo effect was operational. Reilly and Halliday (1985) reported that small doses of alcohol that produced a BAC of 0.02–0.05 g/dL exerted differential effects on tasks related to archery; no effects were shown on strength and endurance, but they observed slower reaction times and a decrease in hand steadiness (factors that might impair performance) and a smoother release of the arrow (which could enhance performance). Unfortunately, no performance data were collected. Thus, the data are not clear relative to an ergogenic effect upon precision shooting performance.

Aerobic Endurance. Alcohol appears to have no beneficial effect, and possibly a detrimental effect, upon energy sources during prolonged aerobic exercise tasks. Only limited amounts of free-fatty-acids may be produced from hepatic metabolism of alcohol, and the acetate released appears to be a very minor energy source during exercise (Lundquist et al., 1973). Januszewski and Klimek (1974) and Schurch and others (1982) noted that although exercise facilitates the elimination of alcohol from the body, the effect is mediated by increased respiratory and perspiration losses. Juhlin-Dannfelt et al. (1977b) and Schurch (1978) reported that in moderately prolonged exercise tasks (40–60 min) at low to moderate exercise intensities (30–60% of $\dot{V}O_2$max), alcohol ingestion exerted little influence on carbohydrate and fat metabolism. On the other hand, in related studies, Juhlin-Dannfelt et al. (1977a) reported a reduced hepatic glucose output after 3 h of exercise. This may have been caused by a decreased rate of gluconeogenesis because the processing of alcohol in the liver may reduce gluconeogenetic substrate (Jorfeldt & Juhlin-Dannfelt, 1978). Juhlin-Dannfelt et al. (1977a) suggested that this decreased gluconeogenesis could possibly contribute to hypoglycemia.

In more prolonged exercise tasks, hypoglycemia may develop as carbohydrate stores become depleted, a condition which may be aggravated by alcohol (Schurch et al., 1981). Hypoglycemia, in association with alcohol intake, may impair temperature regulation in a cold-air environment when consumed before (Graham 1983; 1981a; 1981b; Graham & Dalton, 1980) and after (Haight & Keatinge, 1973) prolonged exercise. Graham and Dalton (1980) concluded that several adverse effects of alcohol ingestion, e.g., impaired carbohydrate metabolism and temperature regulation, are potential dangers in mild exercise of recreational intensity as well as in exhaustive exercise.

M. H. Williams (1972; 1974; 1985) has reviewed the effect of alcohol upon physiological responses to endurance exercise, noting that the effects reported during submaximal exercise were inconsistent. A number of investigators reported significant increases in oxygen consumption, heart rate, and muscle blood flow during a variety of mild to moderate intensity exercise tasks, which would be indicative of an impaired performance, but these finding were not confirmed by others using similar submaximal exercise protocols. During maximal exercise, Williams noted that the effects reported were more consistent; alcohol appears to exert no significant effect upon maximal levels of oxygen uptake, heart rate, stroke volume, cardiac output, arteriovenous oxygen difference, blood pressure, peripheral vascular resistance, or peak lactate, although in one study (Blomqvist et al., 1970) a decreased maximal pulmonary ventilation was reported. Of particular interest since Williams' review has been research examining the effect of alcohol on LVEF which, as noted above, may be decreased at rest following alcohol consumption. However, exercise tends to counteract this effect on LVEF and on other physiological variables influenced by alcohol at rest. Several recent studies (Kelbaek et al., 1988; Kelbaek et al., 1987) have shown that moderate alcohol consumption has no significant effect upon LVEF during exercise, but a higher BAC, e.g., 0.20 g/dL, reportedly causes a 6% reduction in LVEF during exercise at 75 percent of $\dot{V}O_2max$ (Kelbaek et al., 1985).

M.H. Williams (1985) reviewed the earlier research and concluded that small to moderate doses of alcohol exert no significant influence upon performance tests of aerobic endurance. Some recent research supports this conclusion. For example a small dose of alcohol causing a BAC of 0.05 g/dL, has been reported to have little effect upon time for a 5-mile treadmill run (Houmard et al., 1987). On the other hand, McNaughton and Preece (1986) observed a detrimental effect in both an 800 m and 1,500 m run, the effect being dose-related with increasing BACs from 0.01 to 0.10 g/dL. The overall conclusion is that alcohol would not be a very effective ergogenic aid for athletes involved in aerobic endurance events, and could be ergolytic.

Social Drinking and Athletic Performance

Alcohol is the most commonly used social drug in the world. It has existed from earliest times, and almost all societies include a traditional alcoholic beverage as part of their culture or their religion. In the United States nearly 90% of the adult population have consumed alcohol, while 70% consume it on a regular basis (Schoenborn & Cohen, 1986); although most adults consume alcohol in a rational manner, approximately 10% are classified as problem drinkers. Alcohol consumption by high school seniors and college students reflects similar percentage rates (Johnston & Bachman, 1988; United States Department of Health and Human Services, 1980)

Alcohol use by athletes appears to be no different from that of the general population. Williams and Jackson (1975) noted few differences in alcohol use between high school athletes and nonathletes. A study of alcohol use by student-athletes in colleges and universities revealed that 88% had consumed alcohol within the previous year (Anderson & McKeag, 1985; Wadler & Hainline, 1989). Alcohol use is regarded to be the major drug problem by the National Football League (Sullivan, 1987) and is a major cause of concern for most other professional sports (Samples, 1989).

Several lines of evidence suggest that social alcohol consumption, in moderation, has no beneficial or detrimental effect upon physical performance. Epidemiological data are confusing relative to the relationship between fitness and alcohol consumption. For example, in the Tecumseh Health Study, Montoye and others (1980) reported higher levels of VO_2max in moderate drinkers compared to nondrinkers and heavy drinkers. Marti and associates (1988) reported an inverse relationship between alcohol consumption and performance in a 12 min run, but there were no differences between abstainers and light drinkers who consume less than six drinks per week. Moreover, the significant inverse relationship disappeared with a multivariate analysis that considered the contributory effect of other variables, such as cigarette smoking. In an extensive review of the relationship between exercise and other health behaviors, Blair and his colleagues (1985) concluded that the general relationship between the consumption of alcohol socially and exercise or fitness is rather inconsistent.

For athletes who do drink socially, does alcohol consumption the night prior to competition impair performance? Although not much data are available, it appears that light drinking, i.e., one to two drinks, will not significantly impair psychomotor or other types of physical performance. MacDonald and Svoboda (1979) reported no significant effect of one drink taken nightly for 10 d upon standard tests of strength and power or physiological responses to aerobic exercise when performed the following morning. Somewhat different effects may be observed with heavier drinking. Using a crossover experimental design with substantially greater amounts of alcohol, i.e., approximately eight drinks, Karvinin and others (1962) reported no significant influence upon tests of static strength or power the following morning, even though 9 of the 30 subjects had severe hangovers. However, during a 5-min ride at 250 W, the heart rate was elevated significantly during the first 2 min in the hangover condition; moreover, only nine subjects completed the task while hung over, compared to 15 while sober.

A recent well-designed study revealed that a BAC of 0.10 g/dL may adversely influence psychomotor performance the following morning, as evidenced by impaired performance in 10 pilots undertaking a variety of performance tasks associated with airplane operation (Yesavage & Leirer, 1986). Furthermore, because alcohol is a diuretic, excessive alcohol intake the night prior to competition could induce a state of dehydration the following morning; if this condition persisted prior to a prolonged endurance event conducted under warm environmental conditions, performance could be adversely affected. No research has been uncovered which has investigated this possibility, although beer consumption is common among marathoners the night before the race.

An important consideration involves the postrace ritual, which for many marathoners and other endurance athletes involves the consumption of often prodigious amounts of beer, to celebrate the completion of the event or to help induce relaxation and relief from muscular pain. Although alcohol may confer some anaesthetic effects, it does not appear to be the most effective fuel for rehydration because of its diuretic effects. Moreover, after a race the runner usually has an empty stomach and may be substantially dehydrated, conditions leading to a rapid absorption and concentration of alcohol in the body. Given the effect of small amounts of alcohol on psychomotor activities, drinking beer after a race and subsequent operation of an automobile are contraindicated (Clark, 1989; Williams, 1983).

Some athletes may be prone to alcoholism. Although some alcoholic athletes may continue to function effectively, performance eventually suffers, for such a lifestyle is inconsistent with optimal performance. In general, the physical working capacity of alcoholics is lower than healthy nonalcoholic matched controls, which may be related to a variety of factors, including depressed myocardial function in the alcoholics (Lundin et al., 1986).

MARIJUANA

Marijuana, as commonly used, contains the shredded, dried leaves, flowers, and stems from the cannabis sativa plant. Cannabis sativa contains 426 different chemical entities, and 60 of these are cannabinoids (Dewey, 1986). However, of all the chemicals in marijuana, only delta-9-tetrahydrocannabinol (THC) has psychoactive properties in significant amounts (Agurell et al., 1986).

Although marijuana is usually smoked, it may be taken orally, e.g., as baked in chocolate cookies. In typical smoked marijuana the content of THC varies with the ratio of the flowers (containing more THC) to the leaves and is approximately 0.3–3.0%; in hashish, which is the resin from the female flowers, the THC content is approximately 10% (Agurell et al., 1986). A typical 1.5 g marijuana cigarette with 1.5% THC contains approximately 21 mg THC.

Within minutes of marijuana smoking, THC appears in the blood. The peak physiological and subjective effects occur within approximately 30 min, and may last 2–4 h. When marijuana is consumed orally, it may take 30–120 min for THC to reach peak plasma levels. The average plasma clearance values for THC are high because THC is highly lipid soluble; it rapidly enters the brain and adipose tissues, and is quickly metabolized to other THC metabolites. Metabolites of THC are excreted in both the urine and feces, but fecal excretion is the major excretion route in man (Agurell et al., 1986). The fact that THC may be gradually released by the adipose tissues into the circulation may be related to the psychoactive effects sometimes observed much later than the acute psychoactive period. The terminal half-life of THC is in the range of 24–36 h, but its metabolites may be present in the urine for 4–10 d after a single cigarette and for weeks after cessation of chronic use (Agurell et al., 1986; United States Olympic Committee, 1988).

Theoretical Ergogenic and Ergolytic Considerations

Although marijuana, like alcohol, may elicit both stimulant and depressant effects, there is little documented evidence that athletes have used marijuana as an ergogenic aid. It has not been banned by the International Olympic Committee (IOC) or the United States Olympic Committee (USOC), but it is banned by National Governing Bodies for many sports and may be tested for at their request (United States Olympic Committee, 1988). The National Collegiate Athletic Association (NCAA) does ban the use of marijuana, presumably due to its illegality (National Collegiate Athletic Association, 1988).

Marijuana primarily affects the central nervous system. Although its mechanisms of action are poorly understood (Martin, 1986), it has been hypothesized to influence the activity of numerous brain neurotransmitters, including norepinephrine, serotonin, dopamine, gamma aminobutyric acid, acetylcholine, and endorphins. It has been suggested that marijuana alters synthesis or uptake of one or more of these chemicals by various brain substructures, including the cortex, limbic system, and hypothalamus (Dewey, 1986; Turkanis & Karler, 1981; Wadler & Hainline, 1989) Marijuana may also cause neural membrane perturbation and receptor interactions (Martin, 1986) or influence spinal reflexes (Turkanis & Karler, 1981).

Marijuana is recognized as a psychoactive drug, but the behavioral responses to marijuana are influenced by a variety of factors such as expectancy, preexisting mood, setting in which it is consumed, personality, and previous exposure (Mathew et al., 1989). The dosage of THC also exerts a significant effect upon behavioral responses (Dewey, 1986), as do related factors such as time used for smoking, puff duration, volume inhaled, and the time of holding the breath after smoking (Agurell et al., 1986).

Turkanis and Karler (1981), Martin (1986), and Dewey (1986) summarized the available literature by noting that although any cannabinoid can effect a wide variety of neuropharmacologic responses in the brain, the data generally indicate that THC exerts a relatively nonselective complex mixture of excitatory and depressant effects on the CNS. The effects appear to be dose-dependent. Dewey (1986) noted that the behavioral changes are characterized at low doses by a unique mixture of depressant and stimulatory effects and at higher doses predominantly by CNS depression. Often, CNS stimulation is seen at the higher doses prior to depression, which could be comparable to the biphasic effect reported with alcohol ingestion. Martin (1986) further notes that low doses of THC are capable of producing the psychoactivity that is unique to cannabinoids, whereas higher doses may produce effects that are both specific (psychoactive) and nonspecific (general depression) for cannabinoids; unfortunately it has not been possible to establish the concentration of THC at its site of action that is necessary to produce a given pharmacological effect.

Potential Ergogenic Effects. The psychological stimulant effect of marijuana could be theorized to be ergogenic because euphoria, excitement, and enhancement of the senses are characteristic of the cannabinoid syndrome (Dewey, 1986; Mathew et al., 1989; Wadler & Hainline, 1989). Such effects may be beneficial in sports that rer-quire psychological arousal. Marijuana may also elicit a physiological response characteristic of stimulant drugs. For instance, Renaud and Cormier (1986) suggested that marijuana may be a sympathomimetic agent that possibly causes bronchodilation, increased blood flow to the muscle, and a decrease in the perception of dyspnea. They suggested that these effects may be related to increased plasma norepinephrine levels.

One of the consistent acute effects of marijuana is an elevated resting heart rate (Hollister, 1986). The heart rate increase noted in several recent studies ranged from 18–32 beats/min (Capriotti et al., 1988; Foltin et al., 1987; Steadward & Singh, 1975). The increases were greater than those observed after smoking a placebo cigarette (Chait et al., 1988). The increased heart rate is often used as an indicator of THC psychoactivity (Heishman et al., 1988). Agurell and others (1986) noted that the effects of THC on heart rate appear to be independent of the psychoactive effects, because propranolol can block the heart rate acceleration without altering the marijuana-induced euphoria.

On the other hand, marijuana may also elicit a feeling of calm and relaxation (Wadler & Hainline, 1989) that could benefit performance in sports where excessive anxiety might impair performance.

Potential Ergolytic Effects. Several of the psychological effects elicited by marijuana may be ergolytic. Possible adverse behavioral manifestations include panic attacks, paranoia, anxiety, lethargy, drowsiness, distortion of visual perception, and a decrease in attention span, concentration, and memory (Hollister,1986; Mathew et al., 1989; Wadler & Hainline, 1989).

Although one of the reported effects of marijuana is to induce a state of calm and relaxation (Wadler & Hainline, 1989) that might reduce tension in shooting competition, Dewey (1986) noted that the depressant effects of the psychotomimetic cannabinoids differ from the depression induced by other CNS depressants because they may cause a state of hyperreflexia or hyperstimulation during the depressive portion of the cannabinoid syndrome. Moreover, marijuana may increase anxiety in inexperienced smokers (Mathew et al., 1989). Thus, the use of marijuana may be contraindicated as an ergogenic aid for such sports competition.

Marijuana may also induce physiological responses counterproductive to sports performance. Several adverse effects upon the respiratory system, including bronchitis and brochospasm, have been reported (Hollister, 1986), especially with heavy use (Tashkin et al., 1976). Wu and others (1988) reported a significant increase in carboxyhemoglobin saturation, i.e., nearly a five-fold greater increment in the blood carboxyhemoglobin level, which could impair oxygen transport (Biron & Wells, 1983) and lead to a decrease in aerobic performance (Renaud & Cormier, 1986). Hollister (1986) also noted that orthostatic hypotension could result at high doses.

Effects on Sports-related Performance

Psychomotor Effects. In one of the earliest studies, Clark and Nakashima (1968) noted complex (choice) reaction time was consistently impaired with marijuana use. Heishman and others (1988) reported minimal performance impairment with low doses, but Hollister (1986), summarizing the many studies that have used acute doses of marijuana or THC to study various psychomotor functions, concluded that if the dose of the drug was high enough or the task difficult enough, impairments were shown. Several other reviews have also noted that marijuana or THC elicited significant decrements on a wide variety of psychomotor measures (Bird et al., 1980; Biron & Wells, 1983; Mathew et al., 1989; National Institute of Drug Abuse, 1980; Wadler & Hainline, 1989).

The ergolytic effects of marijuana upon performance may be prolonged. Even 24 h after smoking 19 mg THC, 10 experienced airplane pilots experienced trends toward impairment on a number of psychomotor variables associated with aircraft operation (Yesavage et al., 1985). If these findings could be extrapolated to tennis and other sports involving complex motor skills, marijuana smoking could be contraindicated during the competitive season or at least the day prior to competition.

It should also be noted that although both alcohol and marijuana separately may impair psychomotor performance, the combination of the two social drugs appears to lead to further deterioration of basic psychomotor skills (Bird et al., 1980; Chesher et al., 1976) and of skills related to automobile operation (Perez-Reyes et al., 1988).

Aerobic Endurance. The tachycardia effected by marijuana may impair performance in aerobic endurance tests that are based upon submaximal heart rate responses. Steadward and Singh (1975) reported that acute marijuana smoking decreased physical working capacity as evaluated by the PWC_{170} submaximal exercise test on the cycle ergometer. This test predicts physical working capacity based upon the heart rate response to several submaximal workloads and does not actually measure maximal work output. The effect that marijuana smoking had upon the resting heart rate, increasing it by over 30 beats per minute, could account for the predicted decrease in physical work capacity. Shapiro and associates (1976), using a progressive exercise test, found that marijuana decreased exercise tolerance compared to the control condition. Since this test was also based upon heart rate responses, the authors hypothesized that the effects were due to a marijuana-caused tachycardia, leading to an earlier attainment of peak heart rate compared to exercise alone.

Marijuana does not appear to affect adversely the physiological responses to maximal exercise, but it may impair performance. Shapiro and colleagues (1976) reported that 20 mg of THC had no effect on minute ventilation, oxygen uptake, carbon dioxide production, or respiratory quotient during a submaximal or maximal exercise task. Renaud and Cormier (1986) reported no effect upon peak oxygen uptake, pulmonary ventilation, or heart rate, during a maximal exercise task 10 min after smoking the equivalent of 7 mg THC. However, they found that the marijuana led to a significant 6.2% decrease in time to exhaustion on a cycle ergometer, which the authors suggested was due to a premature attainment of maximal heart rate and possible adverse effects of carbon monoxide.

Social Use and Athletic Performance

The use of marijuana for medicinal purposes ar d for its psychoactive effects has a long history, being used over 2,000 y ago by the Chinese and in the early Grecian era. Its use as a social drug gradually evolved westward, being used by the Aztec Indians in Mexico as part of their culture, and eventually gravitated to the United States, where it was declared an illegal drug in 1937. Marijuana consumption was relatively limited until the counterculture revolution of the 1960s, but now its use as a social drug is firmly established and is considered to be the main illicit drug problem in the United States and other Western countries (Hollister, 1986; Mendelson, 1987).

Although marijuana use had increased dramatically throughout the 1960s and 1970s, recent surveys among high school seniors show a significant drop in the past decade; reports of marijuana use within the preceding year decreased from 49% to 36% from 1980 to 1988, while reports of daily use dropped from 9% to 3% (Johnston & Bachman, 1988). Since previous research has shown no appreciable differences between high school athletes and nonathletes relative to marijuana use (Williams & Jackson, 1975), it might be assumed that a decreased use by athletes paralleled the overall decreased use by high school seniors. A recent study emanating from Michigan State University (Anderson & McKeag, 1985), revealed that marijuana use among athletes involved in NCAA competition was 36% during the previous year, i.e., a rate very similar to that of the high school seniors. Wadler and Hainline (1989), reporting results of the Elite Women Athletes Survey, noted that 17% of the respondents had used mariujuana in the past year, while only 3% of Olympic caliber athletes used it prior to competition.

Chronic marijuana use may impair training effects, both psychologically and physiologically. Biron and Wells (1983) noted that an amotivational syndrome may occur, characterized by apathy and loss of motivation. Such an effect may impair the psychological ability to train effectively. Bracker and others (1987), reporting a case study of a college wrestler who smoked marijuana for 5 y and developed unilateral gynecomastia, suggested that the cause may be related to the reported effect of marijuana use to decrease serum testosterone levels. Since adequate levels of testosterone may be necessary for maximizing the training response, physiological adaptations to training may be impaired. In summary, based upon the available research, particularly the potential ergolytic effects of marijuana, the social use of marijuana is contraindicated for athletes in training or competition.

BETA BLOCKERS

The human stress response evolved as a major force in the preservation of the species, but it is also invoked during exercise, particularly during intense exercise. The stress response is mediated primarily via the sympathetic nervous system, which stimulates the release of the catecholamines, i.e., norepinephrine from the sympathetic nerve endings and both norepinephrine and epinephrine from the medullary portion of the adrenal gland. The sympathetic system exerts its effects through various adrenergic receptors—the α-adrenergic receptors and β_1 and β_2 β-adrenergic receptors. Harrison (1985) noted that the adrenergic receptor is a specialized protein in the cell membrane linked to the catalytic moiety of adenylate cyclase, an enzyme that causes the intracellular accumulation of cyclic adenosine 3,5- monophospate (cAMP) and a sequence of events characteristic of the particular cell. Norepinephrine excites mainly the α receptors, but also has a slight effect on the β receptors, whereas epinephrine excites both classes equally well. Shepherd (1985) further notes that the β_1 receptors are activated primarily by norepinephrine released by the sympathetic nerves, and the β_2 receptors are activated by circulating epinephrine from the adrenal medulla. Although the metabolic functions of these receptors are quite complex and many tissues may have several receptor types, the following represent the essential points for this discussion.

The primary response to α-receptor stimulation is peripheral vasoconstriction (Guyton, 1986), although an increased inotropy in the myocardium also may occur (Charlap et al., 1989). Stimulation of β_1 receptors in the heart will increase both the heart rate and contractile force, whereas stimulation of β_1 receptors in adipose tissue will facilitate the release of free-fatty-acids into the blood. Stimulation of β_2 receptors will elicit bronchial dilation in the lungs, peripheral arteriolar vasodilation, glycogenolysis in both liver and muscle, and increased contractility in the muscle (Guyton, 1986; Shepherd, 1985; Wadler & Hainline, 1989).

During exercise, the general response to sympathetic stimulation is an increased cardiac output via an increase in both heart rate and stroke volume, an increased blood flow to the active muscles, a decreased blood flow to the splanchnic organs and inactive muscles, an increased venous return, an increased arterial blood pressure, increased lipolysis and serum free-fatty-acid levels, increased liver glycogenolysis and serum glucose concentration, increased muscle glycogenolysis and contractile force, and increased cellular metabolism throughout the body (Charlap et al., 1989; Guyton, 1986).

These physiological adjustments can support energy production during strenuous exercise. On the other hand, the increased stress on the cardiovascular system, e.g., the increased myocardial oxygen demand due to increased cardiac performance could compromise the health of an individual with cardiovascular disease or hypertension. Thus, medical researchers have developed a variety of drugs to block adrenergic activity in attempts to mitigate the adverse stress response effects on individuals with compromised cardiovascular functions. Drugs such as reserpine were useful, but possessed serious side effects. However, the early 1960s saw the advent of the first beta blockers, drugs that would mitigate the adrenergic effect of the catecholamines with fewer side effects (Harrison, 1985). Propranolol was one of the first to be used extensively, but more than a dozen other generic types have been developed in the intervening years. Kostis and Rosen (1987), Kelly (1985), and Tesch (1985) have noted that there is considerable variation in the phamacodynamic characteristics of the beta blockers currently available. Some beta-blockers possess an ancillary property known as intrinsic sympathomimetic activity (ISA). These ISA agents have partial beta agonistic activity, so the heart rate is attenuated to a lesser extent compared to agents without ISA. Selectivity is another major ancillary property. Nonselective beta blockers block both β_1 and β_2 adrenergic receptors, whereas selective beta blockers, often called cardioselective blockers, block primarily the β_1 receptors with minimal effects upon the β_2 receptors (Kelly, 1985). However, Wadler and Hainline (1989) noted that at high doses the selective beta blockers lose some of their selectivity. Table 9-3 provides a list of some common beta blockers and the major ancillary properties.

Beta blockers are used widely to treat a variety of cardiovascular disorders (Kaplan, 1983; Wilmore, 1988), and are even considered by some to be the first choice of drugs in this regard (Tesch, 1985). Also, because exercise is often prescribed as adjunct therapy in the treatment of cardiovascular disease and hypertension, the interaction of beta blockers and exercise performance has been studied extensively and has been the subject of several major reviews (Chick et al., 1988; Harrison et al., 1985; Tesch, 1985; van Baak, 1988; Wilmore, 1988).

Theoretical Ergogenic and Ergolytic Considerations

Beta blockers may be classified as depressants, although Gengo and others (1987) observed that the precise site of the pharmacologic activity for the sedative effect is not known. Nevertheless, as with alcohol, this tranquilizing effect may be ergogenic in nature. However, these drugs may also possess very potent ergolytic effects for some athletes.

Several groups of athletes, such as ballet dancers, archers, bowlers, marksmen, and ski jumpers, as well as other performance-oriented individuals such as musicians, have been alleged to take beta blockers as a means of reducing anxiety during performance; this could be construed as an ergogenic effect. On the other hand, some athletes may need to take beta blockers to help control hypertension, and they may experience ergolytic effects.

Potential Ergogenic Effects. The major ergogenic application of

TABLE 9-3. *Common Beta Blockers and Major Ancillary Properties*

Generic Name	Beta-1 Selectivity	Intrinsic Sympathomimetic Activity
Acebutolol	Yes	Yes
Alprenolol	No	Yes
Atenolol	Yes	No
Labetalol	No	No
Metoprolol	Yes	No
Nadolol	No	No
Oxprenolol	No	Yes
Pindolol	No	Yes
Propranolol	No	No
Sotalol	No	No
Timolol	No	No

beta blockers has been attributed to its anxiolytic, bradycardic, and antitremor effects (Wadler & Hainline, 1989). Cole (1978) observed that tremor, palpitations, and sweating are symptoms of anxiety, often characterized as a panic attack or stage fright, which could adversely affect performance in precision events. Since excessive catecholamine release may cause tachycardia and muscle tremor and furthur increase anxiety (James et al., 1977), it is not surprising that some athletes have been using beta blockers as an aid to performance (Tesch, 1985). Rogers (1984) reported that beta blockers could be used as an ergogenic aid by athletes in shooting sports. Since the mechanical force of the myocardial contraction may move the body slightly, the bradycardic effect of the beta blockers would provide the shooters with more time to steady their aim between heart beats. Wadler and Hainline (1989) suggested that athletes may use beta blockers to improve hand steadiness.

Some endurance athletes may be using beta blockers to enhance their physiological adaptations to training, and hence to improve performance in competition. Although this topic does not appear to have been adequately researched, the theory is interesting. For example, Kelly (1985) noted that treatment with beta blockers results in an increased density of beta receptors, referred to as receptor up-regulation. He indicated that the long term consequences of the increased beta receptor density are not yet clear, although the suggestion that it is related to a rebound effect of sudden withdrawal from beta blockers is well known. Kelly also indicated that training itself may lead to a decrease in beta receptor density. Thus, one may hypothesize that if beta blockers were used during training, the athlete might increase the number of beta receptors, or at least minimize the loss of these receptors during training. Upon discontinuing the use of beta blockers there may be an exaggerated response to the sympathetic discharge during intense exercise associated with competition. Some associated research supports this theory. Subjects who trained for 14 weeks improved their maximal oxygen uptake, but only after medication with propranolol was stopped at the conclusion of the training period (Ewy et al., 1983; Wilmore et al., 1985A). However, this theory has not been adequately researched relative to any ergogenic potential.

Because of their ergogenic potential, beta blockers are banned by the IOC and the NCAA (National Collegiate Athletic Association, 1988; United States Olympic Committee, 1988.)

Potential Ergolytic Effects. Beta blockers may be ergolytic in a variety of ways. The CNS side effects include tiredness, fatigue, lethargy and depression (Kelly, 1985), all psychological effects that could impair training or competitive performance. Using the Profile of Mood States, Kostis and Rosen (1987) reported a decrease in vigor following the use of pindolol and propranolol.

To most athletes, particularly endurance athletes, the ergolytic effects of beta blockers would be related primarily to the potential blockade of the normal sympathetic or adrenergic response to intense exercise. Given the physiological actions noted previously, beta blockers could attenuate the cardiovascular adjustments to exercise by decreasing cardiac output and reducing muscle blood flow, impairing ventilatory responses, interferring with the optimal utilization of liver glycogen, muscle glycogen, serum glucose, and serum free-fatty-acids, impairing temperature regulation, and adversely affecting potassium metabolism (Eichner, 1989; Opie, 1985). All such effects could facilitate the development of fatigue.

Effects on Sports-related Performance

Although the data available to support an ergogenic effect of beta blockers are limited, the results suggest they may be useful in several sports. On the other hand, substantial research data support an ergolytic effect for other classes of athletes, particularly those involved in aerobic endurance sports.

Psychomotor Performance. Since beta blockers may be classified as depressants, they may be hypothesized to impair psychomotor performance. However, following a review of the available literature, Glaister (1981) and Tesch (1985) concluded that psychomotor performance was not negatively affected by beta blockade. More recent data have supported this conclusion, as Kostis and Rosen (1987) found no significant effects of propranolol upon visual and auditory reaction time or upon results of a complex psychomotor test. On the other hand, in a major review article regarding the neuropsychological side effects of beta blockers, Dimsdale and associates (1989) evaluated 55 studies with 249 observations, noting that the studies contained an extraordinary variety of drug doses and cognitive test batteries. Although the results were generally inconsistent, the authors noted that relative to psychomotor functioning, there is some evidence that beta blockers impair reaction time.

Strength, Power and Local Muscular Endurance. There appears to be little effect of beta blockers on exercise tasks characterized by strength or power, although more prolonged anaerobic exercise bouts may be adversely affected. Kaiser (1984), in a review of his own research, concluded that beta blockers exerted no effect upon muscular strength or 5-s power output. Tesch (1985) reiterated these points relative to sedentary and athletic populations, but indicated that these effects possibly may not be extrapolated to highly competitive strength and power athletes, such as weightlifters or powerlifters. Since glycogen metabolism in the muscle may be impaired by beta blockers, performance in supramaximal tasks relying upon anaerobic glycolysis may deteriorate. Kaiser (1984) reported that anaerobic endurance tasks in the range of 30–60 s were negatively affected by beta blockers. Tesch (1985) also noted that static endurance could be impaired.

Precision Sports. Other than the treatment of cardiovascular disease and hypertension, one of the earliest uses of beta blockers was for treatment of benign essential tremor; in its initial years, Dupont and others (1973) concluded that propranolol was the best drug known for this purpose. Several years later James and colleagues (1977), noting that many musicians have used alcohol and sedatives to stem the adverse effects of anxiety, used a double-blind, placebo study to reveal that oxprenolol could significantly reduce both tremor and nervousness in musicians. These results in musicians were recently confirmed as Brantigan and others (1982) reported that beta blockers reduced the level of anxiety, as measured by the State-Trait Anxiety Inventory, and improved the quality of musical performance as evaluated by judges.

As might be expected, however, beta blockers were applied to sport even earlier. Recognizing that excess anxiety may disrupt performance in precision sports, Imhof et al. (1969) studied the effects of oxprenolol in ski-jumpers. Oxprenolol decreased the emotional heart rate response prior to the jump by 34%, but the authors noted that the elimination of the emotional tachycardia by beta blockade does not necessarily lead to an improvement in physical performance of short duration such as ski-jumping. Videman et al. (1979), also studying ski-jumpers, hypothesized that if the tachycardia is taken as a reflection of excessive sympathetic activity, this may disturb the take-off of the jump, which requires exact timing and a high degree of muscle coordination. They suggested that beta blockade may remove most of the symptoms, and the improvement in six of nine jumpers was significant enough to make an important difference in competition. In this 1979 study they noted that the results provided furthur evidence for the possible use of beta-blocking agents in different situations of emotional tension, but they qualified their findings by suggesting that there were no scientific grounds yet for the use of beta blockers in sports like ski-jumping.

Several studies investigated the effect of beta blockers on pistol shooting competition. Using members of the British National Squad in pistol shooting as subjects, Antal and Good (1980) used two different doses of oxprenolol (40 mg and 80 mg) 60 min prior to shooting. Subjects were tested in both slow and fast shooting, and the heart rate was monitored continuously. During slow fire with the

40 mg dose, the mean score was 2.9 points higher with oxprenolol, with 13 of the 20 subjects firing better. With the 80 mg dose, the score was 3.4 points higher, with 16 of the 20 subjects scoring higher. Nervousness before firing was significantly lower with the 80 mg dose; heart rate decreased 11–16 beats/min. Only the 40 mg dose was tested in the rapid fire, and no beneficial effects were observed. The authors noted that because the shooter makes the decision when to shoot in slow fire, the tension developed is greater; in rapid fire the range warden sets the pace of shooting so the tension is lower. The improvement was seen most in those with the lowest scores, who also had the highest heart rates. Kruse and others (1986), using 33 amateur skilled pistol marksmen as subjects, reported that metoprolol improved shooting performance by 13.4%. Although they noted that the emotional increases in heart rate and blood pressure normally observed in shooting competition were mitigated by beta blockers, there was no correlation between the shooting improvement and changes in heart rate and systolic blood pressure. They suggested that the shooting improvement was an effect of the beta blockers on reducing hand tremor.

For beta blockers to be effective in precision sports, the dose may be a critical factor. Tesch (1985) supported this viewpoint, noting in his review that the individual bowlers whose performance was improved during blockade with oxprenolol had higher heart rates before, during, and after competition as compared with those bowlers whose performance did not benefit during blockade. Additionally, Tesch noted that in pistol shooters who did not improve their total score, the heart rate did not increase during shooting under blockade, while those who did improve had a favorable heart rate increase of 10 beats/min. Videman and others (1979) reported that the three ski-jumpers who failed to improve their performance had greater decreases in the heart rate. Thus, the comment by James and others (1977) that some degree of apprehension may be essential for a good musical performance may also be true of athletes. An excessive depressive effect of beta blockers may be counterproductive in precision sports, as suggested by the familiar inverted U hypothesis relating anxiety to performance.

Aerobic Endurance. The effects of beta blockers upon aerobic endurance have been studied extensively. Although the central nervous system side effects such as a general sensation of tiredness, fatigue, and decreased vigor (Kelly 1985; Kostis & Rosen, 1987) could impair aerobic function, this brief review will focus upon physiological and performance effects. It should be noted, however, that for several physiological and performance variables measured, the research results are not consistent. Wilmore et al. (1985b) offered several explanations for this inconsistency, including mode of exercise, the specific drug, method of administration, time lag between last drug dose and the exercise test, and type of subject population. Moreover, Lowenthal and others (1987) noted that there is marked interindividual variability of beta blocking effects. Nevertheless, several general conclusions appear to be evident relative to the overall effects of beta blockers on aerobic endurance variables, including comparative effects of selective versus nonselective agents.

Physiological Effects. The major physiological processes studied in relation to submaximal and maximal aerobic endurance exercise include heart rate, stroke volume, cardiac output, arteriovenous oxygen difference, muscle blood flow, pulmonary ventilation, and oxygen uptake. The most consistent finding is a significant reduction in exercise heart rate during all levels of exercise, often 50–70 beats/min lower during maximal exercise (Anderson et al., 1985; Bevilacqua et al., 1989; Bugni et al., 1989; El-Sayed & Davies, 1989; Jilka et al., 1988; Morton et al., 1989; Tesch, 1985; Wilmore et al., 1985b).

During submaximal exercise the stroke volume appears to increase under blockade (Joyner et al., 1986; Tesch, 1985). Wilmore (1988) observed that the stroke volume is increased in almost direct proportion to the decrease in heart rate, allowing the cardiac output to remain almost unchanged or only slightly reduced in submaximal exercise, even up to levels of 75% $\dot{V}O_2$max in either hypertensive subjects (Martin et al., 1989) or trained subjects (Scruggs, et al., Research Note). Research by Wilmore's group strongly supports the finding that the stroke volume will compensate for the decreased heart rate during submaximal exercise in order to maintain a normal cardiac output. Some studies have shown reductions in stroke volume (Ades et al., 1989) and cardiac output (Bevilacqua et al., 1989) during submaximal exercise, but oxygen consumption does not appear to be compromised. Tesch (1985) suggested that the arteriovenous oxygen difference may increase to compensate for any change in cardiac output. When observed, decreased oxygen consumption during submaximal exercise may be the result of increased metabolic efficiency associated with a higher R value, i.e., increased reliance on carbohydrate (Tesch, 1985).

Although several studies have revealed no significant impairment of cardiac output (Bevilacqua et al., 1989) or oxygen uptake (El-Sayed & Davies, 1989; Wilmore et al., 1985b) during maximal exercise, most of the key investigators in this area have concluded that physiological functions such as pulmonary ventilation, cardiac output, muscle blood flow and oxygen uptake are impaired by beta blockers during intense, maximal exercise (Golightly & Sutherland, 1985; Kaiser, 1984; MacFarlane et al., 1983; Opie, 1985; Tesch, 1985;

van Baak et al., 1988; Wilmore, 1988). Significant impairments have been especially noted in highly trained runners (Anderson et al., 1985; Joyner et al., 1986). Wilmore (1988), summarizing more than 8 y of research in his laboratory and other available literature, noted that beta blockers may improve maximal physiological functioning in angina patients, have little or no effect upon persons of average or below average fitness, and exert a detrimental effect on the highly trained individual. He suggested that the trained athlete may not be able to compensate for the reduced maximal heart rate by an increased stroke volume, while others may.

Beta blockers may exert other deleterious effects during maximal exercise. Optimal supply and utilization of carbohydrate and fat may be impaired. Opie (1985) and Karlsson (1985) noted that beta blockade may inhibit phosphorylase activity; thus, hepatic glycogenolysis may be impaired, resulting in a more marked decrease of blood glucose during exercise, while a decreased rate of glycogen breakdown in the skeletal muscle may also occur. Although Opie (1985) stated that the evidence for such an inhibition is still only indirect, Lundborg and others (1981) reported decreased blood glucose levels during exercise following beta blockade. Chasiotis and associates (1983) also reported that beta blockers prevented the rise in cAMP and decreased the rate of glycogen degradation normally seen in muscle during exercise. The authors suggested that the effect was related to changes in the phosphorylase-synthetase system. Furthermore, beta blockade reportedly decreases maximal respiratory exchange ratios (Anderson et al., 1985) and impairs lactate production (Tesch, 1985); both of these observations suggest a reduced rate of glycolysis. Additionally, Tesch (1985) reported that the contribution of free-fatty-acids as an energy source in both short term and prolonged exercise is attenuted during beta blockade, an effect which may be more prevalent in exercise-trained individuals (Jesek et al., Research Note).

Problems with temperature regulation and electrolyte balance may also occur as an effect of beta blockade. Freund and others (1987) reported impaired performance in the heat with beta blockade, noting significantly lower skin blood flow and mean skin temperature following propranolol; proper temperature regulation was apparantly being compromised to maintain central venous blood pressure. Adverse effects of propranolol on transfer of heat to the skin reportedly caused elevated core temperatures in both normal (Pescatello et al., 1987) and hypertensive subjects (Pescatello et al., 1990). Crouse and Moritani (1988) reported significant increases in EMG amplitude and significant decreases in mean EMG power frequency in the vastus lateralis following beta blockade. These changes in electromyographical activity were indicative of increased fatigue. Such EMG changes may be related to cellular potassium losses because the rate of rise in serum potassium is significantly higher during beta blockade (Gullestad et al., 1988). Although Lowenthal et al. (1987) noted that the hyperkalemic effects may occur only upon initial treatment, Wilmore (1988) suggested that changes in muscle and plasma potassium concentration with endurance exercise seem to be an important consideration for future research because the constant leakage of potassium from the muscle is accentuated with beta blockade use and may be responsible for fatigue by altering cell membrane potential.

Performance Effects. It is generally recognized that beta blockers may enhance aerobic endurance performance in angina patients (Powles, 1981; Wilmore, 1988). Early research suggested that beta blockers might also be ergogenic for others. Using dogs as subjects, Barnard and Foss (1969) reported that propranolol reduced oxygen consumption and oxygen debt during treadmill running. They raised the interesting point that the dogs had greater mechanical efficiency under the propranolol condition. Following 10 mg of propranolol, healthy boys could perform submaximal and maximal exercise with a significantly lower heart rate and blood lactate, indicative of enhanced oxygen utilization by the muscle (Thoren, 1967). The children also indicated that the work seemed subjectively easier. On the other hand, a review by Furburg (1968) noted that the capacity to perform heavy work decreases among athletes during beta blockade, and Williams (1974) concluded that beta blockers are not ergogenic for endurance athletes.

More recent laboratory studies support the conclusion that beta blockers may impair endurance performance. Beta blockers decreased time to exhaustion at 70% (van Baak et al., 1987) or 50% (Lundborg et al., 1981) of VO_2max, or during a progressive exercise test to exhaustion (El-Sayed & Davies, 1989). Even the use of eye drops containing the beta blocker, timolol, has decreased time to exhaustion in maximal tests (Doyle et al., 1984; Leier et al., 1986).

Additionally, beta blockers have impaired performance in several field studies. These drugs caused slower running times over 2 km (Kaiser, 1984) and 10 km (Anderson et al., 1985). Other experiments and extensive reviews have also concluded that beta blockers may be ergolytic (Juhlin-Dannfelt, 1983; Opie, 1985; Powles, 1981; Schnabel et al., 1983; Tesch, 1985; Wilmore, 1988).

Selective versus Nonselective Agents. Various studies have compared the effects of different beta blockers, particularly nonselective and cardioselective beta blockers and those with ISA, upon physiological responses to exercise. As might be anticipated, the cardioselective and ISA beta blockers, although attenuating some of the sympathetic responses to exercise, generally exerted lesser deleterious effects than the nonselective blockers.

According to Tesch (1985), the cardiovascular effects of beta blockade are achieved equally with both selective and nonselective agents. He noted that the resting heart rate is equally reduced by propranolol and atenolol (β_1 selective) but that the maximal heart rate is decreased more by the nonselective propranolol compared to atenolol. Joyner and others (1986) supported this finding, particularly in trained individuals. Tesch (1985) and Joyner et al. (1986) also observed that the stroke volume response during submaximal and maximal exercise is of similar magnitude when comparing cardioselective and nonselective blockade at equipotent doses.

Kelly (1985) and Wilmore (1988) reported that beta blockers with ISA attenuate the heart rate decrease to a lesser extent, but Wilmore noted that the ISA activity's diminished at higher levels of exercise intensity. In recent research from Wilmore's laboratory, there were no significant differences in cardiac output between propranolol and pindolol up to an exercise intensity of 75% of $\dot{V}O_2$max in subjects who were either hypertensive (Martin et al., 1989) or highly trained (Scruggs et al., Research Note), although the stroke volume was significantly higher and the heart rate somewhat lower with propranolol compared to pindolol. On the other hand, Ades et al. (1989) reported that at 70% of $\dot{V}O_2$max, propranolol decreased cardiac output by approximately 15%, whereas pindolol with ISA did not.

Joyner et al. (1987) reported that ventilatory capacity during maximal exercise was decreased more by propranolol than by atenolol, suggesting that the result was due to an attenuation of tidal volume with nonselective blockade of the β_2 receptor-mediated bronchodilation that normally occurs during exercise. Ades et al. (1989) indicated that muscle blood flow was not adversely affected by either propranolol or pindolol with ISA, but Lowenthal et al. (1987) reported less peripheral vasoconstriction with the cardioselective antagonists.

In total, these differences in physiological responses to various agents suggest that $\dot{V}O_2$max is impaired more with nonselective agents. Although research generally supports this viewpoint, the findings are somewhat inconsistent. In earlier research, Wilmore et al. (1985b) and Kaiser (1984) reported no differences between nonselective and cardioselective agents on $\dot{V}O_2$max, but Lundborg et al. (1981) reported lesser deleterious effects of β_1 blockers. In more recent research from Wilmore's group (Jilka et al., 1988; Joyner et al., 1986) propranolol caused greater reductions in $\dot{V}O_2$max compared to atenolol, particularly so in trained individuals.

Relative to carbohydrate and fat metabolism, Lundborg et al. (1981) reported greater blood glucose decreases under propranolol versus metopolol, and Hespel et al. (1986), comparing a β_1 blocker and a β_2 blocker, found that the β_2 blocker prevented the rise in blood glucose seen during exercise. Tesch (1985) supported this general viewpoint, noting that selective blockers will not reduce the rate of hepatic glycogenolysis. Thus, there could be greater availability of blood glucose during selective versus nonselective blockade. Tesch (1985) suggested that nonselective blockers tend to reduce the rate of muscle glycogen breakdown, but the available data are conflicting. Nevertheless, he did indicate that lactate production is impaired to a greater extent after nonselective than selective blockade.

Tesch (1985) reviewed a number of studies and concluded that the contribution of free-fatty-acids as an energy source in both short term and prolonged exercise is attenuted during both selective and nonselective beta blockade. On the other hand, Hespel et al. (1986) reported that during moderate exercise, the serum free-fatty-acid concentration was lower during β_1 blockade, but under β_2 blockade, the serum triglyceride concentration was not changed. Hall and others (1987) also observed that propranolol reduced the exercise-induced rise in serum free-fatty-acid concentrations, but metoprolol had little effect and produced free-fatty-acid profiles that were similar to those under placebo treatment.

In a summary of the literature, Opie (1985) suggested that cardioselective agents have less effect than nonselective agents in producing metabolic impairment during sustained exercise. Possibly reflective of the smaller adverse effects of cardioselective beta blockers, Tesch (1985) observed a lower rating of perceived exertion (RPE) during exercise under cardioselective blockade when compared to the use of nonselective blockers.

Although endurance performance is impaired by all beta blockers, the adverse effects appear to be fewer with the cardioselective agents (Tesch, 1985). Compared to the nonselective beta blockers, research has shown that the β_1 blockers exert lesser deleterious effects upon time to exhaustion at 50% of $\dot{V}O_2$max (Lundborg et al., 1981) or during progressive maximal exercise tests (Gullestad et al., 1988; Kaiser et al., 1985). Furthermore, Anderson et al. (1985) found that runners averaged 36 min for 10 km on placebo, 39 min on atenolol, and 41 min on propranolol.

Adding ISA to cardioselective beta blockers appears to convey no additional advantage. Two recent studies revealed that although cardioselective beta blockers both with and without ISA impaired performance in maximal endurance capacity tests and submaximal exercise tolerance, there were no significant differences between the two types of drugs (Kullmer et al., 1987; van Baak et al., 1986).

In summary, the fatiguing effects of beta blockers upon aerobic endurance performance have been associated with impaired cardiovascular responses that reduced oxygen and substrate delivery to the muscles, impairment of substrate metabolism in the muscle, and shifts in electrolytes, particularly potassium (Opie, 1985; Gullestad et al., 1988). The mechanism underlying the less adverse effects of cardioselective beta blockers on endurance performance has not been completely elucidated, but has been associated with lesser decreases in maximal heart rate and maximal oxygen consumption (Anderson et al., 1985), less attenuation of maximal ventilation (Joyner et al., 1987), less peripheral vasoconstriction (Lowenthal et al., 1987), and smaller decreases in liver glycogenolysis (Tesch, 1985), blood glucose (Lundborg et al., 1981; Opie, 1985), muscle glycogenolysis (Tesch, 1985), and muscle glycolysis (Kaiser, 1984). Each of these effects may result in fewer subjective complaints (Anderson et al., 1985) and a lower perception of exertional stress during submaximal exercise (Tesch, 1985).

Medical and Social Use and Athletic Performance

Unlike alcohol and marijuana, beta blockers are not classified as social drugs, although a number of performance-oriented individuals, such as musicians, debaters, and others have used beta blockers instead of alcohol to deter the symptoms of stage fright (Brantigan et al., 1982). On the other hand, millions of individuals worldwide use beta blockers for the medical treatment of hypertension, angina and other cardiovascualar disorders (Tesch, 1985). The treatment of these medical disorders is usually multifaceted, and often includes a prescription for aerobic exercise. For example, beta blockers tend to decrease high density lipoprotein cholesterol and increase triglycerides (Lehtonen, 1985), but endurance exercise training may mitigate these effects on the lipid profile (Morton et al., 1989).

Since aerobic exercise is often prescribed as a therapeutic adjunct in the treatment of these medical disorders, and because the sympathetic response to exercise is believed to be important for some of the adaptive responses to exercise training (Tesch, 1985; Williams, R., 1985), an important concern is to minimize the deleterious effects of beta blockers on the training response. Although the subject of whether or not beta blockers prevent an exercise training response is controversial (Chick et al., 1988; Fletcher, 1985; Maksud et al., 1972; Marsh et al., 1983; Sable et al., 1982; Savin et al., 1985;

Wilmore, 1988), it appears that they attenuate the response in some individuals (Ades et al., 1989; Kelly, 1985).

Selective agents appear to have a lesser mitigating effect on the training response (Ades et al., 1989; Tesch, 1985; Wilmore, 1985A). Wilmore (1988) and Tesch (1985) also concluded that cardioselective agents appear to have advantages and should be used with patients who need beta adrenergic blockade and are encouraged to maintain a physically active life-style.

On the other hand, Lowenthal et al. (1987) maintained that with the exception of beta blockers, most drugs taken by patients with cardiovascular disease permit a normal exercise response. In this regard, Eichner (1989) and Lund-Johansen (1987) indicated that it is logical to select an antihypertensive drug that does not reduce exercise capacity when treating physically active patients who have mild to moderate hypertension.

SUMMARY

Although alcohol and beta blockers may enhance performance by reducing tension and tremor in certain precision sports, the overwhelming evidence suggests that these two drugs, plus marijuana, may significantly impair a wide variety of physiological, psychological, and performance variables.

Relative to alcohol, this review supports the general conclusion of the position statement on "The Use of Alcohol in Sports" published by the American College of Sports Medicine (1982) that alcohol has not been shown to improve athletic performance and may actually lead to a deterioration in a variety of events. In those sports where improvement may occur, such as pistol shooting in the pentathlon, alcohol is banned and is therefore illegal. From a medical standpoint, it is important to note that alcohol use contributes to the development of numerous health problems. Drinking more than three drinks per day is associated with cancer, hypertension, hemorrhagic stroke, gouty arthritis, hepatitis, and cirrhosis (National Research Council, 1989; Shils, 1988). Although there is some evidence to suggest that moderate social drinking may convey some health benefits by attenuating the risk of cardiovascular and cerebrovascular disease (Kannel, 1987; Klatsky et al., 1989; Scragg et al., 1987), the relationship of alcohol to the reduced risk of cardiovascular and cerebrovascular disease remains unclear (National Research Council, 1989) On the other hand, moderate social drinking has been associated with increased risk for colorectal cancer (Wu et al., 1987), breast cancer in women (Longnecker et al., 1988; Olson, 1988), osteoporosis (Diamond et al., 1989), and the fetal-alcohol syndrome (Ouellette, 1984).

Marijuana appears to be an ergolytic drug, and its use, even as a social drug, may impair athletic performance. Moreover, its use may be contraindicated for health reasons. Hollister (1986) stated that cannabis is a relatively safe drug as social drugs go, noting that it compares favorably with tobacco and alcohol, but he offered the caveat that the ill effects of those social drugs took a long time to be discovered. Martin (1986) adds that while the cannabinoids do not appear to be highly toxic, it is disconcerting that they seem to exert some alteration in almost every biological sysem that has been studied. Dewey (1986) echoed these thoughts, noting that the state of knowledge is too limited to rule out the possibility that cannabinoids also produce effects on certain peripheral organs. Some adverse health effects have been reported, including a variety of respiratory problems, impairment of cell-mediated immunity, decreased sperm production, and inhibition of ovulation (Hollister, 1986; Wu et al., 1988), not to mention impaired driving ability (National Institute of Drug Abuse, 1980).

Although beta blockers are clearly ergolytic for a wide variety of sports, they may be ergogenic for precision shooting sports. However, like alcohol, their use is illegal for such competition. For athletes with hypertension who must use beta blockers, it is important to select an agent that will produce the least interference with training. Exercise testing appears to be helpful in titrating the dose of beta blocker for such purposes (Powles, 1981).

RESEARCH NOTES

Jesek, J., N. Martin, C. Broeder, E. Thomas, K. Wambsgans, Z. Hofman, J. Ivy, and J. Wilmore. Changes in plasma free fatty acids and glycerol during prolonged exercise in trained and hypertensive individuals taking propranolol and pindolol. Human Performance Laboratory. Department of Kinesiology and Health Education. The University of Texas at Austin, 1990.

Scruggs, K., N. Martin, C. Broeder, Z. Hofman, E. Thomas, K. Wambsgans, and J. Wilmore. β-blockade and stroke volume during submaximal exercise in trained and untrained subjects. Human Performance Laboratory. Department of Kinesiology and Health Education. The University of Texas at Austin, 1990.

BIBLIOGRAPHY

Ades, P. A., E. Wolfel, W. R. Hiatt, C. Fee, R. Rolfe, H. L. Brammell, and L. D. Horwitz (1989). Exercise haemodynamic effects of beta-blockade and intrinsic sympathomimetic activity. *Eur. J. Clin. Pharmacol.* 36:5–10.
American College of Sports Medicine (1982). Position Statement on the Use of Alcohol in Sports. *Med. and Sci. Sports Exerc.* 14 (6):ix-x.

Agurell, S., M. Halldin, J. Lindgren, A. Ohlsson, M. Widman, H. Gillespie, and L. Hollister (1986). Pharmacokinetics and metabolism of -tetrahydrocannabinol and other cannabinoids with emphasis on man. *Pharmacol. Rev.* 38:21–43.

Anderson, R. L., J. H. Wilmore, M. J. Joyner, B. J. Freund, A. A. Hartzell, C. A. Todd, and G. A. Ewy (1985). Effects of cardioselective and nonselective beta-adrenergic blockade on the performance of highly trained runners. *Am. J. Cardiol.* 55:149D-154D.

Anderson, W. A., and D. B. McKeag (1985). The substance use and abuse habits of college student-athletes. Presented to the National Collegiate Athletic Association Council. Lansing: College of Human Medicine, Michigan State University, June.

Antal, L., and C. Good (1980). Effects of oxprenolol on pistol shooting under stress. *Practitioner* 224:755–760.

Areskog, N. (1985). Effects and adverse effects of autonomic blockade in physical exercise. *Amer. J. Cardiol.* 55:132D-134D.

Asmussen, E., and O. Boje (1948). The effects of alcohol and some drugs on the capacity for work. *Acta Physiol. Scand.* 15:109–118.

Barnard, R., and M. Foss (1969). Oxygen debt: effect of beta-adrenergic blockade on the lactacid and alactacid comnponents. *J. Appl. Physiol.* 27:813–816.

Baylor, A. M., C. S. Layne, R. D. Mayfield, L. Osborne, and W. W. Spirduso (1989). Effects of ethanol on human fractionated response times. *Drug Alcohol Dependence* 23:31–40.

Begbie, G (1966). The effects of alcohol and of varying amounts of visual information on a balancing test. *Ergonomics* 9:325–333.

Belgrave, B., K. D. Bird, G. B. Chesher, D. M. Jackson, K. Lubbe, G. A. Starmer, and R. K. Teo (1979). The effect of cannabidiol, alone and in combination with ethanol, on human performance. *Psychopharmacology* 64:243–246.

Bevilacqua, M., S. Savonitta, E. Bosisio, E. Chebat, P. L. Bertora, M. Sardina, and G. Norbiato (1989). Role of the Frank-Starling mechanism in maintaining cardiac output during increasing levels of treadmill exercise in beta-blocked normal men. *Amer. J. Cardiol.* 63:853–857.

Bird, K., T. Boleyn, G. B. Chesher, D. M. Jackson, G. A. Starmer, and R. K. Teo (1980). Intercannabinoid and cannabinoid-ethanol interactions and their effects on human performance. *Psychopharmacology* 71:181–188.

Biron, S., and J. Wells (1983). Marijuana and its effect on the athlete. *Athletic Training* 18:295–303.

Blair, S. N., D. R. Jacobs, and K. E. Powell (1985). Relationships between exercise or physical activity and other health behaviors. *Publ. Health Rep.* 100:172–180.

Blomqvist, G., B. Saltin, and J. M. Mitchell (1970). Acute effects of ethanol ingestion on the response to submaximal and maximal exercise in man. *Circulation* 42:464–470.

Boje, O. (1939). Doping: a study of the means employed to raise the level of performance in sport 1939. *League Nations Bull. Health Org.* 8:439–469.

Bracker, M., R. J. Davies, C. E. Jennings, and R. H. Strauss (1987). College wrestler with unilateral gynecomastia. *Phys. Sportsmed.* 15 (12):115–121.

Brantigan, C. O., T. A. Brantigan, and N. Joseph (1982). Effect of beta blockade and beta stimulation on stage fright. *Amer. J. Med.* 72:88–94.

Bugni, W. J., C. W. Ayers, R. Ashby, P. A. Bittle, and G. Ramirez (1989). Effects of dilevalol on rest and supine exercise hemodynamics in mild to moderate systemic hypertension. *Amer. J. Cardiol.* 63:454–456.

Capriotti, R. M., R. W. Foltin, J. V. Brady, and M. W. Fischman (1988). Effects of marijuana on the task-elicited physiological response. *Drug and Alcohol Dependence* 21:183–187.

Carpenter, J. (1962). Effects of alcohol on some psychological processes. *Quart. J. Studies Alcohol* 23:274–314.

Chait, L. D., S. M. Evans, K. A. Grant, J. B. Kamien, C. E. Johanson, C. R. Schuster (1988). Discriminative stimulus and subjective effects of smoked marijuana in humans. *Psychopharmacology* 94:206–212.

Charlap, S., E. Lichstein, and W. H. Frishman (1989). β-adrenergic blocking drugs in the treatment of congestive heart failure. *Med. Clin. North. Am.* 73:373–385.

Chasiotis, D., R. Brandt, R. C. Harris, and E. Hultman (1983). Effects of β-blockade on glycogen metabolism in human subjects during exercise. *Amer. J. Physiol.* 245:E166-E170.

Cheser, G. B., H. M. Franks, V. R. Hensley, W. J. Hensley, D. M. Jackson, G. A. Starmer, and R. K. Teo (1976). The interaction of ethanol and Δ⁹-tetrahydrocannabinol in man; effects on percetual, cognitive and motor functions. *Med. J. Austral.* 2:159–163.

Chick, T. W., A. K. Halperin, and E. M. Gacek (1988). The effect of antihypertensive medications on exercise performance: a review. *Med. Sci. Sports. Exercise* 20:447–454.

Chui, L., T. Munsat, and J. Craig (1978). Effect of ethanol on lactic acid production by exercised normal muscle. *Muscle Nerve* 1:57–61.

Clark, L. D. and E. N. Nakashima (1968). Experimental studies with marihuana. *Amer. J. Psych.* 125:379–384.

Clark, N. (1989). Social drinking and athletes. *Phys. Sportsmed.* 17(10):95–100.

Cole, J. O. (1978). Drug treatment of anxiety. *Southern Med. J.* 71 Supplement 2:10–14.

Collins, W., D. J. Schroeder, R. D. Gilson, and F. Guedry (1971). Effects of alcohol ingestion on tracking performance during angular acceleration. *J. Appl. Psychol.* 55:559–563.

Crouse, S. F., and T. Moritani (1988). Effects of beta-adrenergic blockade on the EMG during submaximal bicycle exercise. *Med. Sci. Sports Exercise.* 20:S16

Dewey, W. L. (1986). Cannabinoid pharmacology. *Pharmacol. Rev.* 38:151–178.

Diamond, T., D. Stiel, M. Lunzer, M. Wilkinson, and S. Posen (1989). Ethanol reduces bone formation and may cause osteoporosis. *Amer. J. Med.* 86:282–287.

Dimsdale, J. E., R. P. Newton, and T. Joist (1989). Neuropsychological side effects of beta-blockers. *Arch. Intern. Med.* 149:514–525.

Doctor, R., and R. Perkins (1961). The effects of alcohol on autonomic and muscular responses in humans. *Quart. J. Studies Alcohol* 22:374–386.

Doyle, W., P. Weber, and R. Meeks (1984). Effect of topical timolol maleate on exercise performance. *Arch. Opthalmol.* 102:1517–1518.

Dubowski, K. (1985). Absorption, distribution and elimination of alcohol: highway safety aspects. *J. Studies Alcohol* Supplement 10:98–108.

Dupont, E., H. J. Hanssen, and M. A. Dalby (1973). Treatment of benign essential tremor with propranolol. *Acta Neurol. Scand.* 49:75–84.

Eichner, E. R. (1989). Ergolytic drugs. *Sports Science Exchange* 2 (15):1–4.

El-Sayed, M., and B. Davies (1989). Effect of two formulations of a beta blocker on fibrinolytic response to maximal exercise. *Med. Sci. Sports Exercise* 21:369–373.

Ewy, G., J. Wilmore, A. Morton, P. Stanforth, S. Constable, M. Buono, K. Conrad, H. Miller, and C. Gatewood (1983). The effect of beta-adrenergic blockade on obtaining a trained exercise state. *J. Cardiac. Rehab.* 3:25–29.

Fagan, D., B. Tiplady, and D. B. Scott (1987). Effects of ethanol on psychomotor performance. *Brit. J. Anaesthesiol.* 59:961–965.

Fewings, J., M. J. Hanna, J. A. Walsh, and R. F. Whelan (1966). The effects of ethyl alcohol on the blood vessels of the hand and forearm in man. *Brit. J. Pharmacol. Chemother.* 27:93–106.

Fischbach, E. (1972). Problems of doping. *Med Monatsschr.* 26:377–381.

Fletcher, G. F. (1985). Exercise training during chronic beta blockade in cardiovascular disease. *Amer. J. Cardiol.* 55:110D-113D.

Foltin, R. W., M. W. Fischman, J. J. Pedroso, and G. D. Pearlson (1987). Marijuana and cocaine interactions in humans: cardiovascular consequences. *Pharmacol. Biochem. Behav.* 28:459–464.

Forney, R., F. Hughes, and W. Greatbatch (1964). Measurement of attentive motor performance after alcohol. *Percept. Motor Skills* 19:151–154.

Franks, H., V. Hensley, W. Hensley, G. Starmer, and R. Teo (1976). The relationship between alcohol dosage and performance decrement in humans. *Quart. J. Studies Alcohol* 37:471.

Freund, B., M. Joyner, S. Jilka, J. Kalis, J. Nittolo, A. Taylor, H. Peters, G. Feese. and J. Wilmore (1987). Thermoregulation during prolonged exercise in heat:alterations with beta-adrenergic blockade. *J. Appl. Physiol.* 63:930–936.

Furburg, C. (1968). Effects of beta-adrenergic blockade on ECG, physical working capacity and central circulation with special reference to autonomic imbalance. *Acta Med. Scand.* Supplementum 488:1–46.

Gengo, F. M., L. Huntoon, and W. B. McHugh (1987). Lipid-soluble and water-soluble beta-blockers. Comparison of the central nervous system depressant effect. *Arch. Intern. Med.* 147:39–43.

Giles, T., J. Cook, R. Sachitano, and B. Iteld (1982). Influence of alcohol on the cardiovascular response to isometric exercise in normal subjects. *Angiology* 33:332–338.

Glaister, D. H. (1981). Effects of beta blockers on psychomotor performance. A review. *Aviat. Space Environ. Med.* 52:23–30.

Golightly, L., and E. Sutherland (1985). Exercise and β-blocking agents. *Drug Intelligence Clin. Pharmacol.* 19:302–304.

Gould, L. (1970). Cardiac effects of alcohol. *Am. Heart. J.* 79:422–425.

Gould, L., M. Zahir, A. DeMartino, and R. F. Gomprecht (1971). Cardiac effects of a cocktail. *J. Am. Med. Assn.* 218:1799–1802.

Graf, K., and G. Strom (1960). Effect of ethanol ingestion on arm blood flow in healthy young men at rest and during work. *Acta Pharmacol. Toxicol.* 17:115–120.

Graham, T. (1983). Alcohol ingestion and sex differences on the thermal responses to mild exercise in a cold environment. *Human Biol.* 55:463–476.

Graham, T. (1981A). Thermal and glycemic responses during mild exercise in +5 to -15 C environments following alcohol ingestion. *Aviat. Space Environ. Med.* 52:517–522.

Graham, T. (1981B) Alcohol ingestion and man's ability to adapt to exercise in a cold environment. *Can. J. Appl. Sport Sci.* 6:27–31.

Graham, T., and J. Dalton (1980). Effect of alcohol on man's response to mild physical activity in a cold environment. *Aviat. Space Environ. Med.* 51:793–796.

Gullestad, L., L. O. Dolva, E. Syland, and J. Kjekshus (1988). Difference between beta-1-selective and non-selective beta-blockade during continuous and intermittant exercise. *Clin. Physiol.* 8:487–499.

Gustafson, R. (1986A). Effect of moderate doses of alcohol on simple auditory reaction time in a vigilance setting. *Perceptual Motor Skills* 62:683–690.

Gustafson, R. (1986B) Alcohol and vigilance performance: effect of small doses of alcohol on simple visual reaction time. *Perceptual Motor Skills* 62:951–955.

Guyton, A. (1986). *Textbook of Medical Physiology.* Philadelphia: W. B. Saunders.

Haight, J., and W. Keatinge (1973). Failure of thermoregulation in the cold during hypoglycaemia induced by exercise and ethanol. *J. Physiol.* 229:87–97.

Hall, P. E., S. R. Smith, D. B. Jack, and M. J. Kendall (1987). The influence of beta-adrenoceptor blockade on the lipolytic response to exercise. *J. Clin. Pharmacol. Therapeut.* 12:101–106.

Harrison, D. C., W. L. Haskell, and E. Lamdin (1985). A symposium: beta blockers and exercise. *Am. J. Cardiol.* 55:1D-171D.

Harrison, D. C. (1985). Beta blockers and exercise: physiologic and biochemical definitions and new concepts. *Am. J. Cardiol.* 55:29D-33D.

Hebbelinck, M. (1963). The effects of a small dose of ethyl alcohol on certain basic components of human physical performance. *Arch Internat. Pharmacodynam.* 143:247–257.

Hebbelinck, M. (1961). *Spierarbeid en Ethylalkohol.* Brussels: Arsica Uitggaven.

Hebbelinck, M. (1959). The effects of a moderate dose of alcohol on a series of functions of physical performance in man. *Arch. Internat. Pharmacodynam.* 120:402–405.

Heishman, S. J., M. Stitzer, and G. E. Bigelow (1988). Alcohol and Marijuana: comparative dose effect profiles in humans. *Pharmacol. Biochem. Behav.* 31:649–655.

Hespel, P., P. Lijnen, L. Vanhees, R. Fagard, R. Fiocchi, E. Moerman, and A. Amery (1986). Differentiation of exercise-induced metabolic responses during selective β_1- and β_2-antagonism. *Med. Sci. Sports Exercise* 18:186–191.

Hollister, L. E. (1986). Health aspects of cannabis. *Pharmacol. Rev.* 38:1–20.

Houmard, J., M. Langenfeld, R. Wiley, and J. Siefert (1987). Effects of the ingestion of small amounts of alcohol upon 5-mile run times. *J. Sports Med.* 27:253–258.

Huntley, M. (1974). Effects of alcohol, uncertainty and novely upon response selection. *Psychopharmacology* 39:259–266.

Huntley, M. (1972). Influences of alcohol and S-R uncertainty upon spatial localization time. *Psychopharmacology* 27:131–140.

Ikai, M., and A. Steinhaus (1961). Some factors modifying the expression of human strength. *J. Appl. Physiol.* 16:157–161.

Imhof, P. R., K. Blatter, L. M. Fuccella, and M. Turri (1969). Beta-blockade and emotional tachycardia: radiotelemetric investigations in ski jumpers. *J. Appl. Physiol.* 27:366–369.

James, I. M., R. M. Pearson, D. N. Griffith, and P. Newbury (1977). Effect of oxprenolol on stage fright in musicians. *Lancet* 2:952–954.

Januszewski, J., and A. Klimek (1974). The effect of physical exercise at varying loads on the elimination of blood alcohol. *Acta Physiol. Pol.* 25:541–545.

Jilka, S. M., M. Joyner, J. M. Nittolo, J. K. Kalis, J. A. Taylor, T. G. Lohman, and J. H. Wilmore (1988). Maximal exercise responses to acute and chronic beta-adrenergic blockade in healthy male subjects. *Med. Sci. Sports Exercise* 20:570–573.

Johnston, L., and J. Bachman (1988). *The Monitoring the Future Study.* Institute for Social Research. Ann Arbor: The University of Michigan.

Jokl, E. (1968) Notes on doping. In E. Jokl and P. Jokl (Eds.). *Exercise and Altitude.* Basel: S. Karger.

Jorfeldt, L., and A. Juhlin-Dannfelt (1978). The influence of ethanol on splanchnic and skeletal muscle metabolism in man. *Metabolism* 27:97–106.

Joyner, M., B. Freund, S. Jilka, G. Hetrick, E. Martinez, G. Ewy, and J. Wilmore (1986). Effects of beta-blockade on exercise capacity of trained and untrained men: a hemodynamic comparison. *J. Appl. Physiol.* 60:1429–1434.

Joyner, M., S. Jilka, J. Taylor, J. Kalis, J. Nittolo, R. Hicks, T. Lohman, and J. Wilmore (1987). β-blockade reduces tidal volume during heavy exercise in trained and untrained men. *J. Appl. Physiol.* 62:1819–1825.

Juhlin-Dannfelt, A. (1983). β-adrenoceptor blockade and exercise: effects on endurance and physical training. *Acta Med. Scand. Supplementum* 672:49–54.

Juhlin-Dannfelt, A., G. Ahlborg, L. Hagenfeldt, L. Jorfeldt, and P. Felig (1977A). Influence of ethanol on splanchnic and skeletal muscle substrate turnover during prolonged exercise in man. *Am. J. Physiol.* 233:E195-E202.

Juhlin-Dannfelt, A., L. Jorfeldt, L. Hagenfeldt, and B. Hulten (1977B.) Influence of ethanol on non-esterified fatty acid and carbohydrate metabolism during exercise in man. *Clin. Sci. Mol. Med.* 53:205–214.

Kaiser, P. (1984). Physical performance and muscle metabolism during β-adrenergic blockade in man. *Acta Physiol. Scand. Supplementum* 536:1–53.

Kaiser, P., B. Hylander, K. Eliasson, and L. Kaijser (1985). Effect of beta₁-selective and non-selective beta blockade on blood pressure relative to physical performance in men with systemic hypertension. *Am. J. Cardiol.* 55:79D-84D.

Kannel, W. B. (1987). New perspectives on cardiovascular risk factors. *Am. Heart. J.* 114:213–219.

Kaplan, N. M. (1983). The present and future use of β-blockers. *Drugs* 25: Supplement 2, 1–4.

Karlsson, J. (1985). Metabolic adaptations to exercise: a review of potential beta-adrenoceptor antagonist effects. *Am. J. Cardiol.* 55:48D-58D.

Karvinin, E., A. Miettinen, and K. Ahlman (1962). Physical performance during hangover. *Quart. J. Studies Alcohol* 23:208–215.

Kelbaek, H., T. Gjorup, I. Brynjolf, N. Christensen, and J. Godtfredsen (1985). Acute effects of alcohol on left ventricular function in healthy subjects at rest and during upright exercise. *Am. J. Cardiol.* 55:164–167.

Kelbaek, H., T. Gjorup, O. J. Hartling, J. Marving, N. Christensen, and J. Godtfredsen (1987). Left ventricular function during alcohol intoxication and autonomic nervous blockade. *Am. J. Cardiol.* 59:685–688.

Kelbaek, H., T. Gjorup, S. Floistrup, O. Hartling, N. Christensen, and J. Godtfredsen (1988). Cardiac function at rest and during exercise in early and late alcohol intoxication. *Int. J. Cardiol.* 18:383–390.

Kelly, J. G. (1985). Choice of selective versus nonselective beta blockers: implications for exercise training. *Am. J. Cardiol.* 55:162D-166D.

Klatsky, A. L., M. A. Armstrong, and G. Friedman (1989). Alcohol use and subsequent cerebrovascular disease hospitalization. *Stroke* 20:741–746.

Koller, W. C., and N. Biary (1984). Effect of alcohol on tremors. Comparison with propranolol. *Neurology* 34:221–222.

Kostis, J. B., and R. C. Rosen (1987). Central nervous system effects of beta-adrenergic-blocking drugs: the role of ancillary properties. *Circulation* 74:202–212.

Kruse, P., J. Ladefoged, U. Nielsen, P. Paulev, and J. P. Sorensen (1986). β-blockade used in precision sports: effect on pistol shooting performance. *J. Appl. Physiol.* 61:417–420.

Kullmer, T., W. Kindermann, and M. Singer (1987). Effects on physical performance of intrinsic sympathomimetic activity (ISA) during selective beta 1-blockade. *Eur. J. Appl. Physiol.* 56:292–298.

Lang, R. M., K. Borow, A. Neumann, and T. Feldman (1985). Adverse cardiac effects of alcohol ingestion in young adults. *Ann. Intern. Med.* 102:742–747.

Lehtonen, A. (1985). Effect of beta blockers on blood lipid profile. *Am. Heart. J.* 109:1192–1196.

Leier, C., D. Baker, and P. Weber (1986). Cardiovascular effects of opthalmic timolol. *Ann. Intern. Med.* 104:197–199.

Lieber, C. S. (1983). Alcohol-nutrition interaction. *Contemp. Nutr.* 8 (12):1–2.

Longnecker, M. P., J. A. Berlin, M. J. Orza, and T. C. Chambers (1988). A meta-analysis of alcohol consumption in relation to risk of breast cancer. *J. Am. Med. Assn.* 260:652–656.

Lowenthal, D. T., Z. V. Kendrick, R. Chase, E. Paran, and G. Perlmutter (1987). Cardiovascular drugs and exercise. *Exercise Sport Sci. Rev.* 15:67–94.

Lundborg, P., H. Astrom, C. Bengtsson, E. Fellenius, H. von Schenck, L. Svensson, and U. Smith (1981). Effect of β-adrenoceptor blockade on exercise performance and metabolism. *Clin. Sci.* 61:299–305.

Lundin, L., R. Hallgren, J. Landelius, L. Roxin, and P. Venge (1986). Myocardial and skeletal muscle function in habitual alcoholics and its relation to serum myoglobin. *Am. J. Cardiol.* 58:795–799.

Lund-Johansen, P. (1987). Exercise and antihypertensive therapy. *Am. J. Cardiol.* 59:98A-107A.

Lundquist, F., L. Sestoft, S. Damgaard, J. Clausen, and J. Trap-Jensen (1973). Utilizaton of acetate in the human forearm during exercise after ethanol ingestion. *J. Clin. Invest.* 52:3231–3235.

MacDonald, G., and M. Svoboda (1979). The effect of a 10-day period of alcohol consumption on selected measures of physical performance. Abstracts of Research Papers. Washington, DC: AAHPERD.

MacFarlane, B. J., R. L. Hughson, H. J. Green, D. J. Walters, and D. A. Ranney (1983). Effects of oral propranolol and exercise protocol on indices of aerobic function in normal man. *Can. J. Physiol. Pharmacol.* 61:1010–1016.

Maksud, M. G., K. D. Coutts, F. E. Tristani, J. R. Dorchak, J. H. Barboriak, and L. H. Hamilton (1972). The effects of physical conditioning and propranolol on physical work capacity. *Med. Sci. Sports* 4:225–229.

Markiewicz, K., and M. Cholewa (1978). The influence of ethyl alcohol, coffee and tobacco on free fatty acid, triglyceride, and glucose levels in serum during exercise and restitution. *Acta Med. Pol.* 19:373–385.

Marsh, R. C., W. R. Hiatt, H. L. Brammell, and L. D. Horowitz (1983). Attenuation of exercise conditioning by low dose beta-adrenergic receptor blockade. *J. Am. Col. Cardiol.* 2:551–556.

Marti, B., T. Abelin, C. E. Minder, and J. P. Vader (1988). Smoking, alcohol consumption, and endurance capacity: an analysis of 6,500 19-year-old conscripts and 4,100 joggers. *Preventive Med.* 17:79–92.

Martin, B. R. (1986). Cellular effects of cannabinoids. *Pharmacol. Rev.* 38:45–72.

Martin, N., C. Broeder, E. Thomas, K. Wambsgans, K. Scruggs, J. Jesek, Z. Hofman, and J. Wilmore (1989). Comparison of the effects of pindolol and propranolol on exercise performance in young men with systemic hypertension. *Am. J. Cardiol.* 64:343–347.

Mathew, R. J., W. H. Wilson, and S. R. Tant (1989). Acute changes in cerebral blood flow associated with marijuana smoking. *Acta Psychiat. Scand.* 79:118–128.

McNaughton, L., and D. Preece (1986). Alcohol and its effects on sprint and middle distance running. *Brit. J. Sports Med.* 20:56–59.

Mendelson, J. H. (1987). Marijuana. In Meltzer, H. Y. (Ed.). *Psychopharmacology: The third generation of progress.* New York: Raven Press.

Mezey, E. (1985). Metabolic effects of alcohol. *Fed. Proc.* 44:134–136.

Mitchell, M. (1985). Alcohol-induced impairment of central nervous system function: behavioral skills involved in driving. *J. Studies Alcohol,* Supplement 10:109–116.

Montoye, H. J., R. Gayle, and M. Higgins (1980). Smoking habits, alcohol consumption and maximal oxygen uptake. *Med. Sci. Sports Exercise* 12: 316–321.

Morton, A., P. R. Stanforth, B. J. Freund, M. J. Joyner, S. M. Jilka, A. A. Hartzell, G. A. Ewy, and J. H. Wilmore (1989). Alterations in plasma lipids consequent to endurance training and beta-blockade. *Med. Sci. Sports Exercise* 21:288–292.

Moskowitz, H., and M. Burns (1971). Effect of alcohol on the psychological refractory period. *Quart. J. Studies Alcohol* 32:782–790.

Moskowitz, H., and S. Roth (1971). Effect of alcohol on response latency in object naming. *Quart. J. Studies Alcohol* 32:969–975.

Moskowitz, H., M. Burns, and A. F. Williams (1985). Skills performance at low blood alcohol levels. *J. Studies Alcohol* 46:482–485.

National Collegiate Athletic Association (1988). *The 1988–1989 NCAA drug testing program.* Mission, KS:NCAA Publishing.

National Institute on Drug Abuse (1980). *Marijuana and health.* Eighth annual report to the U. S. Congress. DHHS Publication No. (ADM)81–945. Washington, D. C.: U. S. Government Printing Office.

National Research Council (1989). *Diet and Health.* Washington, D. C.: National Academy Press.

Nelson, D. (1959). Effects of ethyl alcohol on the performance of selected gross motor tests. *Research Quart.* 30:312–320.

Olson, R. (Ed.) (1988). Alcohol consumption and breast cancer. *Nutr. Rev.* 46:9–10.

Opie, L. H. (1985). Effect of beta-adrenergic blockade on biochemical and metabolic response to exercise. *Am. J. Cardiol.* 55:95D–100D.

Ouellette, E. (1984). The fetal alcohol syndrome. *Contemp. Nutr.* 9: March, 1–2.

Pennington, R. and M. Knisely (1973). Experiments aimed at separating the mechanical circulatory effects of ethanol from specific chemical effects. *Ann. New York Acad. Sci.* 215:356–365.

Perez-Reyes, M., R. E. Hicks, J. Bumberry, A. R. Jeffcoat, and C. E. Cook (1988). Interaction between marihuana and ethanol: effects on psychomotor performance. *Alcoholism* 12:268–276.

Perman, E. (1958). The effect of ethyl alcohol on the secretions from the adrenal medulla in man. *Acta Physiol Scand* 44:241–247.

Pescatello, L., G. Mack, C. Leach, and E. Nadel (1990). Thermoregulation in mildly hypertensive men during β-adrenergic blockade. *Med. Sci. Sports Exercise* 22:222–228.

Pescatello, L., G. Mack, C. Leach, and E. Nadel (1987). Effect of β-adrenergic blockade on thermoregulation during exercise. *J. Appl. Physiol.* 62:1448–1452.

Pikaar, N. A., M. Wedel, and R. J. Hermus (1988). Influence of several factors on blood alcohol concentrations after drinking alcohol. *Alcohol* 23:289–297.

Powles, A. C. (1981). The effect of drugs on the cardiovascular response to exercise. *Med. Sci. Sports Exercise* 13:252–258.

Reilly, T., and F. Halliday (1985). Influence of alcohol ingestion on tasks related to archery. *J. Human Ergol.* 14:99–104.

Reinus, J. F., S. Heymsfield, R. Wiskind, K. Casper, and J. T. Galambos (1989). Ethanol: relative fuel value and metabolic effects in vivo. *Metabolism* 38:125–135.

Renaud, A. M. and Y. Cormier (1986). Acute effects of marihuana smoking on maximal exercise performance. *Med. Sci. Sports Exercise* 18:685–689.

Rivers, W. (1908). *The Influence of Alcohol and Other Drugs on Fatigue.* London: Edward Arnold.

Rogers, C. C. (1984) Shooters aim to score with beta-blockers. *Phys. Sportsmed.* 12 (6):35.

Rohrbaugh, J. W., J. M. Stapleton, R. Parasuraman, H. W. Frowein, B. Adinoff, J. Varner, E.

Zubovic, E. Lane, M. Eckardt, and M. Linnoila (1988). Alcohol intoxication reduces visual sustained attention. *Psychopharmacology* 96:442–446.

Rundell, O. H., and H. Williams (1979). Alcohol and speed-accuracy tradeoff. *Human Factors* 21:433–443.

Sable, D. L., H. L. Brammell, M. W. Sheehan, A. S. Nies, J. Gerber, and L. D. Horowitz (1982). Attenuation of exercise conditioning by beta-adrenergic blockade. *Circulation* 65:679–684.

Samples, P. (1989). Alcoholism in athletes: New directions for treatment. *Phys. Sportsmed.* 17 (4):192–202.

Savin, W. M., E. P. Gordon, S. M. Kaplan, B. F. Hewitt, D. C. Harrison, and W. L. Haskell (1985). Exercise training during long-term beta-blockade treatment in healthy subjects. *Am. J. Cardiol.* 55:101D–109D.

Schewe, G., H. Knoss, O. Ludwig, A. Schaufele, and R. Schuster (1984). Experimental studies on the question of the marginal value of alcohol-induced unfitness to operate a vehicle in the case of bicyclists. *Blutalkohol* 21:97–109.

Schnabel, A., W. Kindermann, O. Salas-Fraire, J. Cassens, and V. Steinkraus (1983). Effect of β-adrenergic blockade on supramaximal exercise capacity. *Internat. J. Sports Med.* 4:278–281.

Schoenborn, C., and B. Cohen (1986). Trends in smoking, alcohol consumption, and other health practices among U. S. adults, 1977 and 1983. *Advancedata* 118:1–16, June 30.

Schurch, P. (1978). The effect of alcohol on metabolism during a 1-hour bicycle ergometer test. *Med. Welt.* 29:169–171.

Schurch, P., J. Radinsky, R. Iffland, and W. Hollmann (1982). The influence of moderate prolonged exercise and a low carbohydrate diet on ethanol elimination and on metabolism. *Eur. J. Appl. Physiol.* 48:407–414.

Schurch, P., A. Reinke, J. Radimsky, E. Spieckermann, and W. Hollmann (1981). The stability of blood glucose under physical stress in relation to carbohydrate reducing diet, alcohol and training. *Schweiz Sportmed.* 29:77–80.

Scragg, R., A. Stewart, R. Jackson, and R. Beaglehole (1987). Alcohol and exercise in myocardial infarction and sudden coronary death in men and women. *Am. J. Epidemiol.* 126:77–85.

Shapiro, B., S. Reiss, S. Sullivan, D. Tashkin, M. Simmons, and R. Smith (1976). Cardiopulmonary effects of marijuana smoking during exercise. *Chest* 70:441.

Shephard, R. J. (1972). *Alive Man: The Physiology of Physical Activity.* Springfield, IL: C. C. Thomas.

Shepherd, J. T. (1985). Circulatory response to beta-adrenergic blockade at rest and during exercise. *Am. J. Cardiol.* 55:87D–94D.

Shils, M. (1988). Nutrition and diet in cancer. In M. Shils and V. Young (Eds.) *Modern Nutrition in Health and Disease.* Philadelphia: Lea and Febiger.

Sidell, F., and J. Pless (1971). Ethyl alcohol blood levels and performance decrements after oral administration to man. *Psychopharmacologia* 19:246–261.

S'Jongers, J., P. Willain, J. Sierakowski, P. Vogelaere, M. DeRudden, and G. Van Vlaendenen (1978). Effet d'un placebo et de faibles doses d'un betainhibiteur (oxprenolol) et d'alcohol etylique, sur la precision du tir sportif au pistolet. *Brux. Med.* 58:395–399.

Sollman, T. (1956). *Manual of Pharmacology.* Philadelphia, Saunders.

Steadward, R. D., and M. Singh (1975). The effects of smoking marihuana on physical performance. *Med. Sci. Sports* 7:309–311.

Stratton, R., K. Dormer, and A. Zeiner (1981). The cardiovascular effects of ethanol and acetaldehyde in exercising dogs. *Alcoholism* 5:56–63.

Stromberg, C., A. Suokas, and T. Seppala (1988). Interaction of alcohol with maprotiline or nomifensine: echocardiographic and psychometric effects. *Eur. J. Clin. Pharmacol.* 35:593–599.

Sullivan, J. (1987). Unrestricted drug: Leagues just say no to alcohol-abuse sanctions. *Newsday.* December 22.

Tang, P., and R. Rosenstein (1967). Influence of alcohol amd Dramamine, alone and in combination, on psychomotor performance. *Aerospace Med.* 39:818–821.

Tashkin, D. P., B. J. Shapiro, Y. Lee, and C. E. Harper (1976). Subacute effects of heavy marihuana smoking on pulmonary function in healthy men. *New Engl. J. Med.* 294:125–129.

Tesch, P. A. (1985). Exercise performance and β-blockade. *Sports. Med.* 2:389–412.

Tharp, V., O. Rundell, B. Lester, and H. Williams (1974). Alcohol and information processing. *Psychopharmacologia* 40:33–42.

Thoren, C. (1967). Effects of beta-adrenergic blockage on heart rate and blood lactate in children during maximal and submaximal exercise *Acta Paediat. Scand.* Supplementum 177:123–125.

Turkanis, S. A., and R. Karler (1981). Electrophysiologic properties of the cannabinoids. *J. Clin. Pharmacol.* 21:Supplement 8, 9: 449S–463S.

United States Department of Health and Human Services (1980). Promoting health/preventing disease: Objectives for the nation. Washington, D. C.: U. S. Government Printing Office.

United States Olympic Committee (1988). USOC Sports Medicine & Science Division. *USOC Drug Education Program: Questions and Answers.* Colorado Springs:USOC.

van Baak, M. (1988). Beta-adrenoreceptor blockade and exercise. An update. *Sports Med.* 5:209–225.

van Baak, M., F. Koene, and F. Verstappen (1988). Exercise haemodynamics and maximal exercise capacity during beta-adrenoreceptor blockade in normotensive and hypertensive subjects. *Br. J. Clin. Pharmacol.* 25:169–177.

van Baak, M., R. Bohm, B. Arends, M. van Hooff, and K. Rahn (1987). Long-term antihypertensive therapy with beta-blockers: Submaximal exercise capacity and metabolic effects during exercise. *Internat. J. Sports Med.* 8:342–347.

van Baak, M. A., F. T. Verstappen and B. Oosterhuis (1986). Twenty-four hour effects of oxprenolol Oros and atenolol on heart rate, blood pressure, exercise tolerance and perceived exertion. *Eur. J. Clin. Pharmacol.* 30:399–406.

Videman, T., T. Sonck, and J. Janne (1979). The effect of beta-blockade in ski-jumpers. *Med. Sci. Sports* 11:266–269.

Vogel, W. H., and P. Netter (1989). Effect of ethanol and stress on plasma catecholamines and their relation to changes in emotional state and performance. *Alcoholism* 13:284–290.

Wadler, G. and B. Hainline (1989). *Drugs and the Athlete.* Philadelphia: F. A. Davis.

Williams, M. H. (1990). *Lifetime Fitness and Wellness.* Dubuque, IA: Wm, C. Brown Publishers.

Williams, M. H. (1985). *Nutritional Aspects of Human Physical and Athletic Performance.* Springfield, IL: C. C. Thomas.

Williams, M. (1983). Alcohol Is it the new fuel for distance runners? *Runners World.* 18:74.

Williams, M., and C. Jackson (1975). High school athletes shun drug boosts, survey shows. *Phys. Sportsmed.* 4:(2) 58–62.

Williams, M. H (1974). *Drugs and Athletic Performance.* Springfield, IL: C. C. Thomas.

Williams, M. (1972). Effect of small and moderate doses of alcohol on exercise heart rate and oxygen consumption. *Res. Quart.* 43:94–104.

Williams, M. (1969). Effect of selected doses of alcohol on fatigue parameters of the forearm flexor muscles. *Res. Quart.* 40:832–840.

Williams, R. S. (1985). Role of receptor mechanisms in the adaptive response to habitual exercise. *Am. J. Cardiol* 55:68D-73D.

Wilmore, J. H. 1988. Exercise testing, training, and beta-adrenergic blockade. *Phys. Sportsmed.* 16 (12):45–51.

Wilmore, J. H., G. A. Ewy, B. J. Freund, A. A. Hartzell, S. M. Jilka, M. J. Joyner, C. A. Todd, S. M. Kinzer, and E. B. Pepin (1985A). Cardiorespiratory alterations consequent to endurance exercise training during chronic beta-adrenergic blockade with atenolol and propranolol. *Am. J. Cardiol.* 55:142D-148D.

Wilmore, J. H., B. J. Freund, M. J. Joyner, G. A. Hetrick, A. A. Hartzell, R. T. Strother, G. A. Ewy, and W. E. Faris (1985B). Acute response to submaximal and maximal exercise consequent to beta-adrenergic blockade: implications for the prescription of exercise. *Am. J. Cardiol.* 55:135D-141D.

Wolf, S. (1963). Psychosomatic aspects of competitive sports. *J. Sports Med.* 3:157–163.

Wu, A. H., A. Paganini-Hill, R. K. Ross, and B. Henderson (1987). Alcohol, physical activity and other risk factors for colorectal cancer: a prospective study. *Brit. J. Cancer* 55:687–694.

Wu, T., D. P. Tashkin, B. Djahed, and J. E. Rose (1988). Pulmonary hazards of smoking marijuana as compared with tobacco. *New Engl. J. Med.* 318:347–351.

Yesavage, J. A., and V. Leirer (1986). Hangover effects on aircraft pilots 14 hours after alcohol ingestion: a preliminary report. *Am. J. Psychiat.* 143:1546–1550.

Yesavage, J. A., V. O. Leirer, M. Denari, and L. E. Hollister (1985). Carry-over effects of marijuana intoxication on aircraft pilot performance: a prelimninary report. *Am. J. Psychiat.* 142:1325–1329.

DISCUSSION

WILMORE: What's very perplexing is the mechanism by which beta blockers cause fatigue. In our studies, we found that excellent runners (30 min for 10 km and well below 60 min for 10 mile runs), when taking beta blockers and running at only 45% of their $\dot{V}O_2$max, crash and burn in a matter of 60 min or less. In other words, they can't even go out and do a simple training run. This is very confusing to us. The whole issue of the potential of an ergogenic effect in endurance athletes by causing up-regulation of beta receptors is also interesting. In this context, we took about 22 of the best runners in the Tucson area, and every two weeks had them compete in 10 km races where there were prizes awarded. This study was all counter-balanced and randomly designed with treatments of placebo, atenolol, and propranolol. Whenever a placebo trial followed two weeks of treatment with a beta blocker, we never did see an enhancement in performance. Therefore, my guess is that the up-regulation ergogenic concept for explaining the potential ergogenic effect of beta blockers is not viable. People perform so poorly while training on beta blockers that this approach would have negative consequences generally.

EICHNER: Is there really a negative effect of beta blockers on aerobic training? One group presented evidence that beta blockade doesn't attenuate the training effect so much as merely masking the training effect. They suggested that if you stop the beta blockers for 4 d at the end of training and then retest the subjects, $\dot{V}O_2$max seems quite comparable to that for the placebo group.

WILMORE: We've had three training studies now, and it is very clear on the cardio-selective drug, atenolol; there is no masking. They have about a 20% improvement of $\dot{V}O_2$max, which matches the placebo treatment, after 15 weeks of training. With the one study on sotalol, the training effect was totally masked until we took them off of the drug. With propranolol, they got about a 12% improvement in $\dot{V}O_2$max while they were on the drug, but that went up to 20% one week after they stopped taking the drug. So, we have found no attenuation in terms of training response. Another interesting thing is that even in the sotalol study, while subjects were on beta blockers, their performances improved tremendously. These were individuals who were untrained at the beginning and couldn't even run half a mile without stopping to walk. But by the end of the study, they were running sub-eight minute miles for five or six miles—a phenomenal improvement in performance. And yet, while they were still on the drug, their $\dot{V}O_2$max had not changed.

HEIGENHAUSER: We were very interested in the effects of beta blockers on potassium. We found that very low doses (20 mg) of propranolol caused elevations of plasma potassium, yet there was no detriment in performance. If the dosages were increased to around 360 mg, this produced the same effects on potassium but decreased performance. The potassium does not seem to play a role in performance with beta blockers. On the other hand, we observed a dramatic change in mood for subjects who were treated with beta blockers that could cross the blood-brain barrier. These subjects just don't seem to want to do anything, including normal daily activities.

COGGAN: The concept that training may reduce beta receptor density is not supported for skeletal muscle. Sanders and Williams have shown that training in rats increases beta receptor density of skeletal muscle. Also, we just published a human training study in which we didn't get either an increase or a decrease in beta receptor density in muscle. So I am curious about the origin of this concept that training reduces beta receptor density.

WILLIAMS: In Kelly's review of the literature in 1985, he proposed the idea. I agree with you that other research has suggested that training may actually increase beta receptor density.

WILMORE: From the literature it is my impression that the attenuation of peak ejection fraction is not a consistent response in normal individuals under beta blockade. In fact, in healthy normals, ejection fraction is probably not affected unless they are given massive drug doses. I can believe that this effect occurs in the individual with underlying coronary disease, but probably not in normals. Our findings are that the patient population, particularly angina patients, will increase their $\dot{V}O_2max$ while on beta blockers. The highly endurance-trained athletes will substantially reduce their $\dot{V}O_2max$ values, and those people in the middle tend not to have much of an attenuation.

HEIGENHAUSER: What dosages are you talking about, Jack? We had to get up around 360 mg before we had any effect on $\dot{V}O_2max$ in a progressive exercise test. The receptors had to be very well blocked before we got an effect. If we were down around 40–80 mg, there was very little effect. We also measured cardiac outputs during the entire tests, and we did not find any effect on the cardiac output until we got to a maximum cardiac output with very high drug doses.

WILMORE: Our doses of propranolol, for example, were 180 mg/d; atenolol was 100 mg/d; these were about half of what you used. I don't think it is a timing difference, but the mode of administration may be a problem. We've looked at 24 h vs 7 d responses, and they basically track very nicely.

HEIGENHAUSER: We found a lot of individual variability in results for people on propranolol. In some individuals, even doses down around 80 to 100 mg/d have a drastic effect and cause a maximal blockade, whereas we had to give up to 720 mg before we maximally blocked one of our subjects.

LOMARDO: George Sheehan a few years ago claimed that runners should rehydrate with beer. Has any research been done on this issue?

WILLIAMS: I'm not aware of any research along that line, John. I have been around a lot of distance runners, and I think they are drinking beer more for the relaxation effect rather than for any rehydration purposes.

EICHNER: Another theoretical point about the use of alcohol after the race is that in some people, at least, alcohol causes ultrastructural damage to the muscle mitochondria and myofibrils. It would be worth investigating whether alcohol slows the rate of restocking of muscle with glycogen after a race.

CLARKSON: We gave alcohol shortly before eccentric exercise and then several periods after the exercise, and we saw no difference in rate of recovery.

LOMARDO: A lot has been made of the lipid solubility factor in the storage of marijuana in tissue. The suggestion has been that individuals who lose fat will release marijuana that has been stored in that fat in amounts that can raise their THC levels. That has been suggested by people in weight loss clinics as well as by individuals who are cutting weight to play a sport. Is there any research on this?

WILLIAMS: I know that has been hypothesized, but I don't think there are any published studies.

10

Ergogenics for Bicycling

Chester R. Kyle, Ph.D.

INTRODUCTION
HUMAN MECHANICAL AND METABOLIC ENERGY
   Mechanical Power Output
   Energy Input
   Overall Thermal Efficiency
   Efficiency During Exercise
BIOMECHANICS IN CYCLING
   Ergometers and Human Power Output
   Optimal Pedal RPM
   Optimal Crank Length
   Optimal Saddle Height
   Pedal Forces and The Most Efficient Pedaling Style
   Alternate Pedaling Motions
   Vibrations
   Heat Reflectivity
AERODYNAMICS
   Aerodynamic Drag
   Drafting
   Frontal Area
   Smoothing
   Streamlining
   Aerodynamic Clothing and Helmets
   Wheels
   Improved Components and Equipment
   The Effect of Winds on Bicycle Speed
       Headwinds and Tailwinds
       Cross Winds
   The Effect of Altitude
   The Effect of Passing Automotive Traffic
MECHANICS
   The Rolling Resistance of Tires
   Drive Train Friction and Bearing Friction
   The Effect of Weight on Bicycle Speed
       Weight and Acceleration
       Weight, Hill Climbing, and Rolling Resistance

INTRODUCTION

The act of moving from one point to another requires energy, regardless of the means of transportation. The most efficient type of human transport on land is the bicycle in its various forms (Wilson, 1973; Brooks, 1989). In other words, a bicycle requires less energy per unit mass per unit distance than walking, running, or travel by auto, rail or any other form of land transportation.

The pattern of energy distribution is important in all forms of cycling, but it is of paramount importance in competitive cycling. When a bicyclist is traveling on a level road with no wind, the mechanical power provided by the rider in turning the cranks is used to overcome the external friction forces acting on the bicycle and rider. By modifying bicycle equipment, technique, rider position, or other human factors, the energy required to propel a bicycle at a given velocity can be decreased significantly. This chapter will concentrate on competitive cycling; for simplicity, all statements will refer to cycling on a smooth, hard, road surface with a standard road racing bicycle.

Because man is combined with a machine in cycling, there are numerous ways to improve cycling performance. Probably the most effective and the most arduous is by rigorous training (Spangler & Hooker, 1990). The physical condition of the athlete is the most important factor in making a bicycle go fast and in improving a cyclist's endurance. The methods and intensity of training naturally will depend upon the event and the level of competition and will vary with the individual. Because of the complexity of the topic, training will not be covered here.

Other means of improving cycling performance are related to skill, judgement, technique, and strategy. Knowing how to turn corners rapidly, how to draft (slipstream in the wake of a cyclist in front), how to maneuver in a pack of riders, how to climb uphill, how to pedal and ride to conserve energy, where and when to relax, where and when to break away from other riders, how and when to drink and feed, and how to apply dozens of other fine points cycling can all improve performance. Once again, the topic is too complicated to cover here.

This chapter will discuss two other methods by which racing cyclists may go faster. Both are related to more efficient energy utilization. The first concerns how best to combine the cyclist with the bicycle in order to increase power output. This includes modifying the rider's position, cycling style, cadence, or other important physical variables. The second method is to modify the bicycle or its components, the rider's clothing, or any related manufactured equipment in order to minimize energy losses. Although some of the energy savings described in this paper may seem insignificant, many bicycle races are won by centimeters. In reality, nothing can be ignored that might give a slight advantage to a racer.

HUMAN MECHANICAL AND METABOLIC ENERGY

Human mechanical energy output in most forms of exercise is very difficult to measure or estimate. For example, in running or walking it requires sophisticated mathematical calculations to estimate the effective mechanical energy output, and there is a great deal of controversy about how to approach the problem (Williams & Cavanagh, 1983; Webb, 1988). The distribution between potential and kinetic energy of the limbs and body during a stride, and the energy lost in internal friction and the shock contact with the pavement is uncertain. However in cycling, energy output is much easier to determine, since it may be measured directly using a bicycle ergometer. The bicycle-human system forms an ideal combination for scientific analysis.

The other chapters in this book view the human system from a physiological standpoint. It would be useful to look at the human-bicycle system from a purely engineering viewpoint and to consider the human as a heat engine which powers a land transport vehicle (the bicycle). There are several standard performance characteristics usually presented in elementary thermodynamics or power engineering textbooks, but most important is the basic power capacity of the engine.

Mechanical Power Output

The net mechanical power output of a cyclist may be easily measured using a cycling ergometer or a power meter installed on a road bicycle (Hooker & Spangler, 1989). The external power output depends upon the duration of exercise as well as upon body size, strength, aerobic capacity, muscle characteristics, and other variables. For periods of a few seconds, humans can put out over 1000 W as measured by an ergometer. An Italian sprinter, Renzo Sarti, produced 1644 W for 5 s, (Dal Monte & Faina, 1989), and others have produced about 1500 W for 6 s (Kyle & Caiozzo, 1986). This,

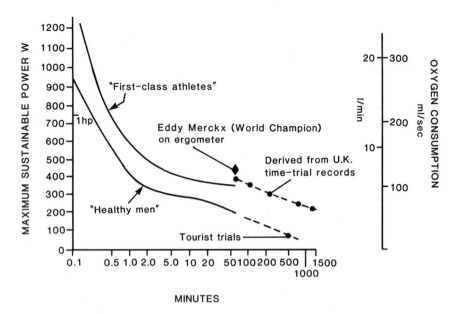

FIGURE 10-1. *Long-duration human power output. From Whitt & Wilson (1982).*

of course, is purely anaerobic power, and power levels drop off steeply with time [see Figure 10-1 (Whitt & Wilson, 1982)].

At the other end of the spectrum, pure aerobic power, the Belgian champion cyclist, Eddy Merckx, produced 455 W for 1 h (Kyle & Caiozzo, 1986). Well-conditioned recreational cyclists can only maintain this power level for slightly over 1 min (Whitt & Wilson, 1982). Most trained, healthy individuals can produce over 700 W for a short period, and about 180 W for 1 h (Kyle & Caiozzo, 1986; Whitt & Wilson, 1982).

The speed at which a bicycle will travel with a fixed power input is dependent upon the resistance forces against the bicycle. Figure 10-2 shows the power required to propel a bicycle at various speeds versus the body weight of the cyclist (Swain et al. 1987; Sjøgaard et al., 1982).

Energy Input

The other side of a standard thermal efficiency equation is the heat equivalent of the fuel input. In this case it would be the energy value of the daily food intake. The total energy in food and drink consumed by trained cyclists varies enormously, depending upon

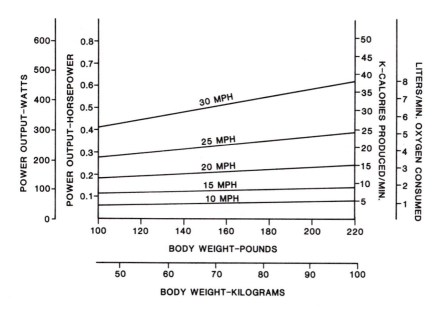

FIGURE 10-2. *The effect of body weight and speed upon power output, energy, and oxygen consumption in cycling. The curves represent a cyclist of normal body type riding a racing bicycle in a crouched racing position at an optimal pedal rate of from 60 to 80 rpm. The energy required to travel a constant speed increases with body weight, but this is compensated for by increased muscle mass and absolute power. The curves were developed from work by Swain et al. (1987) and Slogaard (1982).*

the required exercise intensity. Intake of 2,000 to 3,000 kcal/d is usually sufficient to support recreational cycling. However, for periods of intense competitive exercise exceeding 2–3 h, racing cyclists continually feed to maintain their blood glucose levels and to prolong the time of exercise until they fatigue (Burke, 1990; Coggan, 1990; Coyle, 1989). In the 3,000 mile Race Across America, cyclists often remain on the bike for 20 h/d or more and eat in excess of 11,000 kcal/d (Kyle, 1989a). Typical food intake is from 6,000 to 8,000 kcal/d during this race, and little weight gain or loss occurs during the race.

The amount of food energy that can actually be utilized to produce muscular work is a fraction of the total consumed. Multiple chemical reactions are required to digest food and convert it into a usable form of energy; these processes consume energy and generate heat. The digestive processes themselves use about 6–10% of the energy content of the ingested food (Whitney & Hamilton, 1984). The increased metabolism during digestion requires heat production equivalent to an increase of about 100 mL/min in oxygen consumption (Guyton, 1986). In all, about 70–80% of the energy taken in as food ultimately results in internal heat production that must be dissipated by cooling (Pugh, 1974).

During exercise, the muscle, tendon, and cartilage fibers and segments move relative to one another, creating internal friction that generates heat. The total mechanical work done by the muscle during cycling includes the work done in pedaling the bicycle plus the work done against internal friction. The combined magnitude of the thermic effect of food and the heat due to internal friction can be reasonably estimated from physiological and ergometric data, but the exact details and functional relations are uncertain.

In cycling, as in other sports, the rate of internal friction and other energy losses increase as the cadence or velocity of contraction goes up. Maximum leg force can be exerted at zero leg speed, and the average leg force will decrease as the leg speed rises. At the extreme, the cadence can be so high that the average leg force is zero. At this point the muscle is still producing a great deal of power, but all of the energy is used to move the limbs, and none is available to produce net force about the bicycle cranks. Somewhere in between the two extremes of cycling cadence, maximal external mechanical power will be produced (Furusawa et al., 1927a,b; Gregor et al., 1979; Gregor & Rugg, 1986; Hill, 1922; Kyle & Caiozzo, 1986). This is exactly the same as in an internal combustion engine; i.e., maximum power is produced at medium speeds, beyond which power declines due to increasing internal friction. The maximum cadence in cycling varies, but is about 200 revolutions/min (rpm) for most riders. Maximum power occurs between 120 and 130 rpm (Kyle & Mastropaolo, 1976).

Figure 10-2 also shows the energy and oxygen consumption in cycling versus body weight and speed (Swain et al., 1987). The energy consumed is fairly constant until about 20 miles/h (mph), when it begins to increase rapidly due to air resistance. The wind resistance is proportional to the square of the speed and is nearly proportional to the frontal area. For larger body size, the frontal area increases at about the 2/3 power of the weight; as could be expected, larger people have a greater wind resistance (Sjøgaard et al., 1982). A more recent study by Hagberg and his group (McCole et al., 1990), shows a similar relation between oxygen consumption, speed, and body weight, although Hagberg's results are about 8% lower at 32 km/h than those of Swain. Hagberg's subjects were all experienced racers, and therefore could have been more efficient in both aerodynamic position and in biomechanical technique than those of Swain. Pugh (1974) also did similar work, but his results were about 7% higher than Swain's. It should be noted that Pugh conducted his study on a hilly course, which would add to the energy expenditure.

Overall Thermal Efficiency

To calculate the overall thermal efficiency of any heat engine, it is necessary to know the total energy input in the form of fuel and the energy equivalent of the net mechanical work output. For athletes it is usually impractical to attempt to calculate the total mechanical work output during their normal daily routine because work output for most activities is difficult to define. However, there is one ultraendurance cycling event, the Race Across America (RAAM), where this calculation is possible because the athletes only rest about 2 h/d. Dividing the total heat equivalent of the daily mechanical power to the pedals by the sum of the total daily food energy input and body fat loss will yield the net overall thermal efficiency for the complete 7–10 d race. Using this method, net efficiencies of 16.9%–20.3% have been calculated for three athletes during the RAAM (Kyle, 1988a). This efficiency includes the metabolic energy consumed during the brief rest periods (RAAM cyclists typically ride for 22–23 h/d). The overall thermal efficiency of human athletes as calculated for the RAAM is remarkably high, considering the best economy-model automobiles have efficiencies of 15–20% (Brooks, 1989).

The above net human thermal efficiency is lower than the usual efficiency calculated for cyclists because it incorporates all energy losses, including those from the process of food digestion and the subsequent energy storage in the tissues.

Efficiency During Exercise

A more common estimate of human efficiency in cycling considers only the energy already stored in the muscles and liver before exercise and uses oxygen consumption to calculate the energy liberated per liter of oxygen consumed. Knowing the ratio of carbon dioxide expired to oxygen consumed, the energy liberated in the muscles can be determined. An efficiency can then be calculated based upon the net mechanical power output as measured by a cycle ergometer (Pugh, 1974; van Ingen Schenau, 1983). Since this does not include the energy losses in the digestive process, this estimate of efficiency (21 to 24%) is higher than that described earlier.

BIOMECHANICS IN CYCLING

Biomechanical studies of cycling have been performed for nearly a century, but positive effects on competitive cycling have been hard to demonstrate. There is no doubt that advances in training methods, and a better understanding of physiology and nutrition for cycling have been very productive. However, the use of biomechanics is still in its development stage and it has yet to prove as fruitful as many other avenues of investigation (including empirical experimentation). On the other hand, many important biomechanical studies of cycling have been completed.

Ergometers and Human Power Output

Since about 1895, cycling ergometers that measure human power output have been very useful in gauging human athletic ability and serving as tools during training to measure adaptive changes in an athlete's state of conditioning. A new generation of computerized electronic ergometers could become an irreplaceable part of a cyclist's training regimen. These ergometers provide for displays of power, speed, cadence, heart rate, and other variables in real time. Historically, the first mechanical cycling ergometer was built around 1880, and studies of human power output have continued every since. Some sample values of human power output measurements spanning nearly a century are given in Table 10-1. With present technology, complete bicycle simulators are possible that can permit a cyclist to ride any course in the world in a laboratory environment. This could prove an invaluable analytical tool to sports scientists.

Optimal Pedal RPM

There are several ways of analyzing the problem of selecting optimal pedaling cadence. One is from the viewpoint of maximum power output over a given exercise duration. This is probably the most important as far as racing is concerned. Another is from the standpoint of maximum metabolic efficiency, a perspective of most interest from a theoretical or academic standpoint. These two approaches give quite similar results. Some sample tests are listed in Table 10-2 and have been plotted in Figure 10-3.

Another potential criterion for optimizing pedaling cadence is minimizing a muscle stress function (Hull et al., 1988.) Hull et al.

TABLE 10-1. *Ergometer Power for Cyclists*

Reference	Power, Time
Sharp (1896)	75 W, continuous
Bourlet (1896)	858 W, 8 s
Blix (1901)	590 W, 30 s
Whitt & Wilson (1982)	455 W, 1 h
Kyle & Caiozzo, (1986)	1506 W, 6 s
Vandewalle et al. (1987)	1413 W, 6 s
Dal Monte & Faina (1989)	1644 W, 5 s

TABLE 10-2. *Optimal Pedal Cadence Versus Power*

USING MAXIMAL POWER OUTPUT AS THE CRITERION			
Reference	Duration	Cadence (rpm)	Power (W)
Bouny (1897)	8 s	115	858
Kyle & Caiozzo (1986)	6 s	109	1105
Kyle & Caiozzo (1986)	12 s	106	1010
Kyle & Caiozzo (1986)	18 s	107	890
Kyle & Caiozzo (1986)	30 s	104	705
Kyle & Caiozzo (1986)	1 min	88	510
Kyle & Caiozzo (1986)	2 min	84	400
Kyle & Caiozzo (1986)	5 min	84	330
Kyle & Caiozzo (1986)	20 min	81	310

USING MAXIMAL METABOLIC EFFICIENCY AS THE CRITERION			
Reference	Duration	Cadence (rpm)	Power (W)
Dickinson (1929)	6 min	33	65
Croisant & Boileau (1984)	6 min	80	235
Coast & Welch (1985)	3 min	52	100
	3 min	59	150
	3 min	66	200
	3 min	71	250
	3 min	79	300
Coast et al. (1986)	30 min	80	85% $\dot{V}O_2$max

reported an optimal pedal speed of 97 rpm for a load of about 200 W. They commented that metabolic efficiency may not be the major consideration in choosing an optimal cadence and suggested that minimizing muscle stress might reduce fatigue and increase endurance.

Optimal Crank Length

The optimal crank length depends upon what type of riding the cyclist intends to do, i.e., sprinting, hill climbing, time trialing, or touring. Every task and every cadence has a different optimal crank length, so any crank length is a compromise. Also, the optimal crank length obviously depends upon the leg length of the individual— taller persons need longer crank lengths to maintain geometrically similar pedaling motions. The researchers cited in Table 10-3 sought to maximize power output or to minimize joint moments and stresses at a given power output. The results are in reasonable accordance with standard practice by competitive cyclists. In the tests, crank lengths from 12 cm to 22.5 cm were investigated, and crank lengths from 15–18 cm were judged to be optimum.

Optimal Saddle Height

For maximum power output while seated, a saddle height setting of about 109% of the leg inseam length has been found to be optimal (Hamley & Thomas, 1967). For metabolic efficiency, a height

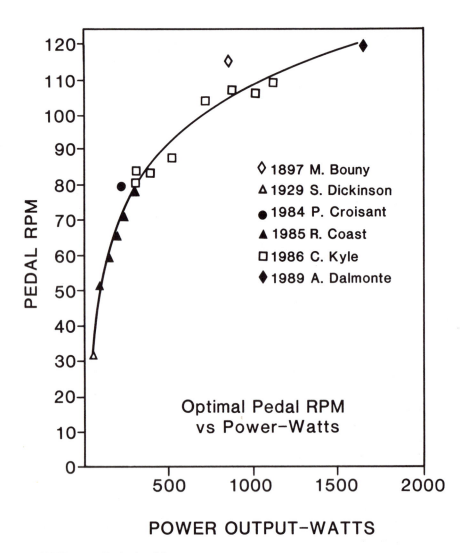

FIGURE 10-3. *Optimal pedal rpm versus power.*

of 105% of the inseam length was found to be optimal (Nordeen-Snyder, 1977). The efficiency curve, however, is fairly flat in the range near the optimal point, permitting a reasonable variation before metabolic changes become noticeable. Most inexperienced cyclists set the saddle height much lower than optimal, however, perhaps because a high seat height makes it hard to mount, dismount, and balance while stopped.

TABLE 10-3. *Optimal Crank Length*

MAXIMIZING POWER OUTPUT (Inbar et al., 1983)		
Leg Length of Cyclist		Optimal Crank Length (mm)
Long legged	No rpm indicated	175
Short legged	No rpm indicated	150

MINIMIZING MUSCLE STRESS FUNCTION (Hull et al., 1988)		
Height of Cyclist		Optimal Crank Length (mm)
Short Man	Optimized for combined	155
Average Man	90, 100, and 110 rpm	165
Tall Man		170

Height of Cyclist/Power	RPM	Optimal Crank Length (mm)
Short Man/200 W	105	170
Short Man/200 W	108	165
Short Man/200 W	110	160
Average Man/300 W	110	175
Average Man/300 W	113	170
Average Man/300 W	116	165
Tall Man/200 W	88	180
Tall Man/200 W	91	175
Tall Man/200 W	93	170

Pedal Forces and the Most Efficient Pedaling Style

A common technique used in many of the above investigations has been to employ an instrumented pedal to measure the normal and tangential pedal forces during cycling. This is one of the oldest methods of biomechanical analysis in cycling. Usually, the purpose of these studies was to try to optimize pedaling technique for greater endurance and lower energy consumption. There is a remarkable similarity between the force diagrams and illustrations shown in studies done in 1896, and those in studies done recently. Some of the past and present investigators who have used a force pedal for biomechanical studies are listed in the references (Bouny, 1897; Broker & Gregor, 1989; Cavanagh & Sanderson, 1986; Dal Monte et al. 1973; Hochmuth, 1967; Hoes et al. 1968; Hull & Gonzalez, 1988; Kunstlinger et al., 1985; Newmiller & Hull, 1988; Sharp, 1896; Soden & Adeyefa, 1979). All of these studies show that the leg does not normally pull up on the upstroke of the pedal, but exerts a positive force during the entire pedal cycle (Figure 10-4). In other words, the active leg helps to lift the opposite leg. Since athletes are extremely adept at maximizing efficiency and minimizing energy consumption, this probably is the best pedaling strategy, although this has not been proven. During sprinting and hill climbing, where high forces are involved, pulling up on the pedals is more common.

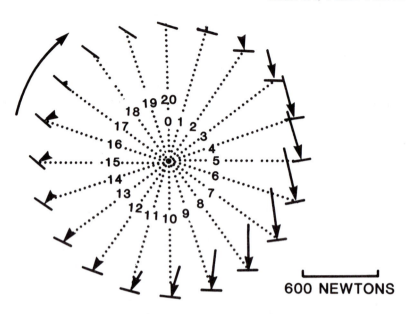

TDC
MEAN ALL RIDERS

600 NEWTONS

LEFT RESULTANT FORCE

FIGURE 10-4. *Pedal force vectors versus crank angle. From Cavanagh and Sanderson (1986).*

Starting in the last century, coaches, athletes, researchers, scientists, and cycling technical buffs have tried to define what constitutes an efficient pedaling style. Many of the forces applied to the pedal do not produce power and are ineffective in transmitting force tangent to the crank arm. Cavanagh and Sanderson (1986), studying elite racing cyclists, attempted to describe a pedaling efficiency function based upon the proportion of the positive pedal forces applied tangent to the crank, assuming that these were the only pedal forces that were productive. Many others have attacked the problem from the same or somewhat different standpoints (Broker & Gregor, 1989; Dal Monte et. al., 1973; Hull et. al., 1988). The result has been a realization that there are many pedaling techniques that seem to work well. Negative or neutral pedal and muscle forces and joint moments may serve a very useful biomechanical purpose. Exactly what this purpose is remains unknown and this is likely to be one of the most productive areas of research in the future.

In pedaling a bicycle, the motion of each segment of the leg during the pedal cycle causes the kinetic and potential energy of foot, lower leg, and thigh to vary continuously. As the angular and linear velocity and elevation of each segment change, the resulting forces in the muscles and joints are due not only to the necessity of applying a pedal force, but also to the requirement for raising and lowering the leg and accelerating and decelerating the limb segments. Using an instrumented pedal to measure pedal forces and applying Newton's equations of motion, it is possible to calculate the muscle and joint forces and moments at each point in the pedal cycle; these data can then be used in an attempt to optimize cycling variables (Hull & Gonzalez 1988). Although promising, this approach has not yet led to direct improvements in competitive cycling performance.

Another technique that could be very useful to racing cyclists has been demonstrated by Broker and Gregor of UCLA (1989). Their study shows that cyclists can alter their pedaling style effectively by using a computerized biofeedback system. The computer displays a cyclist's actual pedal force pattern and compares it to a "template" pattern that the cyclist attempts to follow. With practice, subjects were able to reproduce the template force profile fairly accurately. After the motion was learned, they retained the ability to reproduce the pattern, even when tested two months later. This shows that if an "ideal" pedaling technique can be identified, cyclists can be trained to accurately follow the force pattern by using biofeedback techniques.

Alternate Pedaling Motions

It is common for inventors of alternate pedaling mechanisms, e.g., elliptic sprockets, cam drives, and oval or linear pedal devices, to claim that the metabolic pedaling efficiency will be improved from 10–25%. If this were true, there would be no more standard circular cranks in use. It is possible that an alternate pedaling motion may be found that will produce a metabolic energy savings of 1 or 2%, but anything more than that is unlikely. One study done on elliptical sprockets shows that when they are oriented properly, a 1.5 % energy cost savings could be realized at a power output of 200 W (Henderson et al., 1977).

On the other hand, Harrison (1970) reported little difference in maximal power output between elliptical versus round sprockets. In similar experiments to determine the maximal power possible with oval chainwheels, Kyle (1982) showed that sprockets with an ovality from 1.1/1 to 1.6/1 produce little difference in maximal power output on an ergometer. However, above 1.2/1 in field studies, they have slower acceleration and are inferior for use in 20-min time trials. Since hundreds of alternate drive mechanisms have been invented during the past century, it is regrettable that more of them haven't been tested under laboratory conditions (Miller & Ross, 1980).

Vibrations

Alex Moulton, maker of the Moulton bicycle, has investigated the effect of suspension and shock absorption on the vibration frequencies transferred to the rider in cycling (Moulton, 1973). He found that by filtering the road shock through a spring and damper system on the front and back, the shocks transmitted through the handlebars and seat were attenuated to as little as 1/3 their undamped value at the frequencies of 3—12 Hz that are known to cause fatigue. His suspension system has been twice used successfully by David Bogden in the Race Across America. Bogden experienced no saddle or hand problems as did most other contestants.

Another researcher has measured the frequency of road shocks transmitted through a bicycle frame for a wide variety of European pavements. Schondorf, of the Fachhochschule in Koln, Germany, collected the data for the use of those designing bicycle suspensions (Schondorf & Adams, 1981). Few road bicycles use suspensions, although mountain bikes are beginning to use them in large numbers (Olsen, 1989).

A study of the shock attenuation provided by bicycle gloves containing a gel pad in the palm was recently completed for the Spenco Medical Corporation by E. C. Frederick (1988). Frederick found that gloves significantly dampened the shock transmitted to the wrists from the handlebars (about 0.6 g lower shock transmitted to the wrists when compared to bare hands); however, the differences between several types of cycling gloves was not large.

The affect of vibration damping in a bicycle has been little studied, probably because unlike automobiles, bicycles can obviously function very well on smooth roads without independent suspensions and shock absorbers. However in mountain biking and off-road motorcycling, rough terrain will no doubt make suspensions indispensible for peak performance.

Heat Reflectivity

Larry Berglund, of the John B. Pierce Foundation Laboratory of Yale University, has shown that light-reflective clothing can lower sweat loss and improve cooling in cyclists exercising in direct sunlight . At high noon, the uncovered human body can absorb about 100 W of radiative energy from the sun, and this energy must be dissipated by the body by convective cooling, by radiation, or by evaporative cooling. Bergland found that aluminized fabric was best followed by white and light colored fabric. The aluminized fabric was superior in cooling to bare skin. In other words, the right fabric can cut down on water losses in endurance events (Berglund, 1987).

AERODYNAMICS

Aerodynamic Drag

At speeds lower than 13 km/h, tire rolling friction is the dominant retarding force against a bicycle; however, the wind resistance increases as the square of the bicycle speed, so that above 13 km/h the rolling resistance is overshadowed by wind resistance. In fact, at speeds above 40 km/h, wind drag is responsible for over 90% of the total retarding force on a traditional road racing bicycle (Kyle 1988a). Speeds between 20 and 45 km/h are typical of bicycle recreation, touring, commuting and racing.

Aerodynamic drag in cycling is caused by air pressure and/or friction. Air molecules colliding at an angle with a surface cause a pressure force that can cause drag if the forces are not balanced over the entire surface. This is called pressure drag or form drag because it is related to the shape of an object. Another type of drag is caused by air moving parallel to a surface, resulting in shear forces due to air viscosity. This is called friction drag.

Aerodynamic drag is proportional to the square of the velocity (twice as many molecules collide with the surface twice as fast) (Hoerner, 1965). If the speed is doubled the drag increases by four times. Since power is equal to force times velocity, the power necessary to overcome aerodynamic drag is proportional to the cube of the velocity. If the speed doubles, the power increases by eight times. Small variations in speed can cause very large power increases. For example, doubling the power it takes to go 32 km/h will only speed a bicycle up to about 40 km/h. Because the power output of a human being is limited, bicycles operate in a fairly narrow speed range.

The air drag of an object depends upon the shape and the roughness of its surface. Rough surfaces generate greater shear forces. Smooth surfaces generally have a lower friction drag than do rough ones (Hoerner, 1965). In form drag, the leading edge of a moving body has a higher pressure than the trailing edge, resulting in a retarding force. Bluff or blunt bodies such as cylinders and spheres have very high drag because of the huge low pressure region in their wakes. Streamlined airfoil shapes, on the other hand, have a fraction of the drag of blunt bodies of equivalent size. The air flows smoothly over a streamlined shape without flow separation, resulting in much less energy loss in turbulent mixing. The result of streamlining in cycling is to save energy by disturbing the air as little as possible. A cylinder can have 10–20 times the drag of an airfoil having the same cross sectional area. With bluff objects such as cylinders and spheres, the contribution of shape to the aerodynamic drag is many times greater than surface roughness (Hoerner, 1965); streamlining such objects is very effective in decreasing the aerodynamic drag.

Unfortunately, the human body and most of the parts of a bicycle resemble cylinders and thus have a relatively high aerodynamic drag. The wind resistance of the human body in road racing is responsible for about 2/3 of the aerodynamic friction losses, while the bicycle causes approximately 1/3 (Kyle & Burke, 1984). Naturally, the greatest improvement in cycling performance could be accomplished by improving the aerodynamic drag of the human body. Recently, great advances have been made in producing slick, tight-fitting clothing for cyclists and in changing the rider's posture for maximum aerodynamic benefit (Kyle, 1986; Zahradnik, 1989).

Starting in the early 1980s, the introduction of aerodynamic funny bikes, disk wheels, and aero-components has resulted in a dramatic increase in bicycle racing speeds (Kyle & Burke, 1984; Zahradnik, 1989). Almost every bicycle time trial record in the world has been broken in the past five years. There has been a true revolution in cycling equipment technology. Most of the advances in cycling equipment for time trialing, i.e., solo races against the clock, have been related to lower aerodynamic drag. Aerodynamic wheels, helmets, clothing, and components all have less drag than the traditional equipment they replace. Elbow rest handlebars allow riders to maintain an efficient aerodynamic crouch for long periods, narrow tires have lower air drag than wide ones, and clipless pedals, by eliminating the toe strap and the cage, produce a lower drag than ordinary pedals. Watering systems with tubes that allow the rider to drink without reaching down not only allow a racer to drink frequently without worrying about how to steer with one hand, but they also lower the average aerodynamic drag by eliminating the reach for a bottle. Finger tip shifters have a similar aerodynamic advantage and one that is not so obvious. Index fingertip shifters allow quicker gear changes; therefore, the bike doesn't slow down as much between shifts. By smoothing out speed variations, energy is conserved.

Because aerodynamic drag is proportional to the square of the speed, the mean drag is higher at a variable speed than at a steady speed, even though the average speed is the same.

Drafting

There are four general methods of decreasing wind resistance in cycling. The first and oldest is the practice of drafting or slip-streaming. The most important skill for a beginning cyclist to learn is to follow behind another bicycle closely and safely to benefit from the lower wind resistance and energy consumption provided by drafting. Drafting cyclists consume from 30–40% less energy than those who are leading a pace line or pack (Kyle, 1979). Racing cyclists often follow with a wheel gap of from 15–30 cm, and this is hazardous at any speed. To do this safely, cyclists must never fail to concentrate on the wheel in front and should make sure that wheels never overlap should the rider in front suddenly slow or swerve. Probably the most common accident in a pack is for a drafting rider to touch wheels with the rider in front and crash; broken collarbones and dislocated shoulders are a frequent result.

Figure 10-5 shows the reduction of wind resistance versus spacing for drafting cyclists (Kyle, 1979). Carried to extreme, with a properly designed motorized pace vehicle, 100% of the wind resistance can be removed from a drafting cyclist, and incredible speeds are possible on a bicycle. In fact, by riding in the right spot, a cyclist can extract energy from the wind stream (the trailing vortex behind an auto produces an artificial tailwind). John Howard went 245 km/h (152 mph) riding a bicycle in a special enclosure behind a race car at Bonneville, Utah, on July 20, 1985. Bicyclists have traveled in large groups or used motorized pace machines since the beginning of the sport. Speeds are substantially increased by either method. If riders in a group of cyclists alternate at riding at the front of a pace line, each rider consumes less energy, and the pace line can travel from 2–6 km/h faster than can a single cyclist over the same distance (Kyle, 1979). The larger the group, the faster the cyclists can ride. In Europe, cycle racers sometimes compete behind special pace motorcycles. By drafting, these bicyclists can average nearly 65 km/h for over 160 km, whereas elite racing cyclists in time trials can average only about 40 km/h over the same distance.

Frontal Area

The second method of lowering wind resistance is to decrease the frontal area of the rider and machine. This strategy led to the characteristic egg-shaped cycle racing stance, which lowers the frontal area from about 0.37 m^2 in the upright position to about 0.30 m^2 in the crouched racing position (Nonweiler, 1956). The intent of the newly developed elbow rest handlebars is to permit the rider to assume an even more radical aerodynamic position. The rider's body also forms a more streamlined shape, so the position is doubly ef-

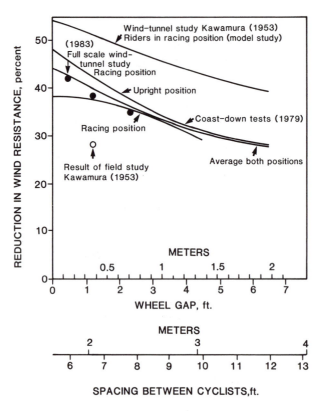

FIGURE 10-5. *Slipstreaming cyclists—reduction in wind resistance with decreased spacing. From Kyle & Burke (1984).*

fective. Figure 10-6 shows the wind resistance of riders in various positions (Kyle & Burke, 1984), and Figure 10-7 shows the total power necessary to propel the same bicycle against the resistive forces. A 20% decrease in drag is possible between an upright riding posture and a crouched racing position. The best, with a 30% drag reduction, is the hill descent position with the hands together on the handlebars, the chin resting on the hands, the pedals in horizontal position, the knees pressing against the top frame tube, and the saddle pressed into the rider's stomach. This riding technique is only practical in descending steep grades without pedaling.

By redesigning the machine to allow the rider to pedal in either a supine or a prone recumbent posture, the frontal area can be reduced and streamlining of the body can be improved even further. However, these riding positions are illegal in conventional bicycle racing; they were outlawed in 1934 by the Union Cicliste Interna-

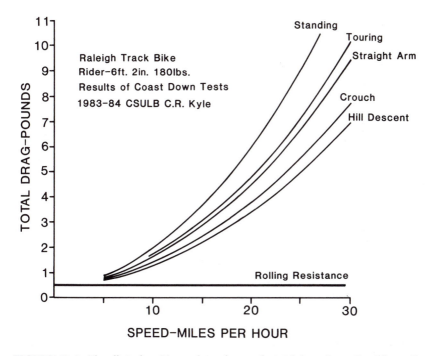

FIGURE 10-6. *The effect of position and speed upon the total drag of a cyclist. The cyclist is tall and thin, so drag and power are higher than normal for the 180 lb. body weight. From coast-down tests at California State University, Long Beach, 1983–84.*

tionale (UCI), the international governing body of conventional bicycle racing. However, recumbent machines are permitted in contests conducted by the International Human Powered Vehicle Association.

By hiding cables and by properly placing other bicycle accessories, the frontal area of the bicycle can be substantially reduced. For example, a vertically mounted bicycle pump has about 20 times the frontal area of a pump mounted horizontally. Also, locating components in the wake of others decreases the effective frontal area and allows the components to draft. Mounting a water bottle behind the seat is better than mounting it in the conventional location on the frame.

Smoothing

The third method of decreasing air resistance is to smooth or round surfaces without substantially altering the vehicle envelope. This means that cables, rods, sharp corners, and unnecessary parts are eliminated or hidden in the frame. Also, skin-tight clothing can

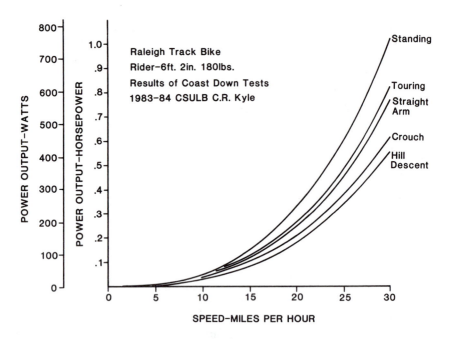

FIGURE 10-7. *The effect of position and speed upon the total power of a cyclist. The cyclist is tall and thin, so drag and power are higher than normal for the 180 lb. body weight. From coast-down tests at California State University, Long Beach, 1983–84.*

be worn by the rider. A standard bicycle is made up of aerodynamically poor shapes, such as cylinders, bolts, springs, chains, sprockets, spokes and levers. The funny bikes of the U.S. Cycling Team smoothed out or eliminated all of these inefficient components (Kyle & Burke, 1984). At first glance, the bike looks fairly conventional, but the modifications dropped the air drag of the bike by 46% and the overall drag of the bicycle and rider by 14% (Kyle, 1987).

Streamlining

The fourth method of reducing wind resistance is to partially or entirely shield the rider and machine with a streamlined shell. By using this method, wind drag can be reduced by more than 80% (Table 10-4), which shows the aero drag and energy consumption possible by recumbent riding positions and streamlining (Kyle et al., 1979; Kyle, 1989b). The best machine shown in Table 10-4 can travel at 32 km/h with 70% less power than a conventional bicycle; this 1978 machine is several generations older than the best human powered vehicles of today.

The drag coefficient is a measure of the aerodynamic efficiency

TABLE 10-4. *Drag & Speed Characteristics of Streamlined Human Powered Vehicles*

Machine	Frontal Area m² (Area in ft²)	Drag Coefficient C_d	Percent Drag Reduction at 32 KPH	Required Power at 32Kph-Watts	Speed With No Power Increase-KPH (Increase-MPH)	Maximum Competition Speed-KPH* (Speed-MPH*)
Bare Bicycle	.50 [5.4]	.78	0	203	32 [19.8]	–
Bicycle Plus Front Fairing I	.50 [5.4]	.60	13%	177	33.5 [20.8]	54.72 [33.9]
Bicycle Plus Front Fairing II	.55 [5.9]	.52	22%	159	34.73 [21.5]	
Palombo Supine Tricycle - Bare	.35 [3.8]	.77	26%	151	34.5 [21.4]	58.21 [33.9]
Van Valkenburgh (Aeroshell) Covers Upper Body	.65 [7.0]	.32	34%	125	36.8 [22.8]	54.22 [33.6]
Aeroshell plus Bottom Skirt	.68 [7.3]	.21	48%	97	39.8 [24.7]	74.85 [46.4]
Palombo Tricycle with Fairing	.46 [4.9]	.28	55%	92	40.9 [25.3]	71.42 [44.3]
Kyle Full Fairing	.71 [7.6]	.10	67%	68	46 [28.5]	74.77 [46.4]
Van Valkenburgh Prone Quadracycle with Fairing	.46 [4.9]	.14	68%	64	46.9 [29.1]	79.47 [49.3]

*Measured at the International Human Powered Speed Championships. From "Predicting Human Powered Vehicle Performance Using Ergonometry and Aerodynamic Drag Measurements" Proceedings, International Conference on Human Powered Transportation, San Diego, 1979. Chester R. Kyle.

of a geometric shape; the lower the number, the better the shape. Poor shapes such as boxes or cylinders have drag coefficients greater than 1.0 (based upon the frontal area). Efficient shapes resembling wing sections or tear drops can have drag coefficients less than 0.1 (Hoerner, 1965). In other words, it would take less than one tenth the amount of energy per unit frontal area to drive a wing section through the air as a box or cylinder. A racing bicyclist has a drag coefficient of about 0.7 to 0.8. Production automobiles are between 0.3 and 0.4, and manufacturers are hoping to lower this to between 0.2 and 0.3 in the future. Completely streamlined human powered vehicles have drag coefficients between 0.1 and 0.14. These machines can go at least 32 km/h faster than the best conventional racing bicycle. The highest speed for a conventional bicycle is about 71 km/h, a record set on a smooth enclosed track by a world champion cycle sprinter, whereas the record for a streamlined human powered vehicles is 105.36 km/h set by Fred Markham at Mono Lake, California, on May 11, 1986. Markham is an excellent athlete, but is by no means a world class cyclist.

Aerodynamic Clothing and Helmets

Modern cycle clothing and helmets have a much lower drag than do conventional clothing and helmets. Table 10-5 shows the results of full scale wind tunnel tests of clothing at the California Institute of Technology (Kyle, 1987). Cyclists were placed in a fixed position on a bicycle in the low speed wind tunnel, and the drag forces were measured at speeds varying from 24 km/h to 56 km/h. A cyclist with a smooth, tight, skin suit had about 240 g less drag at 48 km/h than a did a cyclist wearing a wool jersey. Table 10-6 shows that this would save about 1.83 s/km in a long time trial and result in a lead of 25 m/km against an equal opponent (Kyle, 1990).

The effect of aero helmets is just as spectacular. Table 10-7 shows recent results of wind tunnel tests on racing helmets (Kyle, 1990). Using a good production racing helmet would give a racing cyclist a 19 m lead in one km over an equal opponent wearing a standard helmet.

Table 10-8 shows the results of wind tunnel tests of spinning bicycle wheels. By using two aerodynamic wheels, such as lenticular disks or three spoke composite wheels, a racer could gain a lead of 30 m/km versus an opponent with two conventional 36 spoke wheels (Kyle, 1990). The tests also show that the aerodynamic drag of wide tires is greater than that for narrow ones, that lens shaped disk wheels

TABLE 10-5. *Aerodynamic Drag of Bicycle Clothing at 48 km/h*

Clothing Type	Drag of Bike Plus Rider (g)
Rubberized Skin Suit with Sleeves	2620
Lycra Suit and Tights	2640
Lycra Tights, Wool Long Sleeved Jersey	2860
Tight Polypropylene Warmup Suit	2930

TABLE 10-6. *The Racing Advantage of Aerodynamic Drag Reduction*

Decrease in Drag (g)	Time/km Difference (s/km)	Lead Distance (m/km)	Race Time Difference 1000 m Time Trial (s)	Race Time Difference 4000 m Pursuit (s)
10	0.07	0.95	0.07	0.28
20	0.14	1.90	0.12	0.62
40	0.28	3.80	0.23	1.12
80	0.58	7.80	0.47	2.22
120	0.86	11.6	0.70	3.39
160	1.28	17.2	0.94	4.53
200	1.56	21.0	1.17	5.62
240	1.83	24.8	1.40	6.74

TABLE 10-7. *The Aerodynamic Drag of Bicycle Helmets*

Helmet Tested	Grams Drag 30 mph
1984 U.S. Olympic Aero (Rough Primer Finish)	−8(a)
1986 U.S. Team Aero	−8(a)
Czech Aero	+0(a)
Specialized Prototype Aero	+15(a)
Bell Stratos (Aero)	+36(b)
Giro Aerohead	+41(a)
Manikin, Bald No-Hair	+54(a)
Giro Aerohead, cut off to 30 cm	+61(a)
OGK Aero	+81(a)
Manikin, with Short Hair	+111(a)
Specialized Groundforce	+129(a)
Specialized Airforce	+135(a)
Specialized Microforce	+146(a)
Bell VI Pro	+157(a)
OGK Forza	+162(a)
Standard Leather Strap Helmet	+181(b)
Giro Hammerhead, Lycra Cover	+200(a)

(a) UC Irvine, Feb., 1990, for Specialized, Inc. (b) UC Irvine, Oct., 1985, for Bell Helmet.

are better than flat ones, that wheels with polished surfaces have a lower drag than wheels with a rougher finish, and that standard wheels with flat bladed spokes are better than ones with round spokes. Furthermore, it has been established that with standard wheels, aero shaped rims are superior; and with spoked wheels, the fewer the spokes, the lower the aero-drag.

Improved Components and Equipment

By using aero-components, air resistance can be cut still further. For example, removing the water bottle and cage and placing it behind the seat will cut air drag by about 40 g at 30 mph (Zahradnik & Kyle, 1987). Probably the best job of cleaning up all of the components has been done by Hooker and Spangler (1989). The bicycle they have built has been proven to be almost 1 min faster in 40 km than the best of the time-trial bikes previously tested.

The appeal to improving equipment in order to go faster is that it requires little additional training, skill, or effort—just more money. Racing cyclists often spend hundreds of dollars to remove a single pound from a bicycle and even more to purchase the latest racing system, including clothing, helmets, shoes, pedals, shifters, wheels, etc. Because among equal competitors many events are won by a fraction of a second, equipment can mean winning or loosing. Figure 10-8 shows the progress of the world hour record from 1876 to

TABLE 10-8. *The Air Resistance of Spinning Bicycle Wheels*

27 inch wheels	Drag at 30 mph (6)	10° Yaw Angle*
Dupont/Specialized		
Waxed and Polished, 18 mm tire	112(a)	39(b)
Unfinished Surface, 18 mm tire	126(a)	
Unfinished Surface, 24 mm tire	167(a)	
Aerosports Kevlar Lens Disk, 18mm Tire	115(a)	26(b)
Campy Lens Disk, 18mm Tire	120(b)	
Trispoke, 18 mm Tire	123(a)	115(b)
Aerosports Carbon Flat Disk, 18 mm Tire	123(a)	75(b)
Aerolite 16 Aero-Bladed Spokes, Aero-Rim 18 mm Tire	140(b)	
Wheelsmith 24 Aero-Bladed Spokes, Aero-Rim 18 mm Tire	147(b)	
Wheelsmith 28 Aero-Bladed Spokes, Aero-Rim 18 mm Tire	173(a)	
Wheelsmith 28 Aero-Oval Spokes, Aero-Rim 18 mm Tire	175(a)	
USCF 18 Round Spokes, Aero-Rim, 18 mm Tire	206(c)	
Wheelsmith 36 Round Spokes, Standard Rim 18 mm Tire	258(b)	
26 inch wheels		
Aerosports Carbon Flat Disk, 18 mm Tire	109(c)	
Wheelsmith 32 Round Spokes, Flat Rim 22 mm Tire	208(a)	
24 inch wheels		
Huffy Special Carbon Flat Disk, 18 mm Tire	112(c)	
Aerosports 18 Aero-Bladed Spokes, Aero-Rim 18 mm Tire	127(c)	
USCF 16 Aero-Bladed Spokes, Aero-Rim 18 mm Tire	137(c)	
Wheelsmith 24 inch, 28 Round Spokes, Flat Rim 22 mm Tire	182(a)	

(a) UC Irvine Feb. 1990, for Specialized. (b) UC Irvine, June, 1988, for Specialized/Dupont (c) UC Irvine, Dec., 1985, for USCF.
* The apparent wind direction is at 10° to the bike axis.

1984, and it directly illustrates the importance of equipment. From 1876 until 1900 was an era where equipment was responsible for rapidly improving the record. The modern bicycle, the pneumatic tire, and drop handlebars were all developed in this period. Then came the era of the ever-improving athlete who used event-specific training methods. During this period from 1900 to 1972 the record advanced much more slowly, mostly due to a series of super athletes appearing on the scene. With Francesco Moser in 1984 and his aerodynamic funny bike developed by Antonio Dal Monte of Italy (Dal Monte et al., 1986), a new era of rapid equipment development was introduced.

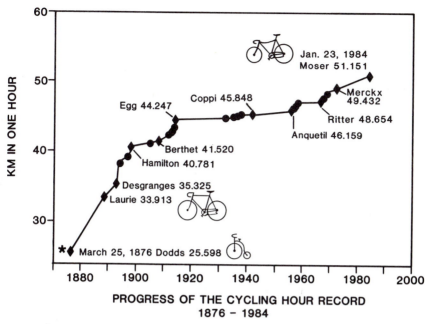

PROGRESS OF THE CYCLING HOUR RECORD
1876 – 1984

★F.L. Dodds, Great Britain, Cambridge March 25, 1876 25.599km

FIGURE 10-8. *Times for the world bicycle one hour record 1876–1990. The first rapid advance was due to equipment improvement (1876–1900). The next advances were basically due to better athletes, better training methods, and record attempts at high altitude (1900–1972). The last advance was due to disk wheels and aerodynamic clothing and equipment (1972–1990).*

The Effect of Winds on Bicycle Speed

Headwinds and Tailwinds. It is well known that headwinds and tailwinds can affect the speed of a bicycle. To maintain a constant rate of energy expenditure, a cyclist must speed up or slow down at a velocity equivalent to about half the wind speed in tailwinds or headwinds, respectively (Kyle, 1973). In other words, if a rider can maintain a 30 km/h bike speed on the level with no wind, he would slow down to about 25 kph facing a 10 km/h headwind or speed up to about 35 km/h with a 10 km/h tailwind. On an out-and-back time-trial course, the net time would not be the same as with no wind. Table 10-9 shows that if a rider can maintain 32 km/h on a level, 1 km out-and-back course with no wind, that with equal effort, he will cover the course more slowly with any wind (Kyle 1988a).

Cross Winds. In 1983, we performed wind tunnel tests at Texas A & M University for the U.S.A. Cycling Team while developing

ERGOGENICS FOR BICYCLING   **397**

TABLE 10-9. *The Effect of Wind on Bicycle Speed on a 1 km Out/1 km Back Circuit Course (Equal Distances with and Against the Wind)*

	Wind Speed (km/h)			
	0	4	8	16
Speed With Wind (km/h)	32	34	36	40
Speed Against Wind (km/h)	32	30	28	24
Average Speed (km/h)	32	31.88	31.50	30.00
Time (min:s)	3:45	3:45.9	3:48.6	4:00

TABLE 10-10. *The Effect of Yaw Angle on Aerodynamic Drag*

Bicycle	Yaw angle*	Drag (kg)**	Difference
Standard Track Bike	0°	3.63	
with rider	10°	3.81	+ 0.30 kg
Aero Bike with 450 mm	0°	3.45	
wheels plus rider	10°	3.39	− 0.06 kg

* The wind angle relative to the bicycle axis. This is equivalent to an 8.5 kph cross wind with a 48 kph bike speed.
** The drag force was measured parallel to the axis of the bike and the wind was constant at *48 km/h* along the axis of the bike. The same rider, in an identical position was used on both bikes.

the team bikes for the 1984 Olympics. Table 10-10 shows the results of tests on two bicycles with the same rider. One was a standard track bike with round tubes and standard 700C wheels and rims, and the other was an aero-bike with airfoil shaped tubing, aero rims on the wheels, and aero handlebars. There were no round tubing sections on the aero-bike. The drag of the standard bike increased when the bikes were rotated at an angle to the wind. However, the drag of the aero bike decreased slightly.

Using a modified equation from Kyle (1989c), the effect of cross winds on bicycle speed in an out-and-back time-trial course was calculated, and the results are shown in Table 10-11. The modified equation gives the aerodynamic drag on a bicycle with a head wind or tail wind:

[1] $$D = W(Crr_1 + Crr_2V) + A_3(V + V_w)^2,$$

where **D** is the drag (N), **W** is the weight (kg), Crr_1 is a static rolling resistance coefficient, Crr_2 is a dynamic rolling resistance coefficient that includes wheel bearing losses and dynamic tire losses, **V** is the speed (m/s), V_w is the wind velocity (m/s) with head winds being positive, and **A3** is a combined aerodynamic drag factor that may be calculated from:

[2] $$A_3 = 1/2\ _pC_dA$$

TABLE 10-11. *Effect of Head Winds, Tail Winds and Cross Winds in an Out and Back 40 km Time Trial.*

Bicycle Type	Wind Speed (km/h)	Wind Angle (°)*	Bike Speed (km/h)	Time for 40 km Out and Back (Min:Sec)	Time Difference (s)
Standard Track Bike					
No Wind	0.00	0°	40.00	60:00	0
Head & Tail Wind	6.95	0° & 180°	39.66 avg.	60:31	+31
Cross Wind	6.95	90°	39.44	60:51	+51
Aero Bike					
No Wind	0.00	0°	40.69	58:59	−61
Head & Tail Wind	7.21	0° & 180°	40.34 avg.	59.30	−30
Cross Wind	7.21	90°	40.86	58:44	−76

* The angle 0° is a head wind along the course. The listed cross winds cause a 10° apparent wind angle with respect to the bicycle.

where $_p$ is the air density (kg/m^3), C_d is the aerodynamic drag coefficient (about 0.7 to 0.9 for bicycles), and **A** is the projected frontal area (m^2). The methods used in the computation are described in Kyle (1989c).

Some quite remarkable results come from the calculations. With both the standard bike and the aero bike, a wind directly along an out-and-back circuit course will cause a slower time trial. The higher speed with a tailwind does not make up for the lost time against the headwind. It can be seen from Table 10-10 that a pure cross wind causes the aerodynamic drag to increase with a conventional bike. This is because the airflow pattern over the body and the bicycle changes, and thus the pressure distribution on the surface is different. Also, the effective wind angle is no longer parallel to the bike, and certain components and cables no longer draft in the wake of others. The result is a higher drag coefficient. What is even more interesting is that with a standard bike, a pure cross wind causes a slower time trial than the same wind directly along the course.

With an aero bike, the opposite is true, with a cross wind the time is even faster than with no wind at all. When the effective wind is at an angle to the direction of bicycle travel, the airfoil shape develops some lift at right angles to the wind (Figure 10-9). The resulting forward thrust component has the effect of lowering the drag, as shown by the wind tunnel tests. In this case the wheel acts like a sail and actually extracts some propulsive energy from the wind. Therefore, on a circuit course with a cross wind, a bike with disk wheels and an aero frame might theoretically be faster than if there were no wind at all.

Figure 10-10 shows the results of a mathematical model of the effects of cross winds at various angles to the course in an out-and-

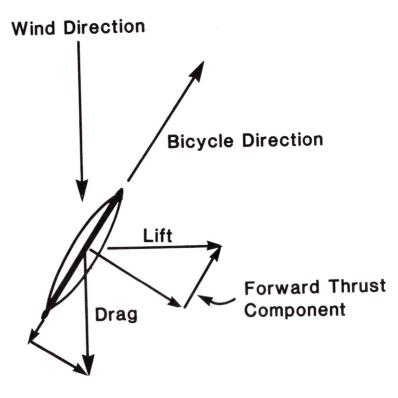

Wind Direction

Bicycle Direction

Lift

Forward Thrust Component

Drag

FORCES ON AN AERO WHEEL

FIGURE 10-9. *Forces on an aero wheel.*

back time trial (Norris, 1987; Flower, 1987). The model assumes that a cyclist can complete a 40 km time trial in 60 min with no wind. In theory, any steady wind at any angle to the course will cause slower times. This is the general experience in practice.

The Effect of Altitude

Figure 10-11 shows the effect of altitude on bicycle speed (Kyle & Burke, 1984). The air density decreases with elevation, and air resistance also decreases in direct proportion to the density (Hoerner, 1965). In theory, bicycle speed should increase substantially with higher elevations, as is shown in the upper curve on Figure 10-11. However, actual records at Mexico City, (elevation about 2,200 m) seem to be only between 3% and 5% higher than at sea level, rather than the 8% predicted by the theory. The difference is due to a decrease in aerobic power because of the rarified atmosphere.

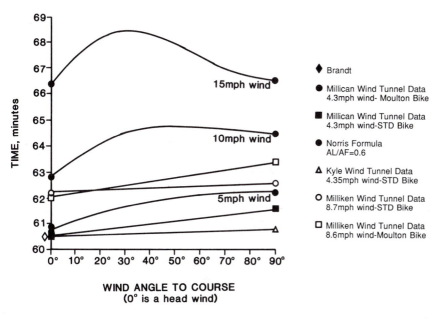

FIGURE 10-10. *The effect of cross winds on a 25-mile time trial.*

Legend:
- ◆ Brandt
- ● Millican Wind Tunnel Data 4.3mph wind- Moulton Bike
- ■ Millican Wind Tunnel Data 4.3mph wind-STD Bike
- ● Norris Formula AL/AF=0.6
- ▲ Kyle Wind Tunnel Data 4.35mph wind-STD Bike
- O Milliken Wind Tunnel Data 8.7mph wind-STD Bike
- □ Milliken Wind Tunnel Data 8.6mph wind-Moulton Bike

WIND ANGLE TO COURSE
(0° is a head wind)

The Effect of Passing Automotive Traffic

Figure 10-12 shows the effect of passing traffic (Kyle & Burke, 1984). The curves are the result of observations by a very consistent time trialist along a very straight and level stretch of highway using a bicycle speedometer accurate to 0.1 kM/h. Speed increases from 0.5 to 5 km/h were common as various motorized vehicles passed with about 1–2 m of side clearance. Large autos caused about a 1 km/h increase, while vans and pickup trucks increased speed about 2 km/h. Large highway trucks raised the speed by 3 km/h or more. The increase lasted about 10 s.

When a strong cross wind was blowing, almost no effect was measurable. When passing traffic slowed, approaching the speed of the cyclist, the duration of the effect increased until it sometimes persisted as long as the cyclist was drafting beside the motor vehicle. Naturally, when traffic was heavy, the overall speed increase was greater. If a steady stream of traffic was passing, speed increased from 5–8 km/h. Because of the obvious influence of passing traffic on cycling speed, time trial records should be certified only on a course free from auto traffic.

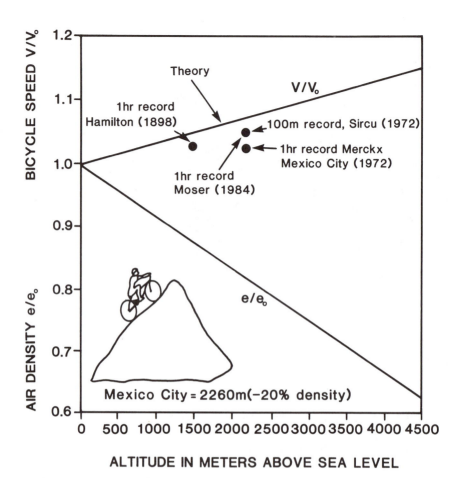

FIGURE 10-11. *The effect of altitude on air density and cycle speed. From Kyle & Burke (1984).*

MECHANICS

By changing or improving the mechanical design of the bicycle, the efficiency of energy utilization can be improved. Such factors as tire rolling resistance, bearing and drive train friction, weight, and stability are critical in allowing a bicycle to function efficiently.

The Rolling Resistance of Tires

Tire rolling resistance is due basically to the deformation of the tread and sidewalls of the tire and the resulting loss of energy in internal friction. Even with perfectly smooth pavement, this deformation will cause losses in speed, although rough pavement will

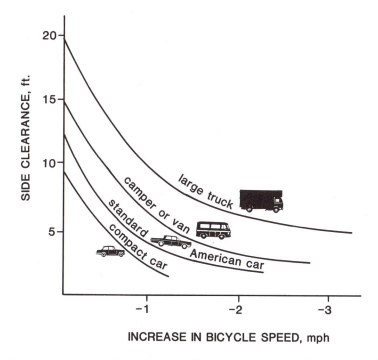

FIGURE 10-12. *Estimated effect of passing traffic on cycle speed. From Kyle & Burke (1984).*

naturally increase the losses. Rolling resistance is a direct function of the weight carried by the tire. Increasing the weight on a tire will increase the deformation; as a result, the rolling resistance is directly proportional to weight. Depending on the design of the tires and the road surface, the retarding force caused by tire friction can vary from about 0.22% to 0.5% of the weight on the tires (Kyle & Burke, 1984).

As mentioned previously, wind resistance is the dominant retarding force in cycling. Even though tire friction is small compared to wind drag, better tire designs have been responsible for significant improvement in cycle racing performance (Kyle, 1988b; Berto, 1988). A good racing tire can weigh as little as 130 g and hold a pressure as high as 15 atmospheres. The tires with the lowest rolling resistance have extremely thin walls, thin smooth tread, and thin tubes. The rubber used in the most efficient tires is natural latex, since it is very resilient and has a low energy loss when flexed. The best wall materials are made from thin threads of silk, nylon, or Kevlar, since they have a high strength to weight ratio and are extremely flexible, thus minimizing both weight and hysteresis losses.

ERGOGENICS FOR BICYCLING **403**

There are probably no huge breakthroughs to be made in tire design that will improve performance by quantum leaps.

Table 10-12 shows the rolling resistance coefficient of typical touring and racing tires (Kyle & Burke, 1984; Kyle, 1988a, 1988d). By multiplying the rolling resistance coefficient by the total weight on the tires and dividing by 100, the resistance to motion may be calculated. As shown in Table 10-12, rolling resistance is a strong function of tire pressure. As the tire pressure increases, the deformation of the tire is less, so the rolling resistance decreases. In racing, competitors will carry as high a pressure as practical in the tires to decrease rolling resistance. Typical pressures range from 8 to 10 atmospheres in road races and from 10 to 15 atmospheres in track races.

Another factor affecting rolling resistance is wheel and tire diameter (Table 10-12). With identical tire construction, as the wheel size decreases, the tire must deform progressively more to support an equal weight, so tires with smaller wheels have an unavoidable higher rolling resistance, even on perfectly smooth pavement. On rough pavement they are at a double disadvantage, i.e., to over-

TABLE 10-12. *The Rolling Resistance of Bicycle Tires*

		Surface		
Tire Type	Pressure Atm	Linoleum	Smooth Concrete	Asphalt
Tubular Tires				
Continental Olympic 27 in × 19 mm	6.8	0.19*	0.17*	0.22*
Continental Olympic 24 in × 19 mm	6.8	0.26	0.23	0.27
Clement Colle Main 27 in × 19 mm	6.8	0.16		
Clement Colle Main 24 in × 19 mm	6.8	0.21		
Clement Colle Main 20 in × 19 mm	6.8	0.29		
Wired on, "Clincher" Tires				
Specialized Turbo S 700C	6.8	0.26		0.29
Specialized Turbo S, Kevlar 700C	6.8	0.23		0.27
Touring Tire, 700 × 25 C	6.8	0.31		0.35
Touring Tire, 700 × 25 C	8.2	0.28		
Knobby Tread Tire 27 in × 2-1/4 in	3.1	1.30		
Knobby Tread Tire 20 in × 2-1/4in	3.1	1.70		
Avocet Fastgrip 20 in × 1-3/4in	5.4	0.40		
Avocet Faqstgrip 20 in × 1-3/4in	6.8	0.37		
Avocet Faqstgrip 20 in × 1-3/4in	8.2	0.32		
Same Tire Worn Tread	6.8	0.30		
Avocet Fastgrip 26 in × 1-3/4in	6.8	Glass = 0.30		0.35
		Rough Macadam = 0.54		
Moulton 17 in × 1-1/4in	5.4	0.34		
Moulton 17 in × 1-1/4in	6.8	0.30		0.39
Moulton 17 in × 1-1/4in	8.2	0.27		

* The rolling resistance coefficient in percent. To get the resistance to motion, multiply the weight on the tire by the coefficient divided by 100.

come irregularities in the pavement requires a greater propulsive force than with a large wheel, and the friction losses are correspondingly greater (consider a roller skate trying to go over a rock that is half the size of the wheel).

Another factor of lesser importance is velocity. Tire rolling friction remains fairly constant with speed, but there is some variation. As the speed increases, shock contact with the pavement increases, and dynamic deformation of the tire increases. This causes greater internal losses that are manifested as heat and increased tire temperature. This effect however is minor, because bicycle tires operate at high pressure, and dynamic losses are small. Tests on a 17 × 1.25 inch Moulton Tire at the General Motors tire test facility in 1987 indicated that the increase in retarding force due to velocity is: F (kg) = W(0.0000105V), where W is the total load on the tire (kg), and V is the forward velocity (m/s) (Kyle, 1988d). Technically, a similar term should be added to the rolling resistance given in Table 10-12. However, the velocity effect is unknown for most bicycle tires. In general it is ignored, and the rolling resistance is assumed to be constant.

Drive Train Friction and Bearing Friction

Bearing and drive train losses are small, from 2–5% of the human energy input to the crank. The losses are proportional to the power level, with the highest losses occurring at the highest power input (Kyle & Caiozzo, 1986). The remaining energy input is consumed in overcoming tire friction and wind resistance. There are probably no major improvements to be made in decreasing bearing and drive train friction losses. However, even very small improvements can be important in racing; therefore, there will always be some changes in components by those seeking to lower the friction losses (Kay, 1988). Bearing friction is similar to tire rolling resistance, i.e., it is proportional to the load on the bearing and proportional to the rotational velocity. Richard Kay of the Champion Bearing Company has measured bicycle wheel bearing friction in a vacuum (Kay, 1988) and reports the following friction for two different sealed bearing types used in bicycle hubs:

$T = W(227 + 3.83N)10^{-6}$ for Champion Ball Bearings with one metal shield and one Teflon seal and,

$T = W(773 + 6.30N)10^{-6}$ for Suntour bicycle hub bearings with one metal shield and one rubber seal. In the two equations, W is the load on the bearing (kg), N is the rpm of the wheel, and T is the torque on the bearing (Nm). From the above it can be shown that tire rolling friction is from 30 to 60 times as large as bearing friction and that wind resistance is several hundred times as high.

Therefore, it would be very difficult to detect the effect of improvements in bearings on bicycle speed with any ordinary instrumentation because the small energy losses due to bearing friction are far overshadowed by wind and rolling resistance. However, the difference between the two bearings in Kay's study represents an extra climb of about 10 m in a 160 km race, so racers would still want the best bearings available. If Kay's data and similar comparisons among commercially available components were published, cyclists could make more logical choices on equipment purchases. Unfortunately, such tests are almost non-existent.

The Effect of Weight on Bicycle Speed

Weight has a triple effect in slowing a bicycle down. First, it retards acceleration. Races are never at a constant speed; there is always a continual shift in position and speed among riders in a pack—especially in corners. The ability to accelerate quickly is critical to a bike racer. Second, weight slows speed in climbing. Lifting extra weight over a hill takes energy that is never recovered on the descent (Kyle, 1988a, 1988c). Third, weight adds to the rolling resistance of tires. Extra weight causes added deformation in the tread and sidewalls of a tire and, thus, increased rolling resistance. Removing weight from a bicycle has been an historic aim of bicycle design.

Weight and Acceleration. Because adding weight to a bicycle increases the inertia, it will slow the rate of acceleration. In bicycle track events, where the acceleration phase is a large part of the total event time, acceleration is highly important. The times in Table 10-13 were calculated by Kyle (1988a) to estimate the effect of weight on a 1000 m time trial and on the 4000 m individual pursuit. The listed acceleration and race times include the adverse effect of weight on rolling resistance. The acceleration times tell how long it takes to reach the top speed at a constant power output.

Adding a small amount of weight does not change the top speed appreciably. However, it does take longer to reach a given speed. The distance traveled during the acceleration phase is greater with

TABLE 10-13. *The Effect of Weight Upon Track Time Trial Races*

Total Weight Rider + Bicycle (kg)	1000−m Time (s)	4000−m Time (s)	Acceleration time 1000−m 60 km/h	Acceleration time 4000−m 50 km/h
81.7	63.38	292.97	14.47	16.7
82.6	+0.08	+0.20	+0.17	+0.18
83.5	+0.16	+0.40	+0.34	+0.38
84.4	+0.24	+0.60	+0.50	+0.58

higher weight; consequently, less distance remains to the finish, and proportionately less time is spent at top speed. The peculiar result of this calculation is that the difference in total race time does not agree with the difference in acceleration time as shown in Table 10-13, especially over the shorter distances.

Although weight is important, it is not nearly as important as aerodynamics. Comparing the times in Table 10-6 with those in Table 10-13, it can be seen that increasing a bicycle's weight by 2.8 kg will have only as much effect on the time as increasing the aerodynamic drag by about 20–40 g. In longer events, aerodynamics would be even more predominant. Therefore, considerable weight can be added to a bicycle to gain an aerodynamic advantage.

Weight, Hill Climbing, and Rolling Resistance. Figure 10-13 shows the effect of adding weight to a bicycle when climbing hills (Kyle, 1988a). With the same power as traveling on level pavement, the bicycle obviously slows when climbing and speeds up when descending hills. One might ask whether the higher speed on the descent will make up for the loss in time on the ascent. Using the equations listed in Kyle (1988a) or in Figure 10-13, it can be shown

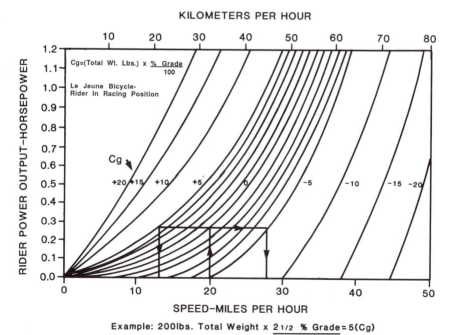

FIGURE 10-13. *The effect of hills on speed. From Kyle & Burke (1984).*

from Table 10-14 that on equal slopes with a 1 km climb and 1 km descent, any type of grade will slow a bicycle down. Also, adding less than 1 kg to the weight of the rider/cycle will slow the bicycle, even on a level course, because of the increase in rolling resistance. Thus, under any circumstances, weight is harmful in competitive cycling.

Bicycle Stability

The factor most affecting bicycle stability is a property of the steering geometry, the trail (Figure 10-14). If the steering axis is projected until it intersects the ground, the distance from this point to

TABLE 10-14. *The Effect of a Hilly Circuit Course Upon Bicycle Speed, 1 km Uphill and 1 km Downhill*

| | Total Weight of Rider + Bike | | | | | | | |
| | 81.7 kg | | | | 82.6 kg | | | |
Slope (%)	Speed Uphill (km/h)	Speed Downhill (km/h)	Time (min:s)	Average Speed (km/h)	Speed Uphill (km/h)	Speed Down (km/h)	Time (min:s)	Average Speed (km/h)
0	32.19	32.19	3:43.7	32.19	32.17	32.17	3:43.8	32.17
2	23.54	41.17	4:00.4	29.95	23.45	41.25	4:00.8	29.90
5	14.45	53.46	5:16.5	22.75	14.32	53.66	5:18.4	22.61
10	8.01	70.46	8:20.5	14.38	7.93	70.79	8:24.6	14.27

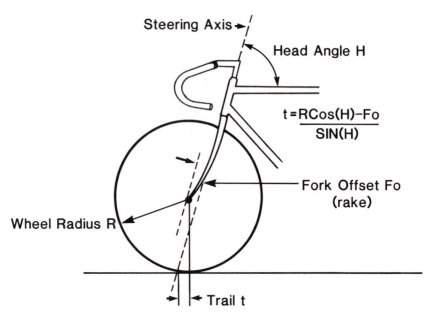

Steering Axis

Head Angle H

$$t = \frac{RCos(H) - Fo}{SIN(H)}$$

Fork Offset Fo (rake)

Wheel Radius R

Trail t

FIGURE 10-14. *Bicycle steering geometry.*

the center of the tire contact patch is the trail, with positive trail being towards the rear. Normally, bicycles have from 4.4–7.0 cm of trail (Jones, 1970; Whitt & Wilson, 1982).

With negative or slight trail, the bike is very sensitive and requires a light and practiced touch to steer. It shows no tendency to self correct and cannot be ridden without hands. As the trail increases, it becomes easier to balance and steer, and tracking improves. Within a certain trail range, the required steering torque is reasonable, the bicycle feels responsive, and no-hands riding becomes easy. Beyond this valley of good response, as trail increases, steering becomes heavy and slow, although it is extremely stable and tracks very well.

In time trials, stability is important because slight variations in steering angle cause the tires to scrub on the pavement, and the rolling resistance increases with each change in direction. This has the effect of a slight braking force with every turn. Also, biomechanically, if a bike is difficult to steer, the rider cannot concentrate totally on producing maximum power and efficiency. The problem is even more acute with front disk wheels. The aerodynamic center of pressure of the wheel is 150 mm ahead of the front axle in a 700C wheel (Edwards, 1986); with unsteady crosswinds, unpredictable steering torques develop that can be very hard to control. By increasing the trail to 8–10 cm (this can be done by reversing the forks), the bike becomes manageable in even strong winds.

Alternate Bicycle Drive Systems

The bicycle drive system has always presented a challenge to inventors seeking to improve it. However, after more than 100 y of development, the sprocket and chain drive system remains firmly entrenched as almost the only method used commercially on bicycles. Why? The major reason is that it is has been optimized for more than a century to carry a few hundred watts in power efficiently and reliably. The chain and sprocket drive provides multiple gear changes; it is light weight, inexpensive, silent, and simple. Although thousands of other bicycle drive mechanisms have been invented, none has totally matched these criteria; to miss even one is usually enough to doom the device from the start. Gear boxes, cam systems, and lever drives almost always fail to be accepted due to high weight, high cost, low efficiency, or other disadvantages.

One device that has made a frequent appearance is an oval chainwheel. In 1894, Charles Skovell was granted U.S Patent No 515449 on the device, and dozens of patents have been issued since. Non-circular chainwheels such as the Shimano Biopace are slight modifications of the normal system and cause periodic variations in the angular velocity of the crank from 2 to 7%. This changes the effective gear ratio in a predetermined manner during the pedal cycle. Manufacturers' claims to the contrary, there is little reliable scientific evidence that the oval chainwheel provides any biomechanical or mechanical advantage over a round chainwheel. Round front sprockets are still the overwhelming choice of racers in any branch of cycling. Miller and Ross (1980) offered a theoretical method of optimizing the shape of a non-round chainwheel to improve cycling performance, but their computer method is unproven.

FUTURE RESEARCH

The problem with applying scientific study methods to cycling is that the enormously complex web of physical variables is completely interrelated. For example, body motion mechanics, position, crank length, pedal platform height, seat height, handlebar height and width, frame geometry, bicycle speed and stability, pedal cadence, power output, frame flex, and bicycle weight, are so interdependent that if one variable is changed, it affects several others, making a study of one variable in isolation impossible.

In other fields where daunting complexity exists, statistics often prove useful in making sense out of confusing data. One of the most promising approaches in cycling would be to use the vast laboratory comprising active racers and recreational cyclists to perform statistical studies of the effect of manipulating variables on performance. This approach is underutilized at present but could be applied if reliable and up-to-date computer data bases could be generated. For example, a central store of past and current world records in cycling is extremely difficult to locate. This valuable information might help to isolate factors leading to the improved performance.

Because of the complexity of scientific analysis, most of the important advances in cycling to date have been empirically developed by coaches, athletes, manufacturers, and inventors. However, analytical instrumentation is improving at an explosive rate. With rapidly developing computer and instrumentation technology, plus improved methods of analysis, answers may soon be forthcoming on many historic questions.

BIBLIOGRAPHY

Berglund, L. (1987). Evaporative weight loss as a measure of absorbed radiation in the human. *8th Conference of Biometeorology and Aerobiology*, American Meteoroligical Society, Boston MA.
Berto, F.J. (1988). Testing bicycle tires. *Bike Tech* October, 1988, 7:5:1–5.

Blix, M. (1901). To the question of human working power. *University Program*, Lund, Sweden.

Bouny, M. (1897). Etudes experimentales variations de la puissance d'un cycliste en function de la cadence. *Revue du Touring Club de France*. Sept. 1897. In: C. Bourlet, *Bicycles et Bicyclettes*, Paris: Gauthier-Villars, 1898.

Bourlet, C. (1896). *Il Nouveau Traite des Bicycles et Bicyclettes le Travail*. Paris: Gauthier-Villars.

Broker, J.P., and R.J. Gregor (1989). Biomechanical feedback and cycling kinetic patterning. *Proceedings, First IOC World Congress on Sport Sciences*, Oct. 28-Nov. 3, 1989, Colorado Springs, CO. p.283.

Brooks, A.N. (1989). Energy consumption of high efficiency vehicles. *Cycling Science* 1:1:6–9.

Burke, E.R. (1990). Sports drinks. *Cycling Science* 2:1:14–17.

Cavanagh, P.R., and D.J. Sanderson (1986). The biomechanics of cycling: studies of the pedaling mechanics of elite pursuit riders. *Science of Cycling*. Human Kinetics Publishers, Champaign IL.

Coast, R.J., and H.G. Welch (1985). Linear increase in optimal pedal rate with increased power output in cycle ergometry. *Eur. J. Appl. Physiol.*:53:339–342.

Coast, R.J., R.H. Cox, and H.G. Welch (1986). Optimal pedaling rate in prolonged bouts of cycle ergometry. *Med. Sci. Sp. Exer.* 18:2:225–230.

Coggan, A.R. (1990). Carbohydrate feeding during prolonged cycling to improve performance. *Cycling Science* 2:1:9–13.

Coyle, E.F. (1989). Carbohydrates and cycling performance. *Cycling Science* 1:1:18–21.

Croisant, P.T., and R.A. Boileau (1984). Effect of pedal rate, brake load, and power on metabolic responses to bicycle ergometer work. *Ergonomics* 27:6:691–700.

Dal Monte, A., A. Manoni, and S. Fucci (1973). Biomechanical study of competitive cycling. *Medicine and Sport, Biomechanics III*, 8:434–439.

Dal Monte, A., M. Faina, and P. Faccini (1986). Italian developments in human powered vehicles. *The Proceedings of the Third International Human Powered Vehicle Scientific Symposium*. International Human Powered Vehicle Association (IHPVA), Indianapolis, IN.

Dal Monte A., and M. Faina (1989). Human anaerobic power output. *Cycling Science* 1:1:13. UCI Congress on the Medical & Scientific Aspects of Cycling. Abono Terme Italy June 19–21, 1989.

Dickinson, S. (1929). The efficiency of bicycle pedalling as affected by speed and load. *J. Physiol. (Lond.)*:67:242–255.

Edwards, E. (1986). Aerodynamic stability of front disk wheels. *Report to the USOC Sports Equipment and Technology Committee*. Colorado Springs, CO.

Flower, R.G. (1987). Technical note on crosswinds. *Bike Tech* 6:4:13–15.

Frederick, E.C., (1988). A comparison of the road shock absorption capacity of cycling gloves. *Report of Exeter Research*, Brentwood, N.H.

Furusawa, K., A.V. Hill, and J.L. Parkinson (1927a). The dynamics of sprint running. *Proc. R. Soc. Lond.* B102:29–42.

Furusawa, K., A.V. Hill, and J.L. Parkinson (1927b). The energy used in sprint running. *Proc. R. Soc. Lond.* B102:43–50.

Gregor, R.J., V.R. Edgerton, J.J. Perrine, D.S. Campion, and C. DeBus (1979). Torque-velocity relationships and muscle fiber composition in elite female athletes. *J. Appl. Physiol.*:Respirat. Environ. Exercise Physiol. 47:388–392.

Gregor, R.J., and S.G. Rugg (1986). Effects of saddle height and pedaling cadence on power output and efficiency. *Science of Cycling*. Human Kinetics Publishers, Champaign IL.

Guyton, A.C. (1986). *Textbook of Medical Physiology*. Saunders 7th Ed.

Hamley, E.J., and V. Thomas (1967). The physiological and postural factors in the calibration of the bicycle ergometer. *J. Physiol.* 191:55–57.

Harrison, J.Y. (1970). Maximizing human power output by suitable selection of motion cycle and load. *Human Factors*. 12:3:315–329.

Henderson, S.C., R.W. Ellis, G. Klimovitch, and G.A. Brooks (1977). The effects of circular and elliptical chainwheels on steady state ergometer work efficiency. *Med. Sci. Sp.* 9:4:202–207.

Hill, A.V. (1922). The maximal work and mechanical efficiency of human muscles and their economical speed. *J. Physiol. (Lond.)* 56:19–41.

Hochmuth, G. (1967). *Biomechanik Sportlicher Bewingen*. Wilhelm Limpert Verlag, GMbH. Frankfurt.

Hoes, M.J.A.J.M., R.A. Binkhorst, A.E.M.C. Smeekes-Kuyl, and A.C.A. Vissers (1968). Measurement of forces exerted on pedal and crank during work on a bicycle ergometer at different loads. *Int. Z. Ang. Physiol. ein. Arb.* 26:33–42.

Hoerner, S.F. (1965). *Fluid Dynamic Drag*. Hoerner Fluid Dynamics, Brick Town N.J.

Hooker G., and D. Spangler (1989). Scientific performance testing. *Cycling Science* 1:1:2–5.

Hull, M.L., and H. Gonzalez (1988). Bivariate optimization of pedaling rate and crank arm length in cycling. *J. Biomech.* 21:10:839–849.

Hull, M., H. K. Gonzalez, and R. Redfield (1988). Optimization of pedaling rate in cycling using a muscle stress based objective function. *IJSB* 4:1:1–20.

Inbar, O., R. Dotan, T. Troush, and Z. Dvir (1983). The effect of bicycle crank-length variation upon power performance. *Ergonomics* 26:12:1139–1146.

Jones, D.E.H. (1970). The stability of a bicycle. *Physics Today,*:34–40, April, 1970.

Kay, R. (1988). The new ball bearings. *Bike Tech,* October, 1988, 7:5:10–13.

Kunstlinger, U., H.G. Ludwig, and J. Stegemann (1985). Force kinetics and oxygen consumption during bicycle ergometer work in racing cyclists and reference-group. *Eur. J. Appl. Physiol.* 54:58–61.

Kyle, C.R. (1973). Factors affecting the speed of a bicycle. *Report no. 1,* Mechanical Engineering, Calif. State Univ., Long Beach CA. Nov. 2, 1973.

Kyle, C.R., and J. Mastropaolo (1976). Predicting racing bicyclist performance using the unbraked flywheel method of bicycle ergometry. *Biomech. Sport Kinanthropom.* 6:211–220. F. Landry and W. Orban (Eds.), Miami Symposia Specialists.

Kyle, C.R. (1979). Reduction of wind resistance and power output of racing cyclists and runners traveling in groups. *Ergonomics* 22:4:387–397.

Kyle, C.R., V.J. Caiozzo, and M. Palombo (1979). Predicting human powered vehicle performance using ergometry and aerodynamic drag measurements. *Proceedings of the International Meeting on Human Powered Transportation.* New York: Metropolitan Association of Urban Designers and Environmental Planners. 200–224.

Kyle, C.R. (1982). Experiments in human ergometry. *Transactions of the 1st Human Powered Vehicle Scientific Symposium.* Indianapolis, Indiana: International Human Powered Vehicle Assoc. 74–76.

Kyle, C.R., and E.M. Burke (1984). Improving the racing bicycle. *Mech. Engineer.* 109:6:35–45.

Kyle, C.R. (1986). Athletic clothing. *Sci. Amer.* 254:3:104–110.

Kyle, C.R., and V.J. Caiozzo (1986). Experiments in human ergometry as applied to the design of human powered vehicles. *Internat. J. Sport Biomech.* 2:6–19.

Kyle, C.R. (1987). The wind resistance of racing bicycles, cyclists and athletic clothing. *Report to the USOC Sports Equipment and Technology Committee.* March 10, 1987.

Kyle, C.R. (1988a). The mechanics and aerodynamics of cycling. *Medical and Scientific Aspects of Cycling.* Eds. E.M. Burke and M.N. Newsom, Human Kinetics Books, Champaign IL.

Kyle, C.R. (1988b). Power output and energy consumption. *Bicycling:*194–199, May, 1988).

Kyle, C.R. (1988c). How weight affects bicycle speed. *Bicycling:*186–190, May, 1988.

Kyle, C.R. (1988d). The Sunraycer wheels, tires, and brakes. *G.M. Sunraycer Case History.* Published course notes for Ae107a, Graduate Aeronautical Laboratories, California Institute of Technology.

Kyle, C.R. (1989a). The human machine. *Bicycling:*196–200, May.

Kyle, C.R. (1989b). Designing efficient human powered vehicles. *Ties,* Drexel University, Philadelphia PA.

Kyle, C.R. (1989c). The aerodynamics of handlebars and helmets. *Cycling Science,* 1:1:22–25.

Kyle, C.R. (1990). Wind tunnel tests of bicycle wheels and helmets. *Cycling Science.* 2:1:27–30.

McCole, S.D., K. Claney, J.C. Conte, R. Anderson, and J.M. Hagberg (1990). Energy expenditure during bicycling. *J. Appl. Physiol.* 68:748–853.

Miller, N.R., and D. Ross (1980). The design of variable ratio chain drives and ergometers—application to a maximum power bicycle drive. *Proceedings of the International Conference on Medical Devices and Sports Equipment.* Eds. Shoup & Thacker, ASME, N.Y. 49–56.

Moulton, A. (1973). The Moulton bicycle. *Cambridge University Friday Evening Discourse,* The Royal Institution, London, 23 Feb. 1973.

Newmiller, J., and M.L. Hull (1988). A mechanically decoupled two force component bicycle pedal dynamometer. *J. Biomech.* 21:5:375–386.

Nonweiler, T. (1956). The air resistance of racing cyclists. *Report No. 106.;* Oct. 1956. The College of Aeronautics, Cranfield, England.

Nordeen-Snyder, K. (1977). The effects of bicycle seat height variation upon oxygen consumption and lower limb kinematics. *Med Sci. Sp.* 9:113–117.

Norris, L. (1987). Crosswind drag, a new analysis. *Bike Tech* 6:2:14–15.

Olsen, J.N. (1989). The mountain bike, where to from here? *Cycling Science* 1:1:10–13.

Pugh, L.G.C.E. (1974). The relation of oxygen intake and speed in competition cycling and comparative observations on the bicycle ergometer. *J. Physio.* (Lond.) 241:795–808.

Schondorf, P., and K.J. Adams (1981). Load spectras for bicycles. *Technical report of the Fachhochschule,* Cologne Germany.

Sharp, A. (1896). *Bicycles and Tricycles.* MIT Press, Cambridge MA. Reprint 1896 ed.

Sjøgaard, G., B.Nielsen, F. Mikkelsen, B. Saltin, and E.R. Burke (1982). *Physiology in Bicycling.* Mouvement Publications, Ithaca, N.Y.

Soden, P.D., and B.A. Adeyefa (1979). Forces applied to a bicycle during normal cycling. *J. Biomech.* 12:527–541.

Spangler, D., and G. Hooker (1990). Scientific training and fitness testing. *Cycling Science* 2:1:23–26.

Swain, D., J.R. Coast, P.S. Clifford, M.C. Milliken, and J.S. Gundersen (1987). Influence of body size on oxygen consumption during bicycling. *JAP* 62:2:668–672.

Vandewalle, H., G. Peres, J. Heller, J. Panel, and H. Monod (1987). Force-velocity relationship and maximal power on a cycle ergometer. *Eur. J. Appl. Physiol.* 56:650–656.

van Ingen Schenau (1983). Differences in oxygen consumption and external power between male and female speed skaters during supra maximal cycling. *Eur. J. App. Physiol.* 51:337–345.

Webb, P. (1988). The work of walking a calorimetric study. *Med. Sci. Sp. Exer.* 20:4:331–337.

Whitney, E., and E.M. Hamilton (1984). *Understanding Nutrition.* Wert Publishing Co., St. Paul MN.

Whitt, F.R., and D.G. Wilson (1982). *Bicycling Science.* MIT Press, Cambridge MA.

Williams, K.R., and P.R. Cavanagh (1983). A model for calculation of mechanical power during distance running. *J. Biomech.* 16:115–128.

Wilson, S.S. Bicycling Technology (1973). *Scientific American.* 228:March 1973, 81–91.

Zahradnik, F. (1989). Lemond's leading edge. *Bicycling:*9:30–34, Nov., 1989.

Zahradnik, F., and C.R. Kyle (1987). Aerodynamic Overhaul. *Bicycling:*72–82, June, 1987.

DISCUSSION

COSTILL: I have always been fascinated by watching competitors in track and field and other sports who pay little or no attention to aerodynamics. Some of the bouffant hair styles of female runners appear to be remarkable examples of poor aerodynamics. I often wonder how much faster they might be had they done some streamlining. In swimming, on the other hand, suits are nearly non-existent, and many swimmers shave their body hair to reduce some of the drag. Please comment on how important some of these factors are in activities of much lower velocity than cycling.

KYLE: Oddly enough, shaving legs, when measured in the wind tunnel, does lower the wind resistance significantly in a human being. There is a good reason for cyclists shaving their limbs, and there is a good reason for runners to shave theirs. Air resistance accounts for only 6–8% of the total energy cost at low speed running, say 12–14 mph, but 6–8% is a lot. If you could lower the wind resistance on a runner just 2–4%, it would make a difference of anywhere from a few centimeters in the 100 m dash to 30 m in a marathon.

In swimming, the drag is lower when you shave your limbs because it decreases the turbulence in the vicinity of the limbs, and fabric can be optimized for smooth suits, especially for women. Tight fitting swimming caps can also reduce drag significantly. We recommend that women sprinters in track should also wear a smooth, tight cap, but some of them are so much better than the competition that they don't really need that extra edge.

I just thought of an anecdote related to this topic that might be interesting. I was responsible for the funny looking uniforms with the hoods that were worn by the US track team in 1988. They were a disaster. The hurdler won a gold medal wearing the uniform, but the 4 × 400 m relay team was disqualified. They wore the uniforms for the first time the day of the race. The coaches put alternate runners in the qualifying heat because they knew they could qualify, but they passed the baton out of the zone. The runners claimed that the hoods impaired their hearing. This is one point I would like to make—in competition, one should never adopt new equipment that is unfamiliar to the athletes.

NADEL: I understand that if in the 1990 Tour de France Laurence Fignon had not had his ponytail exposed, he would have improved his time by a 8 s, enough to win the race.

KYLE: His aerodynamic errors accounted for more than a minute in lost time. His ponytail accounted for about 8 s, but he also failed to use an aero helmet, and he did not have the elbow rest handlebars; those factors are worth more than 8 s.

NADEL: Is heat dissipation substantially compromised by wearing aero-dynamic clothing that covers more of the skin surface?

KYLE: Where you have fabric covering the skin, sweat saturates the fabric and tends to evaporate more uniformly with less dripping, so there may be a positive effect on evaporative heat loss by having the fabric close to the skin. If the fabric wicks properly and transfers the liquid to the surface of the fabric, and if the fabric is very thin, any reduction in evaporative cooling should be minimized. The overall effect of fabrics that reflect solar radiation and produce a fairly efficient evaporative cooling, e.g., lycra-type fabrics, does not seem to be bad for cooling.

WILMORE: We did a trial last summer in which we had full body garments on cyclists exercising at about 34° C in an environmental chamber. During 90 min we recorded temperature, voluntary fluid intake, and sweating rate. We tested three different whole body suits and compared them to riding with-light weight shorts. We found no differences in any of these measures. That study was not conducted outside, but it seems to address the issue of evaporation with cycle suits.

NADEL: When we tested elite cyclists for the Daedalus project, we found that the mechanical efficiency, that is, the relationship between the oxygen uptake and the mechanical power output, varied extremely widely, more widely than I ever imagined. The range was 18–31%. What this implied to us is that you can trade off poor mechanical efficiency or mechanical economy for a large maximal oxygen uptake or vice versa if you want good performance. Indirectly, these cyclists knew that. Some of them knew that they had very high maximal oxygen uptakes, but yet they could be beaten by a cyclist with a lower $\dot{V}_2max$ but a greater mechanical efficiency. Could you comment on this?

KYLE: I think that is one of the areas for the greatest possibility of improvement in cycling because there should not be this tremendous variability. I do not think that physiologically the bodies of elite cyclists are that much different, and yet there is a tremendous variation in their efficiency.

COYLE: In Ethan Nadel's project, the cyclists were cycling in a non-familiar, semi-recumbent position. This was a novel task, so the 18–32% variability in economy may represent differences in learning this unfamiliar task. When cyclists are experienced and are positioned correctly with the right seat height, frame size, handlebars, etc., the variation in efficiency is much less, that is, 22–25% at 80 rpm, which most long distance cyclists use most of the time. What exactly contributes to that we are not sure. One possibility may be that muscle fiber composition could account for a small part of that difference in efficiency, but that has never been documented.

KNUTTGEN: Ethan, did you also measure efficiencies on the traditional cycler ergometer of these same people for which you have the wide variation in mechanical efficiency?

NADEL: We did it on only one of our subjects. It was not a goal of our project to speak to this question because, frankly, we really did not find this out until analysis afterwards. In the one person for whom we had the foresight to do this, cycling economy in the upright position was the same as in the recumbent position. The differences in efficiency may provide an explanation for how in an elite crowd you cannot really predict performance on the basis of maximal oxygen uptake when the range of these scores is small.

KNUTTGEN: Whether you calculate efficiency as gross efficiency or net efficiency is an important consideration. Many years ago at the University of Copenhagen we calculated efficiencies by subtracting out the energy cost of no-load cycling at the particular rpm. In that way you find that humans can actually get up to a net efficiency of about 40%.

KYLE: This is typical of an internal combustion engine if you don't consider the drive train, tire losses, and other factors. Its efficiency is then about 36%.

KREIDER: In our Tour de Norfolk study we brought six professional cyclists in and had them ride 100 miles/d for 4 d straight. We were able to use Velodyne race simulators in which the cyclists mounted their own bicycles on the ergometer. Their efficiency was about 25–28% using their own bicycle. Using their own bicycles, efficiency may be greater than we expect.

GISOLFI: When these runners or cyclists put on tights to increase aerodynamic performance, does the fabric limit movement?

KYLE: Lycra is so light that it requires very little tension to maintain the integrity of the fabric, and I doubt if it has any effect on movement. It certainly does not seem to.

ROBERTSON: When one calculates metabolic efficiency during upright cycling as a function of peddling rate at a fixed power output, a parabolic relationship is usually seen. The optimal rate in hackers like myself is down around 60 to 80, and in fairly competitive individuals it seems to be up around 80 to 100. Does this same phenomenon occur for recumbent cycling? Is there a different set of efficiencies as a function of the type of cycle and the training state?

KYLE: There could be an effect. We had six students whom we tested both in a prone position and then in the standard cycling position. We studied the maximal power output over different time periods from 6 s to 25 min and found for the shorter time periods where they were forced to sprint at high rpm that the prone position was the worst. It was down about 8% in maximum power production. The supine was down about 4%, but that difference between prone and supine positions was possibly a training effect because those who were most familiar with peddling in the supine position had no drop in power whatsoever from about 30 s and higher and tended to pedal at the same rpm as in the upright position.

COYLE: We should define net efficiency as a change in oxygen uptake for a change in power. But efficiency is also used loosely as a term related to muscle fatigue. In some of the cyclists we have tested using instrumented pedals, we see that they adopt a strategy that may not be physically efficient, i.e., they began pulling and pushing on a pedal and not producing much torque, but we think they do this to reduce their muscle fatigue. In other words, they are willing to use certain muscle groups and a certain portion of the range of motion and to expend extra energy that helps reduce the fatigue of other muscle groups that may be the limiting factor in that performance. I think the ultimate goal is not necessarily to improve metabolic inefficiency per se but to reduce overall fatigue. The strategy for doing that becomes very complex.

SAWKA: One of the things we noted with upper body exercise in working with a very small skeletal muscle mass was that people could do a lot more work at higher rpm. Perhaps with a very small muscle mass you can increase the rpm, thereby reducing peak tension, and, therefore, improve muscle perfusion for a given power. In cyclists is there any relationship between leg strength or muscle cross sectional area and the rpm that they select?

KYLE: Yes, the fastest track cyclists in the world use the highest rpm, and they choose the gear arbitrarily. Normally, they weigh

188–220 lbs. and have huge thighs. Also, they typically have a very high proportion of fast twitch muscle fibers. At the other end of this spectrum is the long distance cyclist, who has to have not only endurance but also the power to sprint at the end of the race. A track cyclist is very special type of a animal.

COGGAN: Cycling is somewhat unique because it demands both an extreme aerobic endurance and extreme short-term power production. Several studies have suggested a possible interference between training for strength at the same time one is training for endurance. In my case that was probably the limiting factor in my performance. I was never able to train both ways and achieve high levels of both power and endurance at the same time.

HEIGENHAUSER: With respect to the force-velocity curve and the curve of efficiency versus the ability to produce maximal power, where are cyclists on those curves generally when they are doing long distance races? The rpm that produces greatest power may be different than the rpm that produces greatest mechanical efficiency.

KYLE: In road racing, cylists can drop their power or energy consumption by more than 30% by dropping back into the pack. It's a very complex strategy. They operate most of the time at a low energy output—about 60% of $\dot{V}O_2$max. All of a sudden, when they get up to the front, they are sometimes at 110% $\dot{V}O_2$max. So they store energy when they are back in the pack and pay it off when they are in the front. Finally, when they break away from the pack, they often cycle at 85–92% of $\dot{V}O_2$max. I don't know if I can answer your question about the efficiency curve.

HEIGENHAUSER: What I can gather from some of the studies is that when cycling for 30 s, cyclists' maximum power output is 800 w, but their maximum power in a test of $\dot{V}O_2$max is only about 600 w. So there is quite a difference between the power they can produce for 30 s and that which they can produce during a typical $\dot{V}O_2$max test. NADEL: Specific power (W/kg) is probably more relevant than total power output. The cyclists may be very large or very small, and so it's the W/kg that we should be talking about to bring these people all together.

COGGAN: I don't think expressing power production or $\dot{V}O_2$max relative to body weight is a very good predictor because much of cycling is contested on the flat; unless the terrain becomes very hilly, it is an advantage to be large. That shows up in the body weights of the best cyclists. There are very few 110–120 pounders who can compete; it is very rare for someone to be a successful competitive cyclist unless he has a $\dot{V}O_2$max of 5 L/min or higher. A cyclist's $\dot{V}O_2$max may be 70 mL/kg x min for a total of 4.2 L if he weighs

60 kg, but that cyclist will not make it to category I. There is an advantage for being large unless the race is up in the mountains.

CONLEE: Is there a certain body size or body dimension that is optimal for a competitive cyclist?

KYLE: It's event specific. Cyclists in time trials typically weigh between 150–180 lbs. The reason is that their frontal area goes up about as the 2/3 power of their weight, and so the heavier person has a higher energy density. However, because the lighter person has a higher power to body weight ratio than the heavier person, there is an optimal body size that turns out to be 150–180 lbs. for time trials. For sprinting, where massive, explosive, high-velocity forces are necessary, the body weight could be anything; typically sprinters are very heavy, from 180–220 lbs. For hill climbing, because the lighter person has a higher power per unit mass ratio, the best cyclists typically weigh 130–140 lbs.

ROBERTSON: You noted that in drafting there is a distinct advantage to getting the front wheel fairly close to the competitor's rear wheel. That is also the case in automobile racing, except that you cannot get so close as to take the air from the leader's engine or you wind up with a heating problem. Is there an analogy with the human? Is there an advantage to at least keeping a little distance for purposes of cooling?

KYLE: Well, no because the heat dissipation into the atmosphere is so low with the human being that it doesn't make a bit of difference. You'd think that the person in front in cycling might benefit by drafting, as is true in automobile racing; but what happens in automobile racing is that the gap becomes very small—just a few inches. Changes in air pressure distribution are at the rear of the front automobile; because they are so close together, both automobiles essentially become one object that is two car lengths long, and the net drag of both cars is lower. In cycling, there is no benefit in front; you cannot even tell when somebody is on your wheel. The only reason the trailing cyclist has thermal regulation problems is that the wind velocity for convective cooling is less, and that's important.

COYLE: Regarding the optimal body weight for time trials, I suggest that it should be larger than 150–180 lbs. The best time trialist, i.e., one who rides 40 km on the level, is simply the person who can put out the most power in one hour—not power per kg body weight and not necessarily power per unit surface area, although that would seem to make sense. But the person who is 50% heavier may have a surface area which is only 10% larger when cycling, so it helps to be bigger. Theoretically, I expect that we should seek out our biggest people who have some chance to improve their endurance capability and just see what are the highest maximal power outputs that they can maintain.

KYLE: That is a really practical approach. We might gain some good insight by doing that.

Index